HEALING
Spices

HEALING
Spices

How to Use 50 Everyday and Exotic Spices
to Boost Health and Beat Disease

Bharat B. Aggarwal, PhD
with
Debora Yost

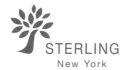

STERLING
New York

STERLING
New York

An Imprint of Sterling Publishing
387 Park Avenue South
New York, NY 10016

© 2011 by Bill Gottlieb
Edited and Packaged by Bill Gottlieb, Good For You Books

10   9

Distributed in Canada by Sterling Publishing
^{c}/o Canadian Manda Group, 165 Dufferin Street
Toronto, Ontario, Canada M6K 3H6
Distributed in the United Kingdom by GMC Distribution Services
Castle Place, 166 High Street, Lewes, East Sussex, England BN7 1XU
Distributed in Australia by Capricorn Link (Australia) Pty. Ltd.
P.O. Box 704, Windsor, NSW 2756, Australia

Sterling ISBN 978-1-4027-7663-2

For information about custom editions, special sales, premium and
corporate purchases, please contact Sterling Special Sales
Department at 800-805-5489 or specialsales@sterlingpublishing.com.

DEDICATED TO

the Sages, Rishis, Scientists, Gurus, Acharyas, and my parents—
whose wisdom continues to inspire me!

Acknowledgments

From Bharat Aggarwal, PhD:
I would like to thank Dr. Chitra Sundaram for her assistance in researching the medical literature on spices; Ms. Alamelu Vairavan, the co-author of *Healthy South Indian Cooking*, for her encouragement and for educating me how to cook with spices; my wife, Uma Aggarwal, for "Adding Spice to my Life"; and my two sons, Rishi and Manoj Aggarwal, for being supportive and team players. I would also like to thank my sister, Kamlesh Goyal, who is always adding new dimension to my thinking about spices and their benefits. Above all, I would like to thank the thousands of patients suffering from various chronic diseases who have expressed curiosity about the uses of spices. I would also like to thank McCormick Spices in the United States and Ottogi Corporation in Korea, two of the world's biggest suppliers of spices, for contributing more to my knowledge of spices.

From Debora Yost:
With Dr. Aggarwal, I would like also like to thank Dr. Chitra Sundaram and Alamelu Vairavan. Also, thanks to my dear friends and superb cooks Nancy Wilson, Sharon Esterly, and John Lehman, for assisting us with some of the more challenging recipe creations. I offer a special thanks to friend and cook extraordinaire Susan Banfield, for taking me on fun-filled culinary adventures through the Indian and Asian marketplaces of North Jersey. I am forever grateful to my husband, Nick Yost, the spice of my life, for his patience during long hours of writing and for helping me explore the world of spice almost nightly as we taste-tested the recipes in this book. And last, but not least, I want to thank my former colleague at Rodale Books and longtime and cherished friend Bill Gottlieb, for his superb editing and his encouraging support. Thanks for bringing me into this book. As always, we made a great team.

From Bill Gottlieb:
Thanks to all the superb professionals who joined with Good For You Books in creating this book: Bharat Aggarwal, PhD, a world-class scientist devoted to the health and well-being of humankind; Dr. Aggarwal's co-author, Debora Yost; the designer, Peter Holm, of Sterling Hill Productions; the illustrator, Michael Gallatly; the project manager and proofreader, Rose Young; the copyeditor, Megan Anderson; the photography editor, illustration researcher, and indexer, Denise Getz; and the literary agent, Chris Tomasino, of Tomasino Literary Agency. It was a pleasure and a privilege to have worked with such skilled individuals who—without ever meeting together face-to-face—formed such a creative and productive team. Thank you!

CONTENTS

PART THREE ◆ Special Spice Combos

PART FOUR ◆ Spices as Natural Medicines

PART FIVE ◆ Resources

Introduction:

From My Laboratory to Your Kitchen

Spices have been in my life—in my diet, in my medicine cabinet, and in my thinking—since I was a youth growing up in Punjab in northern India. And now—as Professor of the Department of Experimental Therapeutics at the University of Texas M.D. Anderson Cancer Center—spices are the subject of many experiments in my laboratory, where my colleagues and I are discovering the molecular and biochemical secrets behind the therapeutic power of these ancient medicines, and conducting human studies to put those secrets to use in the battle against cancer.

When I was growing up in India, spices were the main medicines my family used for everyday healing, in keeping with the tradition of *Ayurveda*, India's system of natural healing, which employs spices, herbs, and healthful lifestyle to prevent and treat disease.

But more than medicine, spices were, well, *spices*. Knowing how to creatively combine and cook with spices is part of family culture in India, a domestic art that comes naturally to us, as if it were a part of our DNA. It is a great honor in India to cook for guests—and it is a delight for the guests, since the best food in India is found in homes, not restaurants.

So you can imagine my culinary misery when, in 1973, after earning my master's of science in biochemistry in India, I traveled to the University of Louisville to earn my PhD in biochemistry. It was impossible to find restaurants that served spicy vegetarian foods or markets that sold the spices I craved! Well, a professor had told me about Berkeley, California, a much more "liberal" environment where one could find just about anything—including other vegetarians and exotic spices. In no time, I was on a Greyhound bus heading to California and enrollment at the University of California, Berkeley, where I eventually earned my PhD. And, indeed, Berkeley was America's promised land of spices: I was able to find the foods and spices to recreate the vegetarian way of life I had always known and loved.

My first real job after graduating from Berkeley was a gem. I was hired by Genentech—one of the first companies specializing in genetic engineering—to find gene-based treatments for cancer. During my nine fascinating years at Genentech, I made some important scientific discoveries, including isolating *tumor necrosis factor* (TNF), a Jeckyl-and-Hyde protein that is critical for regulating the immune system but also plays a role in triggering the inflammation underlying cancer and many other chronic diseases.

And as I worked at Genentech—a pharmaceutical company where there wasn't any interest in investigating spices as a treatment for disease—my fragrant friends were never far from my mind (or my meals!).

I recalled the brilliant yellow powder called turmeric that my mother used daily in virtually every meal. She'd also sprinkle it on a cut when I fell and hurt myself. Or put it on my forehead when I had a fever. If I was nauseous, she gave me ginger to make me feel better. If I couldn't sleep, she gave me coriander in warm milk. On sweltering summer days, she made our family a refreshing drink out of kokum, an Indian spice that would cool us off as instantly and magically as if we were all standing under a waterfall. (You'll find the recipe on page 152.) It seemed like almost every spice in our giant spice cabinet was a food *and* a medicine.

And the spices that were used as folk remedies by my mother were also part of the *materia medica* of the ancient medical texts of India,

China, and Tibet. I often wondered: Just how potent *are* these spices? Could curcumin, the active ingredient in turmeric, or garcinol, the active ingredient in kokum, be powerful enough to help slow or stop tumor growth? (I later discovered that the answer to both of these questions is *yes*.)

My twin interests in unraveling the biochemical secrets of cancer's lethal intrusion and researching the healing power of spices led me in 1989 to Houston and the Department of Experimental Therapeutics at the University of Texas M.D. Anderson Cancer Center.

There, during the 1990s, I discovered that curcumin *is* active against cancer. One experiment after another led to a greater understanding of its potential. Yes, it *is* capable of attacking breast cancer . . . colon cancer . . . and pancreatic cancer. And now the positive results of this research are being tested in clinical studies with cancer patients.

At first, my experiments on "traditional folk medicine" didn't get much attention at the highly conventional M.D. Anderson. When I first mentioned to an oncologist that a compound in an ordinary Indian spice had anti-cancer properties that I'd never seen in any other substance, I was politely shooed out of his office.

A few months later, however, I attended a conference in India with John Mendelsohn, MD, president of M.D. Anderson and one of the most influential oncologists in the United States. While there, he attended my presentation on the healing potential of curcumin and then talked to me afterward. "I had *no* idea that the science behind your results was so solid," he said. We talked more on the long flight home. By the time we returned to Houston, he had decided he wanted to launch human studies on curcumin and cancer.

Today, dozens of human studies on curcumin have been completed, and many more are underway. Research shows that curcumin may help treat a range of health problems, including heart disease, Alzheimer's disease, arthritis,

prostate problems, inflammatory bowel disease, psoriasis, and, of course, various cancers, including colorectal, breast, pancreatic, bladder, oral, cervical, and stomach.

Discovering the tremendous healing capacity of turmeric and curcumin got me hooked on investigating spices in my laboratory. We moved on to experiments with many other spices and their compounds: the garcinol in kokum, the zerumbone in ginger, the ursolic acid in oregano, the quercetin in onions, the capsaicin in red chile, the ellagitannins in pomegranate, to name a few. And one by one, we found, *yes*, spices and their compounds *are* powerful healers.

Back in 1995, when I started investigating turmeric, there were less than 50 published scientific studies on the healing potential of spices. Today, there are thousands. Worldwide, researchers have linked culinary spices to the prevention and treatment of more than 150 health problems. Spices, they have found, contain compounds that fight oxidation and inflammation, the two processes underlying most chronic diseases. And studies that analyze dietary patterns and disease—so-called population or epidemiological studies—have linked high spice intake to low rates of chronic disease.

These studies haven't escaped the attention of the FDA and National Institutes of Health (NIH)—but our government isn't acting fast enough to inform the public that the typical American diet is sorely lacking in spices. They aren't even mentioned in the USDA's food pyramid! That's why I wrote this book.

Simply including more vegetables, fruits, and other whole foods in your diet *can't* win the fight against disease, because the real secret to preventing disease and prolonging life is a diet rich in whole foods *and* spices. And spices—by the pinch and the teaspoon—may be more important than the foods they flavor! Open a bottle of oregano or fry fenugreek in a pan—that powerful, intoxicating aroma is the scent of health and healing!

Although many Americans have become more interested in spicy cuisine (attested to by the many ethnic restaurants in the US), most don't take full advantage of the wonderful world of spices, either for their culinary appeal or their healing potential. The main reason, I believe, is that Americans aren't taught how to use them to their full capacity.

It doesn't have to be that way.

Healing Spices finally gives spices their much-deserved attention. It is the first book to present in everyday language the scientific facts about the curative power of spices. *And* it gives you everything you need to know to put more of those spices into your diet.

I cook with spices every day. Turmeric, red and green chile, coriander, cumin, ajowan, amchur, green and brown cardamom, cinnamon, clove, onion, garlic, and ginger—every one of them is in my daily diet. And they can be in yours, too—cooking with spices is a skill you'll develop quite easily, with the information and instructions in this book. And once you do, you'll add new and delicious flavors to your diet.

Please, don't go another day without adding spice to your life. Do you want to prevent heart disease, type 2 diabetes, Alzheimer's, and cancer? (Who doesn't?) Well, add more garlic, cinnamon, and turmeric to your meals. And don't forget the other 47 spices discussed in this book!

The spice trade—in pepper, clove, cinnamon, and other spices considered as precious as gold—has fueled the world's economy from ancient times, with nation battling nation for control of spices and the spice routes that brought them to market. My hope is that this book will help open up a new (and far more peaceful!) "spice route"—the one from the market to your kitchen to your mealtime table.

I'd like to close with a quote attributed to Charlemagne, the eighth-century king, conqueror, and spice lover, which sums up my feelings about healing spices: "Spices, the friend of physicians and the pride of cooks."

May spices be the friend of your health and the pride of your kitchen!

Bharat B. Aggarwal, PhD
January 2011

PART ONE

The Healing Power
of Spices

Ancient Medicines, New Discoveries

The Proof Is Positive—Spices Can Heal

Spices

Wars were fought over them, kingdoms were lost because of them, and new lands were discovered in search of them. In ancient times and for centuries to follow, spices were often more precious than gold.

But before they were money, spices were medicines. Turmeric, cloves, cinnamon, coriander, ginger, and black peppercorns—healers all—are among the oldest spices, with their use dating back to the world's first civilizations. Sanskrit writings from the India of 3,000 years ago describe the varied therapeutic uses of spices, and ancient medical texts from China are filled with remedies using spices for hundreds of ailments.

Spices Throughout History

Spices originated in India, Indonesia, and other parts of south and southeast Asia and—as anciently as 2600 BCE—were imported from Asia to the countries of the eastern Mediterranean, such as Syria and Egypt.

The Egyptians revered spices—literally—using cinnamon and cassia for mummification, and putting them in the tombs of pharaohs as a necessary accompaniment in the afterlife.

The Romans saw spices as the ultimate luxury item. They perfumed palaces and temples with them. At banquets, heaps of spices were on display to enthrall guests, and were used to flavor foods and wines. Even legionnaires headed off to battle wearing spice-scented perfumes. In the first century, Roman officials were outraged when the Emperor Nero burned a year's worth of precious cinnamon on his wife's funeral bier. In the fifth century, the raiding Visigoths agreed to call off their siege of Rome for a bounty of gold, silver—and pepper.

In the 8th to the 15th centuries, the spice trade was controlled by the Republic of Venice, which became fabulously wealthy as a result—with Arabs playing the role of middlemen, zealously guarding the secret sources of most spices, to keep demand and prices high. In the late 15th century, Portugal and Spain sought to break that monopoly—and the sea voyage of Christopher Columbus, looking for a new Western route to the "Spice Islands," inadvertently "discovered" the Americas.

As Columbus sailed west, others sailed east. Over the following centuries, the Spanish, Portuguese, Dutch, French, and British colonized the countries that were the source of spices. By the 17th century, the spice-trading Dutch East India Company was the richest corporation in the world, with 50,000 employees, 30,000 soldiers, and 200 ships. Spices, says an article in *The Economist*, are the "world economy's oldest, deepest, most aromatic roots."

By the 18th century, spices were grown around the world and in large quantities—and spices had become one among many commodities in world trade.

In the 21st century the dramatic history of spices is repeating itself—in terms of *scientific* exploration. Modern medical and nutritional researchers are discovering unimaginable riches of *health* in the spices that have been such an integral part of human history.

The Jewels of the Plant Kingdom

Spices contain an abundance of *phytonutrients*, plant compounds that bestow health and promote healing in a variety of ways. Most of them are powerful antioxidants that control and disarm the *reactive oxygen species* (also known as "free radicals") that can damage cells, causing illness and aging. Phytonutrients are also anti-inflammatory—and chronic, low-grade inflammation has been linked to the development of many of our most debilitating and deadly health problems, such as cardiovascular disease, cancer, type 2 diabetes, and Alzheimer's disease. Spices also derive their healing power from their large concentration of *volatile oils*, the compounds that supply their pungent aromas. (*Volatile*, a word used by chemists, means a rapidly evaporating oil that doesn't leave a stain and that smells like the plant it's from.)

Epidemiological studies that explore the link between diet and health show that populations eating a diet rich in spices have lower rates of certain diseases. The United States, for instance, has three times the rate of colon cancer as India, which is well known for its spicy cuisine. India also has one of the world's lowest rates of Alzheimer's disease. Greece, well known for a healthy diet rich in garlic, onions, rosemary, and marjoram, enjoys a low rate of heart disease. Spain, the country that consumes the most saffron, has low levels of the "bad" LDL cholesterol that clogs arteries and increases the risk of heart disease.

But, you might ask, can't you get all of those phytonutrients from fruits and vegetables? Quite simply, no. Spices contain many *unique* phytonutrients. Here are just a few examples:

- *Curcumin* has potent anti-cancer properties, and studies show it can fight dozens of other diseases. Its only source: the spice turmeric.
- *Thymoquinone*, a powerful immune booster, is found only in the Indian spice black cumin.
- *Piperine*, the compound that makes you sneeze when you eat black pepper, protects brain cells and has a dozen other healing actions.
- *Carbazole alkaloids*, which fight type 2 diabetes, colon cancer, and Alzheimer's disease, are found only in curry leaf, an Indian spice.

- *Galangal acetate*, which eases arthritis, is found only in galangal, an Asian spice.
- *Diosgenin*, found in fenugreek, can douse inflammation and kill cancer cells.
- *Anethole*, found in both anise and fennel, relaxes menstrual cramps and can quiet a colicky baby.
- *Eugenol*, which gives clove its distinctive aroma, is a powerful natural painkiller.
- *Rosemarinic acid* makes rosemary one of the most powerful antioxidants on earth.
- *Gingerol*, a compound in ginger, tames nausea.
- *Hydroxycitric acid*, abundant in the Indian spice kokum, powerfully inhibits appetite (and is already a leading ingredient in many weight-loss formulas).
- *Capsaicin*, found only in chiles, can help relieve the symptoms of arthritis and psoriasis.

As you'll read in *Healing Spices*, these and other compounds have many different mechanisms of action, along with their antioxidant and anti-inflammatory powers. Many spices are powerful battlers of microbes—bacteria, viruses, and fungi. They limit the release of histamine, the biochemical that causes allergic symptoms. They strengthen the disease-fighting immune system. They regulate blood sugar and insulin levels, preventing or treating diabetes. They calm nerves, easing anxiety and pain. They boost metabolism, burning calories. They play hormone-like roles, balancing, strengthening, and regenerating the body. They relax the muscles of the digestive tract, relieving intestinal ills. With all these abilities and more, they can even slow aging.

How to Use This Book

You can gain the health benefits I just mentioned by eating plenty of spices. How do you do that? Read and use this book!

Healing Spices is a voyage to a wondrous new world of spices, in which you'll discover important and useful knowledge to improve your health—while experiencing an unforgettable culinary and sensory adventure along the way! Even if spices are totally foreign to you, I promise that by the time you finish this book, you'll feel like an old hand.

Just promise me one thing: Don't be intimidated by spices that are unfamiliar to you, or by what appears to be a lot of spices in a recipe. First, these spices may not be as foreign as you think. (I'll say more about that in a moment.) And the fact that a recipe contains a lot of spices doesn't necessarily mean the recipe is hard to make, time-consuming, or fiery-hot. I know that once you've read the entry on any one of the 50 healing spices in this book, all the foreboding and confusion you may have felt about what to do with that spice will have vanished. You'll feel just as confident shaking a little galangal or star anise into a stir-fry as you are sprinkling it with salt and pepper!

This book walks you through each of those 50 healing spices in what I hope is an entertaining and easy-to-follow format. To benefit from *Healing Spices*, you don't have to read this book from the first page to the last. Each spice entry (and chapter) is complete in itself. You may want to start reading about the spices that:

- interest you the most,
- help you manage a health problem you have,
- help guard against a health problem you want to avoid,
- are a part of your favorite ethnic cuisine,
- or simply pique your curiosity.

I just have one suggestion before you get started. Read the next chapter—"The Healing Spice Cabinet"—first. It offers the basics on buying spices and working with them in the kitchen. Contrary to what you may think, putting more spice in your life doesn't require a big investment or special tools. (Yes, you will need a tool to grind spices, but chances are you already have a suitable appliance that will do the job.)

Once you've read Part I—this chapter and the next—it's time for Part II, the 50 chapters that feature each of the healing spices. I've organized them all similarly for ease of use. In each chapter, you'll find sections on:

The healing potential of each spice. I put a spice in this book *only* if there is intriguing or established science showing the spice may help prevent or heal specific conditions and diseases. That science is presented in everyday language—in fact, you might find yourself actually enjoying reading about scientific studies! For quick reference, all of the health conditions potentially affected by each spice are highlighted in a box in the chapter.

Getting to know the spice. I offer the most interesting highlights into each spice's medicinal and culinary history. You may be surprised to discover that a spice you swear you've never tasted is actually a key ingredient in some of your favorite ethnic dishes. Did you know, for example, that galangal is to Thai dishes what garlic is to Italian food? It's practically in everything Thai. Did you know that authentic Mexican cooks are just as passionate about putting cocoa in a sauce or savory dish as they are about chiles? That's why I say the spices you may think are "foreign" to you are probably already in foods you enjoy.

How to buy the spice. You'll get specific advice on making the best purchase—the best form in which to buy a spice in order to derive the most flavor, the country reputed to be the exporter of the most flavorful variety of the spice, where you can buy the best (sometimes for less), how a particular spice should smell, and even how to examine a spice for flaws and age. You'll also learn how to store a spice for maximum lifespan.

In the kitchen with the spice. This section provides great culinary advice for each spice. It removes all the mystery (but not the magic) from using the spice in cooking, offering specific suggestions on creatively using it to enhance your meals, so you can enjoy the spice's health-giving benefits. It also offers a list of other spices that are good complements, and dishes where the spice shines—indispensable information for creating your own recipes.

A recipe showcasing the spice. For each spice, you'll find a recipe that showcases its special flavor. All the recipes were developed and tested just for this book. Many of the recipes selected are classics, such as: Chicken Oreganata (featuring oregano, of course); Spain's romescu sauce, a tomato-based sauce thickened with pulverized almonds, which is featured in Prawns with Almond Hot Pepper Sauce; or Hungarian Goulash, which wouldn't be authentic without caraway. There are also sparkling originals, such as Roasted Tomato Soup with Fennel and Mint, Pears Poached in Port and Star Anise, and Shellfish in Saffron Broth.

That's what you'll find in the spice-by-spice chapters of Part II. The next part of the book—Part III—gives you even more ideas on how to use many of those spices.

Part III, "Special Spice Combos," is a unique cooking lesson on how to maximize your use of spices, by teaching you about my favorite style of cooking—curry. That's right, curry is neither a spice nor a dish. It is a *method* of cooking, using a variety of spices to produce unique mouth-watering aromas.

I also offer curry spice mixes and pastes from the world's most famous curry-making nations so you can duplicate the tastes on your own. Plus, I offer more than two dozen spice mixes—also among the world's most famous—that you can make ahead, so you can whip up a spice delight with the least amount of effort. I also offer suggestions on the best ways to use these mixes.

Part IV, "Spices as Natural Medicines," is a condition-by-condition reference guide that lists all the spices that have been scientifically shown to have preventive or healing potential for each one of more than 150 health conditions, from acne, arthritis, and anxiety to stroke, ulcers, and wrinkles. In cases where a scientific study successfully tested a therapeutic dosage, that amount is included.

Part V, "Resources," is a buyer's guide that eliminates the legwork in finding some of the more hard-to-find healing spices. Out of the 50 spices in this book, perhaps a dozen aren't likely to be available in even the best stocked grocery store. No problem! Thanks to the Internet, even

What Is a Spice?

Think of coal becoming a diamond. Think of the 0/1 of bytes blossoming into the images you see on the computer screen. Think of a tablespoon of cocoa powder transforming an ordinary glass of milk into a delicious treat. Think of anything *concentrated*—a distillate of the original—that delivers a bounty of whatever the original contained, plus its own unique (and often more delightful) qualities.

That's a spice.

A spice is edible, aromatic, and *dried*, and it comes from a plant's root, bark, stem, bud, leaves, flower, fruit, or seed. Spices come in a veritable rainbow of rich hues—brilliant reds, oranges, browns, greens, blacks, and whites. Unlike herbs, all spices are edible.

A spice is *not* an herb. Herbs are usually leaves, and they're not always edible. For example, cilantro (the herb) is the fresh leaves of a plant; coriander (the spice) is the dried seed of the same plant. When leaves are dried, they become a spice.

(Like all definitions, however, the definition of a spice is not so, well, cut-and-dried. In this book, I've included a few spices that don't *exactly* fit the above definition of a spice, but which are widely used to spice foods. Onion is one example. Lemongrass—a leaf that is used fresh rather than dried—is another. But for the most part, the definition above is the best way to understand what a spice is and what it isn't.)

the most exotic spice is just a click away. By using this guide, all the spices in this book can be in your kitchen nearly overnight. (My recipe testers had no problem getting them and none live in a big city.)

That's *how* to use this book. I know I don't have to explain *why*—spices are an incredibly tasty and healing addition to a healthy, healing lifestyle. Enjoy!

From Mysterious to Mainstream—How to Buy and Store the Healing Spices

Imagine an ice cream sundae without *vanilla*, pesto without *basil*, salsa without *chile*, or paella without *saffron*. You can't, because the spice defines everything about the dish—its taste, texture, and aroma, how it is made, and how it is remembered. Eating would be just about joyless if it weren't for spices—and the best cooks know it. Case in point:

Several years ago, researchers from Cornell University examined more than 4,500 recipes from nearly 100 cookbooks. They found that

IN A SURVEY OF COOKBOOKS

BY FOOD SCIENTISTS,

93 PERCENT OF RECIPES

CONTAINED AT LEAST

ONE SPICE; THE AVERAGE

WAS FOUR.

93 percent included at least one spice, with the ingredient lists averaging four. That average, however, is considered a *minimum* in the cuisines popular for their unique and intense flavors, such as Indian, Indonesian, and Thai. Compared to those cuisines, the typical American diet is bland.

It's not that Americans aren't fond of exotic food. The proliferation of restaurants featuring these and other ethnic cuisines across the United States attests to the growing American interest in spicy fare. So why aren't Americans enjoying more spicy food at home?

They're intimidated! Most of the spices from nations with spicy cuisines are unfamiliar to American palates. Many of them, such as galangal, asafoetida, and black cumin (to name a few), aren't available in typical supermarkets—in fact, it's possible you may never have heard of them! Plus, a long list of spices in a recipe makes a dish seem complicated and expensive.

But enjoying spices at home doesn't have to be intimidating—or complicated, or expensive. The secret to feeling comfortable with spices is *understanding* them—how to buy them, use them, and combine them in ways that quickly transform a bland recipe into a flavor to savor. This book not only offers hundreds of reasons for spicing up your life to help improve health and avoid illness—it also gives you hundreds of ideas for doing it in a very tasty way.

But first, you need to know the basics.

Spices in Cooking and Eating

Contrary to popular belief, spice is not a synonym for hot. In fact, most spices do not add fiery flavor to food. Rather, spices are *aromatic*, which serves several culinary purposes. Spices:

- give food a pleasant, mouthwatering aroma that stimulates the appetite and increases the enjoyment of food.
- blend into new and pleasing taste sensations.
- impart a characteristic flavor, be it sweet, sour, tangy, or hot.

- serve as a natural tenderizer for tough but economical meats.
- add body and texture to a dish, with some acting as thickeners and binders for sauces.
- color a dish, making it appetizing to look at.
- assist the digestive process.

All spices perform several of these tasks. Turmeric and saffron, for example, add both brilliant color and aroma to food. Coriander acts as a thickener, while also giving a dish a nutty flavor. Ginger enlivens taste and aids digestion.

However, sniff any raw spice and you'll detect little, if any, aroma. That's because, with few exceptions, spices are just like any other food—something to *cook*. Most raw spices are dried organic matter—roots, bark, leaves, dried fruit, and the seeds of shrubs and trees. Those raw items are difficult to digest and may leave you with an upset stomach if you try.

In India, where highly spiced foods are a cherished way of life, cooks typically add spices to hot oil at the beginning of food preparation, just before adding other ingredients. This releases the spices' volatile oils, which flood the senses with heady aromas. Spices are again added at the end of cooking. As you read about how to cook with spices (in the culinary sections that accompany each of the 50 healing spices discussed in Part II and in Part III, which is devoted to spice cuisines), you'll develop a sure sense for how to add spices to your at-home meals. And you'll discover that cooking with the healing spices is *easy*. So is the first step: obtaining them.

Finding Spices

All the healing spices are easy to obtain, although it may take some ingenuity to find some of them, depending on where you live. You'll discover that they needn't be expensive, either.

Half of all Americans live within 50 miles of a major city that includes large Asian, Indian, and Latin populations, and most of these cities have at least one Asian, Indian, and Latin grocery store. Those stores are where you'll find some of the more unusual healing spices, such as amchur, cardamom, kokum, galangal, and tamarind. You can find these markets by looking in the phone book or on the Internet, as they generally do not advertise. (And Oriental sections of national and regional supermarkets continue to get more expansive, with many spices that you couldn't find a few years ago—such as fenugreek, lemongrass, star anise, and wasabi—appearing on shelves.)

Many of these markets, particularly the Indian markets, sell spices in bulk, packaged in tins or plastic bags of 14 ounces or more. (Spices purchased in bulk keep best if you remove them from their plastic wrapping and store them in airtight glass containers.) The cost of buying bulk is much less than buying 2.5-ounce bottles of the same spice in a large chain supermarket. Or you can share the cost, splitting the bulk purchase with family or friends.

There are also many spice retailers that sell through the Internet. But compare prices, as spices bought via the Internet are generally more costly than those from a local market. You'll find a helpful list of Internet spice retailers in the "Buyer's Guide" on page 309.

Purchasing and Storing Spices

Spices are typically sold in one- or two-ounce tins or glass containers. Spices sold in bulk generally come in plastic. (Stay away from cardboard packaging, which doesn't preserve freshness.) As mentioned earlier, if the spice isn't sold in tin or glass, it's best to transfer it as soon as you get home into an airtight tin or glass container in order to preserve freshness.

You can purchase spices fresh, dried, whole, cracked, coarsely ground, and finely ground. (You'll learn about how to buy the individual spices featured in this book under the entry for each spice in Part II.) But you'll get the most aromatic pleasure out of your spices if you buy them whole and grind them yourself. That's because whole spices start to "leak" aroma and flavor as soon as they are ground. This is why whole spices have very little, if any, aroma until they are ground.

If you grind your spices, store them in small spice jars that you can purchase at many discount stores, supermarkets, major retailers that sell kitchen equipment, or Internet sites that sell spices.

Store all spices in a cool, dark place. Heat, moisture, and direct sunlight accelerate the loss of flavor and can break down the aromatic chemical components. Ideally, store spices at a temperature between 50° and 60°F. High temperatures can cause spices to cake or harden, and change or lose color.

When using spices, don't let them sit around the stove. Tightly close the container immediately after its use and return it to its cool storage space as soon as possible.

Under ideal conditions, ground spices will keep for about a year and whole spices for two or three years.

Old spices lose flavor and healing power. If a spice in your pantry is past its prime, throw it out. You can test ground spices by opening a bottle and holding it up to your nose—if there is little aroma, toss it. To test whole spices, rub them lightly between your fingers. If they are still fresh, they will release a little volatile oil that you can feel and smell.

Spice Equipment

Cooking with the healing spices requires only a few pieces of equipment.

Mortar and pestle. This common device is essential for crushing spices in small amounts—a teaspoon or less. Chances are you already own one. Make sure the pestle fits snuggly in the mortar. If not, it will make crushing and grinding more difficult. The best mortar and pestles are marble. (Those made of wood retain the aroma of volatile oils, creating an unwanted addition to the aroma of other spices.)

An alternative to a mortar and pestle is a rolling pin—put the spice between two pieces of wax paper and crush it by rolling over it repeatedly with the pin.

Spice grinder. Grinding more than a tiny amount of spice requires an assist from electric power. There are three kinds of appliances suited to the job: a spice grinder, a coffee grinder, or a hand-held mini food processor. You'll get spices ground to a smooth powder in seconds, compared to the task of doing it by hand with a traditional mortar and pestle. And no skill is involved. Just drop the spice in and turn on the appliance. (Make sure to follow the manufacturer's directions.) If you start to detect an odor in the appliance after several uses, grinding sugar or rice should make it disappear.

Small heavy skillet. You will need this for dry roasting, a technique required before grinding many whole spices and seeds. (See below.) The best kind is an old-fashioned, treated cast iron skillet. Not only does it work the best, it's also inexpensive compared to many of today's top-of-the-line pots and pans. A smaller pan is ideal for cooks preparing spices at home.

Roasting Spices

Most (but not all) whole spices benefit from a light, dry roasting before grinding. It's important that you do this properly. The goal is to brown them without burning them. If it's your first try, be prepared to lose a batch or two.

To begin, heat a small heavy frying pan (preferably one made of cast iron) over medium heat until it gets nice and hot, about two minutes. Add the spices. Grab the handle (make sure to use an oven mitt or potholder, as the handle gets very hot) and shake the spices around. At the same time, stir the spices continuously with a wooden spoon so they don't burn. For the first minute or two while the spices are losing their moisture, nothing will happen. As they continue to fry, they will start to smoke. Your nose will sense the fragrance as they start to release their aroma. Continue to fry until they are a deep brown. If they are cooking too fast, turn down the heat. Transfer the spices to a clean plate to cool before grinding.

Spices are generally roasted individually, even if you are making a blend, as they don't brown at the same rate.

The whole process can take anywhere from a few to 10 minutes. The time element depends on the type of spice you are roasting, the amount of spice, and the size of the pan. The larger the pan, the faster the spices will brown.

You'll get plenty of practice in roasting spices when you learn how to make healing spice blends in Part III.

Spices are beautiful to behold, pleasing to smell, and memorable to taste. The spice-by-spice chapters in Part II allow you to explore them one by one, for great health and exquisite flavors.

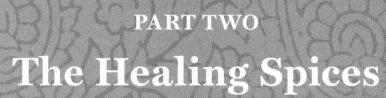

PART TWO

The Healing Spices

AJOWAN   *Nature's Pharmacy*

Ajowan (pronounced aj'o-wen) is a spice that's popular in India—where it's prized not only for its ability to add zest to curries and aroma to breads and biscuits, but also for its power to cure everyday ills. Many Indians are more likely to drink a little *omam* water—ajowan seeds steeped in warm distilled water—than to take an aspirin for a headache, cough medicine for a cold, an antacid for heartburn, or an antihistamine for allergies. And this folk remedy is now getting its scientific due: researchers have identified more than two dozen medicinally active compounds in the tiny crescent-shaped seeds. One of them is as strong as morphine.

Natural Pain Relief

When you chew on raw ajowan seeds, your mouth fills with a hot, bitter flavor that is so intense it momentarily numbs the tongue a bit. (In the kitchen, ajowan is always cooked, which takes the sting away.) That's the *thymol* in ajowan—which can numb pain as well.

In a study by researchers in Iran (where ajowan is a folk remedy for headaches and arthritis), the pain-numbing power of ajowan was compared to morphine in laboratory animals—and ajowan was just as effective! "The present study supports the claims of traditional Iranian medicine showing the *Carum copticum* [ajowan] extract possesses a clear-cut analgesic [pain-relieving] effect," write the researchers in the *Journal of Ethnopharmacology*.

The Secret Ingredient: Choline

Omam water is used as a home remedy for a variety of gastrointestinal ills: easing heartburn, relieving belching and bloating, reducing flatulence, and stopping diarrhea. In one experiment, researchers studied four different omam water solutions (whole seeds soaked in cold water, a warm infusion made with whole seeds, an extract of the powdered seeds soaked in cold water, and roasted seeds steeped in hot water) to find out which worked best and why.

When they gave each of the four preparations to laboratory animals, they discovered that all four helped heal the digestive tract, probably because of the presence of *choline*, a nutrient that aids the brain in sending healing messages to the body. But the roasted seeds had the greatest effect on GI health. When the scientists analyzed the seeds, they found *acetylcholine*, a chemical that controls involuntary muscles, like those that line the gut. Other researchers say the presence of acetylcholine may explain why ajowan so successfully soothes an ailing digestive tract.

An All-Purpose Healer

Asthma, high blood pressure, coughing, bacterial infections—ajowan has been used as a folk remedy for all of them. Researchers are supporting its healing reputation with new scientific evidence:

Asthma. Researchers gave a boiled extract of ajowan to people with asthma. Another group of asthmatics received *theophylline*, a bronchodilator that expands the airways. Every 30 minutes for two hours, the researchers measured lung function. The extract improved breathing ability by up to 32 percent—similar to the drug. Ajowan is comparable to theophylline in opening asthmatic airways, concluded the researchers in the journal *Therapie*.

High blood pressure. Ajowan had the same effect as the calcium channel blocker verapamil (Calan) in decreasing the blood pressure of laboratory animals. The researchers said that acetylcholine probably played a role in the pressure-lowering effect of the spice.

Cough. Iranian researchers found that ajowan works *more* effectively than codeine in suppressing a cough in laboratory animals. The probable reason: once again it's the acetylcholine, calming the contractions that result in coughing.

Bacterial infection. Researchers in India found that ajowan disarmed eight strains of infection-causing bacteria. And in a test of 54 herbs against drug-resistant *Salmonella* bacteria, ajowan was one of those that could kill the germ.

Getting to Know Ajowan

Ajowan (which also goes by the names *carom seeds* and *ajwain*) is a stranger to most American kitchen cabinets but not to American medicine cabinets, where one or more of its active ingredients are used in cough medicines and lozenges. Thymol, its essential oil, is found in toothpaste and mouthwash. And components of the spice are also used to maintain the shelf life of packaged foods and perfumes. Ajowan is a cherished spice not only in the cuisine of India, but also in those of Iran, Pakistan,

Ajowan is an ingredient in many perfumes.

Afghanistan, and North Africa. It has a natural affinity for starchy foods, and is used to perk up the flavor in dishes featuring root vegetables and legumes. In India, it's an essential ingredient in lentil dishes, both for its taste and for its ability to improve digestion and prevent flatulence.

When dining in an Indian restaurant, you might find it in an appetizer fritter called *pakora* or a filled dumpling called *samosa*. It's popular in Indian baked goods, and is found in a wafer-thin Indian flat bread called *pappadam* and in the puffed, pastry-like fried bread *paratha*. In

---

Ajowan may help prevent and/or treat:

Allergies	Flatulence	Infection
Asthma	High blood	Pain
Cough	pressure	
Diarrhea	(hypertension)	

Ajowan pairs well with these spices:

Chile	Oregano
Coriander	Marjoram
Garlic	Mustard seed
Ginger	Turmeric

and complements recipes featuring:

Apples	Pancakes
Breads	Root vegetables
Fish curries	Savory pastries
Legumes	Vegetarian entrees

Other recipes containing ajowan:

Chaat Masala (p. 265)

Afghanistan, ajowan is used in breads and pastries. It's also a key ingredient in the Ethiopian spice blend *berbere*, which is used to flavor vegetable dishes and meat stews.

How to Buy Ajowan

Ajowan is inexpensive but somewhat hard to find. It's available in Indian markets and some specialty spice shops. Use the "Buyer's Guide" on page 309 to find it on the Internet.

The small seeds (the size of celery seeds) are always sold whole, as they are rarely used in ground form. Look for seeds that are light brown, uniform in color, and free of extraneous debris. The freshest seeds will have an herbal aroma. If

Ajowan Parathas

Parathas are Indian pan-fried flatbreads that are often served as an accompaniment to a main meal. They are usually eaten with yogurt and pickles.

2 cups whole wheat flour
1 teaspoon salt
3 teaspoons ajowan seeds
1 teaspoon turmeric
½ teaspoon chili powder
Warm water
½ cup ghee or vegetable oil

1. Put the flour, salt, ajowan seeds, turmeric, and chili powder in a large mixing bowl. Combine thoroughly.
2. Make a well in the center of the flour and add a little water, about 2 tablespoons, and start mixing. Keep adding a little warm water until the mixture starts to get lumpy. Add and mix until you get medium-firm dough.
3. Put the dough on a floured surface and knead back and forth, turning, until the dough is nice and smooth, about 10 minutes. As you knead, the ajowan seeds will release their oils and aroma.

Set the dough aside, covered with a clean kitchen towel, for 30 minutes.

4. Put a little flour on your hands and start to form the parathas by rolling into balls about the size of a golf ball. Make sure they are smooth with no cracks.
5. Lightly flour a rolling pin and roll out the parathas to the size of a crepe. You can stack them by separating them with a piece of waxed paper until ready to use.
6. Heat a heavy skillet or a griddle over medium-high heat and add enough oil to coat. When the oil is hot, add as many parathas as will easily fit without touching. When the dough starts to bubble, turn the parathas. Heat for about 30 seconds, cover the surface with a little oil, and turn again. Continue this process until both sides are crisp and golden brown. Transfer to a warm oven until you're finished with the batch.

Makes about 1 dozen.

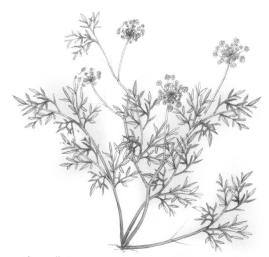

The small ajowan plant is similar to parsley.

stored in an airtight container away from heat and moisture, they will keep for two years or more.

In the Kitchen with Ajowan

Ajowan has a strong thyme and anise-like flavor—and a little goes a long way. The spice always must be cooked to take away the numbing impact of the raw seeds. The longer it cooks, the mellower it gets. To enhance the flavor, first fry it in a little oil until it deepens in color.

The small seeds are chewable, so they don't have to be ground. Ajowan lovers generally prefer the crunch that whole seeds add to a dish. But if you'd rather grind the seeds, dry roast them first. (See page 11 for directions on dry roasting.) The seeds are tender and easily broken with the fingers, so you can get a fine powder using a mortar and pestle.

The spice is best known for the flavor it imparts to breads, savory biscuits, and desserts. It also blends nicely in chutneys, relishes, and pickles. Here are a few ideas for experimenting with ajowan:

- Add it to meat and fish curries, lentil stews, and potato casseroles. Because it mellows with long cooking, feel free to add more than a pinch.

- Dry roast and add it to trail mix or spiced nut blends.
- Add a pinch to homemade bread and pastry doughs. It gives piquancy to the pastry crust of a chicken potpie or other meat pies.
- Sprinkle on top of steamed or stir-fried vegetables.
- Blend roasted seeds into a compound butter for sautéing vegetables.
- Fry it in oil and combine it with garlic, ginger, and turmeric to make a stir-fry.

ALLSPICE *An All-Around Healer*

Allspice. What else would you name a spice that resembles the taste and aroma of so many others!

When put to a blind sniff test, allspice has been erroneously identified as nutmeg, cinnamon, black pepper, and juniper berry, but it's most often mistaken for clove. And it's no wonder. Allspice gets its rich and fragrant aroma from the volatile oil *eugenol*, the same substance that has made oil of clove such a well-known pain desensitizer.

Eugenol, however, isn't all that gives allspice a reputation for being a healing spice. Allspice contains more than two dozen compounds with an even greater variety of healing actions, making it a genuine all-round curative.

Jamaican Me Healthy

If you've ever set foot on the tropical island nation of Jamaica, you have surely experienced allspice at its absolute best—as the spicy secret in the country's signature style of cooking, known as jerking. Allspice is what gives jerk chicken and pork their zing. (Ten-alarm fiery Scotch bonnet chiles give it sting.) Even the best homespun recipe can't match the taste of Jamaica's jerk, because the oh-so-slow jerk cooking you spot at roadside stands all over the country is done over a fire seasoned with the wood and the leaves of the *pimento* tree that produces allspice berries. The small and scrubby evergreen is partial to sandy Jamaican soil and it doesn't grow

prodigiously elsewhere, which is why it is hard to find genuine jerk anywhere else in the world.

When Christopher Columbus first "discovered" dried allspice berries after setting foot on Jamaica in 1494, he quite excitedly thought he'd found peppercorns—the Lotto of its day, considering that pepper was traded as currency at the time.

ALLSPICE IS THE SECRET IN JAMAICA'S SIGNATURE STYLE OF COOKING, KNOWN AS JERKING.

It was an honest (and no doubt a subsequently disappointing) misidentification. Whole allspice berries look like peppercorns—they're just a little larger in size and have a deep reddish-brown hue. Medicinally, allspice possesses antiviral and antibacterial qualities, making it an infection fighter.

It has analgesic and anesthetic properties, so it can offer mild pain relief. Jamaicans were the first to use it as a folk remedy to help alleviate a cold, soothe a stomachache, regulate the menstrual cycle, and relieve indigestion, flatulence, and other digestive woes.

Russian soldiers took advantage of its warming (stimulant) qualities during Napoleon's invasion during the winter of 1812 by sprinkling it in their boots to improve blood flow and help keep their feet warm. Its antifungal qualities have made it a home remedy for athlete's foot, simply by sprinkling powdered allspice between the toes. Used as an essential oil (pimento oil), its anti-inflammatory action has been found to help bring relief to sore muscles and the painful joints of rheumatoid arthritis.

A Powerful Antioxidant

Allspice is loaded with antioxidants. Researchers in Japan found these tiny berries contain 25 active *phenols*, a category of antioxidant. They include ellagic acid, eugenol, and quercetin—all of which fight the oxidative cell damage that can lead to cancer, heart disease, Alzheimer's, and other chronic health problems. Allspice may have other healing powers.

In three separate studies, researchers in Costa Rica found that allspice lowered high blood pressure in laboratory animals. The researchers theorize allspice works by relaxing the central nervous system and improving blood flow in the arteries.

Recently, researchers confirmed what Costa Rican herbalists have known for centuries. Allspice helps relieve the symptoms of menopause. The researchers were investigating allspice and 16 other plants used in herbal medicine as a possible natural alternative to hormone replacement therapy, which increases the risk of heart disease and certain types of cancer. Although the research is preliminary, the scientists think allspice may be a viable natural alternative in the treatment and management of menopause and osteoporosis.

Hard to Duplicate

Allspice is sweetly pungent with a peppery kick, a complex taste that is hard to match. For example, whenever you're out of cinnamon, cloves, or nutmeg, an equal portion of allspice is the perfect substitute, but when you're out of allspice, no single spice will do. To get a close substitute for allspice, combine one part nutmeg to two parts each of ground cinnamon and cloves.

Getting to Know Allspice

You may not realize it, but you are probably already well acquainted with allspice. It is a common flavoring in soft drinks, chewing gum, ketchup, barbecue sauce, pates, terrines, smoked fish, and canned meats. You might even have worn it: allspice is commonly used to fragrance cosmetics and even deodorants. If the label on one of those products says *spice*, you can bet that it's allspice.

Allspice also puts flavor to the liqueurs Benedictine and Chartreuse, and if you've ever had the Jamaican drink called *pimento dram*, you were drinking rum flavored with allspice.

Allspice is also a common ingredient in curries, mulling spices, and, of course, jerk. It is best known, however, as a pickling agent. The Jamaicans were using allspice to preserve freshly slaughtered meat and caught fish long before Christopher Columbus "discovered" it and took it back to Spain. Today, allspice is a key ingredient in the Spanish dish *escabeche*, fish that is first fried, then marinated in a mixture of oil, vinegar, and whole allspice. Moroccans use it in *tagines*, slow-cooked stews made in a clay pot, and in the Middle East it is a key ingredient in *kibbeh*, a dish made with bulgur and chopped meat.

Mexicans use it to spice chocolate, a custom that goes back to the ancient Mayans, and it is a key ingredient in *racado rojo*, a ground spice mixture and popular condiment in the cuisines of Puerto Rico and Mexico's Yucatan. In the

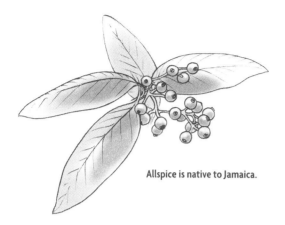

Allspice is native to Jamaica.

United States, it is most commonly used in desserts and is the ingredient that gives pumpkin pie its distinctive flavor. It is the secret ingredient (along with chocolate) in "Cincinnati-style" chili, named after the town that claims to have more chili parlors than anywhere else in the United States.

Allspice never quite attained status as a coveted spice in Europe, although the Germans make good use of it. They use it to flavor fish and meat dishes and in making sausages. It is one of the four spices in the French mix *quatre épices* (p. 271). The English are fond of it in fruited pastries, and the Scandinavians depend on it for making pickled herring. Those little dark balls you see in jars of pickled herring are not pepper, as commonly believed. They are allspice. Columbus wasn't the only one to be fooled by Mother Nature.

How to Buy Allspice
Allspice is the only spice native to the Western Hemisphere. Though it is indigenous to Jamaica, the pimento tree can be found growing wild in the rainforests of South and Central America. Few remain, however, because most were cut down for their berries and efforts to resow them have been difficult.

Making allspice is the leading industry in Jamaica, and Jamaican allspice is considered superior to the spice produced in Guatemala and other nations in Central and South America.

Allspice may help prevent and/or treat:

High blood pressure
(hypertension)
Menopause problems

Allspice pairs well with these spices:

Almond	Cocoa	Mustard seed
Black pepper	Cumin	Nutmeg
Cardamom	Garlic	Onion
Cinnamon	Ginger	Oregano
Clove	Mint	Turmeric

and complements recipes featuring:

Chocolate	Nuts
Curries	Picked vegetables,
Fruit pies and puddings	fruits, and fish
Game	Rice pilafs
Lamb	Seafood
Mulled cider or wine	

Caution: Allspice is an irritant to the skin and can cause a skin reaction in people with eczema. If using pimento (allspice) essential oil, make sure it is well diluted in another oil.

Other recipes containing allspice:

All-American Chili con Carne (p. 110)	Grilled Lamb Patty Pockets with Cucumber Mint Sauce (p. 165)
Apple Pie Spice (p. 271)	
Berbere (p. 267)	
Chesapeake Bay Seafood Seasoning (p. 273)	Jamaican Jerk Marinade (p. 269)
Cocoa Rub (p. 270)	Mulling Spice (p. 273)
	Pickling Spice (p. 272)
Coconut Meatballs with Peanut Sauce (p. 101)	Ras-el-hanout (p. 266)
	Spiced Mixed Nuts (p. 90)

Yucatan Pickled Red Onions

If you've visited Cozumel, Cancun, or any of the other resorts along Mexico's Yucatan peninsula, you've probably come across this relish sitting on tables in restaurants with other condiments. It goes with all kinds of Mexico foods, but you can use it like any onion dressing, including as a topping for hot dogs and burgers.

1 medium red onion, peeled and thinly sliced
8 black peppercorns
1 teaspoon toasted cumin seeds
10 allspice berries
½ teaspoon dried Mexican oregano or other
  oregano
3 cloves garlic, minced
½ teaspoon salt
½ cup white vinegar

1. Place the onions in a medium saucepan, cover with water, and bring to a boil. Drain immediately and rinse with cold water to stop the cooking. Pat the onions dry and put in a glass or ceramic bowl.

2. Put the black peppercorns and toasted cumin seeds in a spice grinder and coarsely chop them. Transfer to a small bowl. Break the allspice berries between your fingers and add to the ground spice. Add the oregano, garlic, and salt and mix together. Add the vinegar and pour the mixture over the onions.

3. The onions will be pickled in 24 hours and will keep for two weeks in the refrigerator.

Makes about 2 cups.

You'll get the most flavor by buying whole allspice, rather than ground, and grinding the spice yourself in small batches. You'll definitely notice the difference if you do a lot of baking.

Whole allspice has a long shelf life and will keep for several years in a dry, dark place. Once ground, allspice will gradually lose its robust flavor, so don't make more than you will use in a few months.

ALMOND   *Heart Guard*

Almond—a spice? You bet!
Though we think of almond as a *nut*, it's really a *seed* from the fruit of the almond tree. And, by definition, a dried seed is a *spice*. Its spicy nature is why almond imparts so much flavor to an array of sweet and savory dishes. It's also why almond has such a storied history as a traditional medicine. So let's rescue almond from the nuthouse (so to speak) and bring it home to the spice cabinet, where it belongs.

As a spice, almond is unique in several ways. Where most spices are virtually calorie-free, almonds are calorie-crowded—one ounce (about 20 almonds) contains 150 to 200 calories. And 78 percent of those calories are from *fat*. But never fear—most of that fat is in the form of "good" monounsaturated fatty acids, which (as you'll see in a moment) research links to a healthier heart. (And even to weight control.)

Almonds also contain other heart-helping nutritional factors. Just one ounce of almonds supply 50 percent of the Daily Value (DV) for vitamin E, a nutrient long touted for aiding circulation. The same ounce provides 25 percent of the DV for magnesium, a heart-calming mineral. The spice is also rich in folate (a B-vitamin linked to lower levels of heart disease), in plant sterols (natural compounds that have a similar composition to cholesterol, helping block its absorption), and in fiber (also linked to lower cholesterol).

Let's look more closely at why almond is one of your heart's best friends . . .

Be a Mono-Maniac—
About the Health of Your Heart

Want to eat a meal that contains the top six nutritional heart protectors? Dine on a serving of fish flavored with garlic and topped with slivered almonds. Don't forget a side or two of vegetables. Drink a glass of red wine with the meal. And for dessert, munch on an apple and a small piece of dark chocolate. Yes, say British researchers (who used statistical evidence from the scientific literature on heart disease to dish up this heart-protecting meal), eating these foods every day would reduce the worldwide rate of "cardiovascular events" such as angina, heart attacks, and stroke by 76 percent and extend life by an average of 6.6 years.

"We selected these foods because each possesses a substance that benefits the heart in a special way," said lead researcher Oscar H. Franco, MD, of the University Medical Center Rotterdam in the Netherlands.

Almond was chosen because two ounces supply the day's requirement of heart-protecting monounsaturated fatty acids (MUFA). Statistically, almond accounted for about 12 percent of the total calculated reduction in heart disease and increase in longevity.

Other findings about almonds and the heart:

Lower cholesterol. A team of world-class nutritional researchers at the University of Toronto tested almonds to see if they could help the hearts of 27 people with high cholesterol. After one month of eating one ounce of almonds a day (about a handful), heart-clogging LDL cholesterol fell by 4.4 percent. Eating 2.5 ounces a day lowered LDL by 9.4 percent. The ratio of "bad" LDL to "good" HDL cholesterol also improved. And almonds decreased the *oxidation* of LDL, one of the first steps in turning dietary cholesterol into artery-clogging blockages.

What accounted for the improvement in the cholesterol profile? The high levels of MUFA, said the researchers. They point out that years of studies show MUFA can increase artery-clearing HDL, improve LDL/HDL ratios, and lower LDL—thereby significantly decreasing the risk of heart disease. And when you're consuming *more* MUFA from almonds, said the researchers, you're also consuming less saturated fat from meat and dairy—and saturated fat is a known risk factor for heart disease.

"Almonds . . . reduce lipid [blood fat] risk factors for coronary heart disease," conclude the researchers in *Circulation*, a journal of the American Heart Association. They recommend them for "inclusion in lipid-lowering diets."

Lower C-reactive protein. C-reactive protein is a biomarker of chronic, low-grade inflammation—and the most up-to-date thinking points to artery-damaging inflammation as *the* process behind the epidemic of heart disease (and many other chronic diseases). The University of Toronto researchers teamed almonds up with several other nutritional components in an approach they call a "Dietary Portfolio" (an analogy to an intelligently varied investment portfolio). The foods—almonds, plant sterols from a heart-healthy brand of margarine, soy protein from soy foods such as tofu, soluble fiber such as that found in oatmeal—lowered high levels of C-reactive protein by 23.8 percent. That was *more* than a statin drug, which research shows can also lower the inflammatory biomarker.

Lower blood pressure. In a similar study of the Dietary Portfolio—this time on 50 people with high blood pressure—eating almonds and the other foods for one year lowered systolic blood pressure (the upper measurement in the blood pressure reading) by 4.2 points and diastolic blood pressure (the lower measurement) by 2.3 points. The researchers then analyzed the diets of the study participants to find out which of the Portfolio foods they actually ate and didn't eat over the course of the year—and discovered that "only compliance with almond intake . . . related

---

EATING ALMONDS CAN LOWER

HIGH BLOOD PRESSURE.

---

to blood pressure reduction." In other words, it was the *almonds* that made the difference, not the plant sterols, the soy, or the soluble fiber. The study was reported in the *European Journal of Clinical Nutrition*.

Almonds lower high blood pressure and increase HDL. And high blood pressure and low HDL are two factors in a condition called the "metabolic syndrome"—which also includes high blood sugar, excess stomach fat, and high triglycerides (a blood fat). Having all or most of these risk factors increases your risk of death from a heart attack or stroke by 74 percent. And metabolic syndrome also is a setup for type 2 diabetes—which itself increases the risk of heart disease six- to seven-fold! Almonds to the rescue . . .

Mastering the Metabolic Syndrome

Researchers at the City of Hope National Medical Center in California conducted a study on weight loss that also measured the parameters of the metabolic syndrome. Sixty-five overweight people were put on a low-calorie diet formula *and* about 2.5 ounces a day of almonds. Another group used the formula and ate foods equal to the almonds in calories and protein. After six

months, those on the almonds lost 62 percent more total weight, lost 50 percent more belly fat, had 56 percent less body fat, and had an 11 point drop in systolic blood pressure (compared to no change in the no-almond group). The almond group also had an increase in HDL (again, no change in the no-almonds). Of those in the study who already had diagnosed diabetes, 96 percent of those eating almonds reduced their diabetes medications, compared to 50 percent of the no-almonds. Both the almond and no-almond group had positive changes in levels of blood sugar, insulin (the hormone that controls blood sugar), total cholesterol, triglycerides, LDL, and LDL/HDL ratio.

"An almond-enriched low-calorie diet improves a preponderance of the abnormalities associated with the metabolic syndrome," concluded the researchers in the *International Journal of Obesity and Related Metabolic Disorders*.

High-Fat Weight Control

Almonds aren't shy about calories. A handful supplies 150 to 200. Snack on a handful of almonds twice a day, and you're taking in 400 calories—maybe 20 percent of your total intake! But here's the big surprise in the little almond: studies show that people who eat more almonds are much *less* likely to gain weight!

Researchers in Spain analyzed two years of health data in nearly 9,000 people and found that those who ate almonds at least twice a week were 31 percent less likely to gain weight than those who didn't.

Scottish researchers found that adding almonds to the diet for 10 weeks *didn't cause weight gain*—because people started to eat less of other foods. You can eat heart-healthy almonds without risk of putting on the pounds, they concluded.

Scientists in the Department of Foods and Nutrition at Purdue University in Indiana took a close look at the effect of eating almonds, asking a group of 13 healthy volunteers to chew a mouthful of about 10 almonds either 10, 25, or 45 times. Chowing down on the almonds "acutely suppressed" hunger, the researchers note in the *American Journal of Clinical Nutrition*. It also "elevated fullness"—the feeling of satisfaction after eating. The ideal amount of chewing for those benefits: 25 times per mouthful (10 was too few, and 45 was too much).

In addition to controlling your weight, eating almonds will simply make you healthier. In a study reported in the *British Journal of Nutrition*, researchers followed the eating patterns of 81 people. After six months, they were told to keep eating as usual—but add two ounces of almonds a day, an additional 220 calories and 16 grams of fat.

The outcome? Well, they ate the almonds, but they ended up eating *less* calories and *less* fat than they were eating *before* adding almonds. They also ate less sodium, less dietary cholesterol, less trans fats, and less sugar.

Getting to Know Almond

Washington D.C. is famous for apple blossoms—and Majorca for almond blossoms. From January through early March, Spain's largest island is covered in a carpet of geranium-pink flowers from four million almond trees.

Almond is not native to Spain, however, but to western Asia and North Africa. Ancient Egyptians believed the almond had medicinal powers, and they used it to treat everything from

Almond may help prevent and/or treat:	
Cholesterol problems (high total cholesterol, high "bad" LDL cholesterol, low "good" HDL cholesterol)	Insulin resistance (prediabetes)
	Metabolic syndrome
	Overweight
	Stroke
Diabetes, type 2	Triglycerides, high
Heart disease	
High blood pressure (hypertension)	

colds to cancer. India's traditional Ayurvedic physicians used almond to treat digestive, skin, and dental problems. They also ground it into a paste and mixed it with porridge to help patients pass kidney stones.

Today, Majorca is reputed to produce the world's tastiest almonds—and Spanish cuisine has the world's largest collection of almond recipes, ranging from the savory (including soups and sauces) to the sweet (including confections, biscuits, and a variety of desserts). Almond is the basis for Catalonia's famous romescu sauce, a puree that also includes tomatoes, garlic, and red chiles.

The Germans make lavish use of almond. Lübock in the north is world famous for its marzipan, a sugary almond paste that is an ingredient in many cake fillings and confections.

Italians use almond in their universally popular liqueur amaretto. In France, there's the almond syrup *orgeat*, an emulsion of almond, sugar, and water that is used to flavor a mai tai and other cocktails.

In the US, almonds are most popular for making sweets, including butter pastries, cakes, and pralines.

In India, almonds are popular in savory dishes, accenting rice dishes, curries, and vegetable dishes.

In the Middle East, chefs grind almonds into

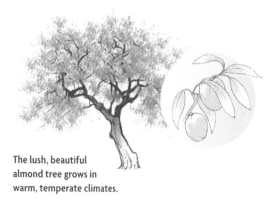

The lush, beautiful almond tree grows in warm, temperate climates.

flour, which they use as a thickener for stews, soups, and gravies.

How to Buy Almond

The almond tree—a lush, beautiful weather-sensitive tree that grows only in warm, temperate climates, such as Spain, Italy, and California—produces the familiar almond: a shell-covered oval seed with off-white flesh covered by thin, brown, leathery skin. Once picked, you can buy almonds in a variety of ways—in the shell, shelled and whole, natural, blanched, with or without their skins, dry roasted, sliced, slivered, diced, and as a paste, powder, butter, oil, or extract.

The freshest almonds are still in the shell. Look for unshelled almonds that aren't split, moldy, or stained. If you buy shelled almonds, get them in sealed bags rather than from open bins, which expose them to air and humidity, dissipating freshness. If buying from bins, look for almonds that are plump and uniform in color. And *smell* them: they should smell sweet and nutty. If the smell is bitter and sharp, they're rancid—the fat in the almond has spoiled.

When purchasing dry roasted almonds, opt for those with no additives or preservatives.

The more intact the almond, the longer the shelf life. Almonds in the shell stay fresh longer than shelled almonds in the skin, which stay fresh longer than skinned almonds, which stay fresh longer than skinned and slivered . . .

As with all spices, keep almond in an airtight container away from excessive heat and direct light. (The cooler the temperature, the longer they'll keep.) You can refrigerate almonds, where they'll stay fresh for several months. They keep in the freezer for about a year.

You can find almonds in all their forms in most markets, specialty stores, Indian and Asian stores, and online. The best almonds come from Spain (Majorca), Italy, and California.

You'll find purveyors of almonds by place of origin in the "Buyer's Guide" on page 309.

Almonds come in two varieties: sweet and

Almond pairs well with these spices:

Ajowan	Cocoa	Sun-dried
Allspice	Coconut	tomato
Anise	Garlic	Vanilla
Chile	Mint	Wasabi
Cinnamon	Nutmeg	

and complements recipes featuring:

Casseroles	Green beans
Chicken	Lamb
Cookies	Pudding
Curries	Salads

Other recipes containing almond:

Black Pepper Rice with Almonds (p. 57)	Sage Sausage and Apricot Stuffing (p. 215)
Garbanzo Beans with Mushrooms and Toasted Almonds (p. 29)	Wasabi Orange Chicken with Toasted Almonds (p. 260)
Los Banos Low-Fat Brownies (p. 97)	

---

bitter. Bitter almonds aren't for sale because they're poisonous. (They're loaded with cyanide, among other toxic compounds.) However, bitter almonds are used to make almond oil, with the poisonous compounds extracted in the oil-making process.

In the Kitchen with Almond

Almond's sweet, buttery taste makes it a natural for almost any sweet or savory dish. Almonds are easy to grind in a spice mill. Give the grinder a few quick pulses until you get the size of crushed nuts desired. (If you let the grinder run, you'll end up with almond butter.)

Raw almonds should be blanched or roasted before using.

You can remove almond skins by blanching

Prawns with Almond Hot Pepper Sauce

This seafood dish is made with romescu *sauce, a signature dish from Spain's Catalonia region. It is traditionally served with grilled seafood. If you have leftover sauce, serve it warmed over penne.*

To prepare the shrimp:
2 pounds jumbo shrimp, shelled and deveined
3 tablespoons olive oil
2 tablespoons fresh ground black pepper
1 teaspoon coarsely ground sea salt
To make the sauce:
⅓ cup blanched, slivered almonds
1 large ripe tomato, seeded
3 cloves garlic, smashed
2 dried red chiles, seeded
½ teaspoon ground red chile (cayenne)
¼ cup red wine vinegar
1 cup extra-virgin olive oil
Salt and freshly ground black pepper to taste

1. Combine the shrimp, the 3 tablespoons of olive oil, pepper, and salt in one layer in a baking dish and set aside while making the sauce.
2. Preheat the oven to 350°F. Line a baking sheet with aluminum foil. Place the almonds in one layer on the foil and bake for 10 minutes or until the almonds color lightly. Cool. Pulverize the almonds in a spice grinder with a few quick turns.
3. Put the tomato, garlic, red chiles, and vinegar in a food processor and process until smooth. Add the almonds and blend with a few quick turns. With the processor running slowly add the 1 cup of olive oil through the feed tube.
4. Increase the oven temperature to 400°F. Put the shrimp in the oven and roast for 10 minutes or until they turn pink and are firm.
5. Serve the shrimp on a bed of hot rice and spoon the sauce, room temperature, over the shrimp. You can also lightly heat the sauce and serve it tepid. Just continually stir the sauce as it heats so it does not separate. You can also serve the sauce chilled in place of traditional cocktail sauce to go with cold, peeled shrimp.

Serves 8 as a first course or 4 as an entree.

the almonds in boiling water until you see that the skins are starting to swell. Rinse under cold water. The skins should come off easily when you pinch the flesh.

To roast almonds, put them on a baking sheet in a 350°F oven for about 15 minutes. Slivered and sliced almonds should be baked about half that time.

To put more almonds in your diet, eat a handful at least five times a week as a snack. Here are other ways to increase almond intake:

- Churn almonds into butter by putting almonds in a spice grinder and letting it run. Eat it with a sliced apple.
- Spread almond nut butter instead of peanut butter or cream cheese on your morning bagel.
- Add a new twist to your kids' PB&J by substituting almond for peanut butter. (They may not even notice the difference.)
- Add slivered or sliced toasted almonds to cereal, yogurt, salads, and sandwiches.
- Make almonds into a cocktail snack by mixing 1 cup of unblanched almonds with 2 teaspoons extra-virgin olive oil, 3 teaspoons of dried thyme, 1 teaspoon of salt, and an egg white. Toast in a 400°F oven for 10 minutes. Sprinkle with fresh thyme.
- Add sliced almonds to chicken or tuna salad.
- Add a drop of almond extract to sweets containing almond.
- Add a few drops of almond extract to whipped cream.

AMCHUR   *Mango with an Extra Pinch of Health*

India's world-famous Madras Marina Beach, on Bengal Bay's northern coastal town of Chennai, is one of the largest and most beautiful beaches in the world. It's a year-round destination, but in late spring it really starts to teem with vacationers, many of whom head as fast as they can to one of the scores of seaside food stalls to snack on the region's famous delicacy—sliced and spiced green mango.

Green mango is the same tropical fruit that Americans enjoy for breakfast, sliced over cereal or pancakes, or chopped into a salsa to complement a Caribbean fish dinner, but with one difference. Americans eat mangoes when they're *ripe*—orange, juicy, and sweet. In India, they eat mangoes when they're *unripe*—green and tart.

Most Americans these days are familiar with mango—it's found in the produce section of supermarkets and is a common ingredient in fusion cuisine. But unless you've traveled to India or Asia, or shopped in an Indian or Asian specialty market, it's unlikely you've experienced mango as a *spice*. The spice—*amchur, am* meaning mango and *chur* meaning powder—is a powder made from unripe, green mango. And like the whole fruit, it's *very* good for you, delivering a concentrated dose of mango's many health-giving nutrients.

Filled with Good-for-You Phytochemicals
As its colorful flesh suggests, mango—like oranges, carrots, sweet potatoes, and other orange-colored foods—is filled with healthful *phytochemicals*, the nutritional compounds that help prevent many chronic diseases, such as heart disease, cancer, and type 2 diabetes. The standout phytochemical in mango is beta-carotene, a powerful antioxidant. But it's rich in several others.

When researchers from the University of Florida measured the phytochemical content of eight tropical fruits, mango was the winner. "We think mangoes have some unique antioxidants, as well as quantities of antioxidants that might not be found in other fruits and vegetables," they commented. And one of the most unique—and most powerful—is *lupeol*.

Anti-cancer. Studies show that lupeol can block the mutation of DNA, one of the main causes of tumor formation—and it does so as an antioxidant, neutering *radical oxygen species* (ROS), hyperactive molecules that run amok, triggering mutations.

And in an animal study on prostate cancer, lupeol battled back against prostate damage, leading researchers to conclude that "mango and its constituents . . . deserve study as a potential chemopreventive agent against prostate cancer."

Prostate health. An animal study also shows the lupeol in mango can reduce an enlarged prostate, a condition called *benign prostate hypertrophy* (BPH) that strikes four out of five men over 50, with urinary symptoms such as urgency, more frequent urination, a weaker stream, straining, and waking up several times a night to urinate. Lupeol, concluded the researchers, "could become an important alternative to treatment of BPH."

Balancing blood sugar. Studies from researchers in Brazil show mango can help normalize blood sugar (glucose) levels, with glucose level in animals fed mango flour 66 percent lower than in non-mango animals.

Reversing gum disease. In other animal research, researchers found that *mangiferin*—another antioxidant from mango—can reduce the inflammation of periodontal (gum) disease and slow the rate of bone loss. "Our results have demonstrated promising therapeutic potential of mangiferin both in the prevention and treatment of periodontitis," they conclude.

Pollution protection. Researchers in India found that mangiferin protected liver cells against the damaging effects of cadmium, a pollutant.

Strengthening the thyroid. In more research from India, animals given extracts of mango had

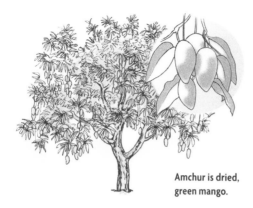

Amchur is dried, green mango.

Amchur may help prevent and/or treat:

Benign prostatic hypertrophy (BPH)	Gum disease (periodontal disease)
Cancer	Heart disease
Diabetes, type 2	Thyroid problems

Amchur pairs well with these spices:

Ajowan	Garlic
Almond	Ginger
Black cumin seed	Fenugreek seed
Black pepper	Mint
Chile	Star anise
Coriander	Tamarind
Cumin	

and complements recipes featuring:

Chickpeas	Marinades
Chutneys	Meats
Curries	Seafood

Other recipes containing amchur:

Chaat Masala (p. 265)	Los Banos Low-Fat Brownies (p. 97)

higher output of several thyroid hormones. Some health experts think that hypothyroidism—low thyroid function—is epidemic in the US, accounting for a wide range of problems, including weight gain and fatigue.

Heart disease. Another team of Indian researchers found that mangiferin helped slow the development of heart disease in animals fed a high-fat diet, reporting their findings in *Vascular Pharmacology*. And a team of Cuban researchers studied a proprietary mangiferin extract called Vimang and concluded that it had "potential" in the treatment of heart disease.

The Indian Mango—Cream of the Crop

There are at least a hundred different varieties of mango, with varying sizes, colors, textures, and tastes. If you thought that a mango you ate today had a different flavor than the mango you ate last week, it's probably not your imagination—especially if one mango came from India and the other didn't.

The mangoes of India are different than the mangoes grown anywhere else in the world: larger, less fibrous—and much sweeter. Among mango connoisseurs, the flavor of the Indian mango is considered to be unsurpassed. (And among Indian mangoes, the Alphonso is considered the best brand.)

Late spring marks the beginning of mango season in India, when the branches of the big, burly trees start to sag from the weight of fist-sized fruit. People buy them by the dozens to eat green, sprinkled with cumin, salt, and sometimes soy sauce. Mangoes are enjoyed just as much in the summertime when they're ripe, but it's the tart taste of the green mango that is truly prized.

Like avocados, mangoes only ripen properly off the tree. In fact, mangoes left too long on the tree are inedible, as worms invade the ripening flesh. It's because they are picked still green that they are ideal for exporting—a big benefit for people in the United States, Europe, and other temperate areas where mangoes don't grow.

Mangoes grow not only in India, but also in Africa, Southeast Asia, the Caribbean, Latin

America, and the Pacific Islands, including Hawaii. But the fruit originated in India, and India is by far the world's largest grower. During the late 17th century, emperors of India's Mogul dynasty ordered the planting of 100,000 mango trees to make sure there would be an unlimited supply of the fruit. To this day, Indians know how to put all those mangoes to tasty use. And one such use is amchur.

Getting to Know Amchur

Amchur is little-known outside of India, but it's a staple in Indian homes. It's made by drying green mango slices in the sun and then pulverizing the dried fruit into a powder. It has a tart and tangy taste, similar to powdered lime. And,

traditionally, it's used in much the same way Americans use lime (and lemon): as a souring agent. In India, it helps sour chutneys (this is why the mango chutney you can buy bottled in Indian and Asian markets is green, something that often puzzles people unfamiliar with the Indian penchant for the unripe mango). It also sours relishes and pickles (green mango pickles are often highly spiced and extremely hot). And it sours curries, especially vegetable curries. Amchur is also a key ingredient in the spice blend *chaat masala*, a sour condiment used to complement curry dishes.

Most notably to aficionados of Indian cuisine, amchur is used to tenderize the meat and chicken cooked in famed Indian *tandoori* ovens. It's one of the ingredients credited for making tandoori

---

Garbanzo Beans with Mushrooms and Toasted Almonds

Chana *means beans in India. This dish is adapted from a popular dish often sold by food vendors in South India. Serve it over basmati rice for a main vegetarian entree. The* sambaar masala *adds extra heat.*

3 tablespoons canola oil
3 cups sliced mushrooms
½ cup sliced almonds
1 teaspoon black cumin seeds
2 cups chopped onions
10 garlic cloves, minced
1 tablespoon grated fresh ginger
1 tablespoon amchur
1 tablespoon ground fenugreek
1 teaspoon *sambaar masala* (p. 265)
   or 1 tablespoon *garam masala* (p. 264)
1 teaspoon ground cumin
3 dried red chiles, seeds removed and diced
1½ cups vegetable stock
2 15.5-ounce cans garbanzo beans (chickpeas)
¼ cup cilantro

1. Heat 1 tablespoon of oil in a medium skillet over medium-high heat. Add the mushrooms and fry, stirring constantly, until the mushrooms release their liquid and it evaporates, about three minutes. Add a few tablespoons of vegetable stock

if the pan gets too dry. Transfer to a plate and set aside.

2. Wipe out the skillet with a paper towel and add another tablespoon of oil. When the oil gets hot, add the almonds and stir-fry until lightly browned, stirring gently, about three minutes. Transfer to a plate and set aside.

3. Heat the last tablespoon of the oil in a medium-sized Dutch oven over medium-high heat. When hot add the black cumin seeds and sizzle for 30 seconds. Add the onions and fry until golden brown, about five minutes, stirring constantly. Add the garlic and ginger and stir five minutes more, stirring constantly. Add the amchur, fenugreek, sambaar masala, ground cumin, and chiles and cook one minute.

4. Stir in the stock, the garbanzo beans, and the reserved mushrooms. Bring to a simmer, cover, and cook for 25 minutes. When serving, sprinkle with the toasted almonds and cilantro.

Makes 6 servings.

dishes succulent and juicy. (It also lowers the pH level of a sauce, keeping it fresher longer.)

AMCHUR IS USED TO TENDERIZE THE MEAT AND CHICKEN COOKED IN INDIAN TANDOORI OVENS.

Amchur is more popular in northern India. Southern Indians prefer tamarind as a souring agent. (Please see the chapter on tamarind.)

How to Buy Amchur

Amchur is sold as a powder or as dried green mango slices. Your best bet is the powder—the dried slices are tough and hard to grind.

When pulverized, green mango turns gray, but the amchur you'll find in the market is tan, thanks to a touch of golden-hued turmeric, another popular spice from India. So don't be put off by a gray color; it has nothing to do with freshness or quality. A grayer amchur only means less (or no) turmeric was added.

Amchur can be purchased at Indian markets or via the Internet. It's sold under the names *amchur*, *amchoor*, or *green mango powder*. It will keep in a cool, dark place in an airtight container for about a year.

In the Kitchen with Amchur

Think of green mango powder as an exotic (and dry) alternative to citrus. It has a tart flavor but is much milder than a lemon. Use it as you would any souring agent, such as in pickles, chutneys, and relishes.

Amchur is excellent in dry spice blends when you need something tart to add balance. Here are a few other ideas for cooking with the spice:

- Use it in marinades with or instead of citrus juice. It works particularly well in marinades for tough cuts of meat.
- For a tangy taste, sprinkle it on steamed vegetables, as you would lemon.
- Sprinkle a little in melted butter served with steamed shrimp or lobster.
- Sprinkle it on meat and vegetable kebobs before grilling.
- Add it to your favorite fruit chutney recipes.
- Sprinkle it in marinated cucumber and onion salads.

ANISEED   *The Ultimate Digestif*

Walk into any tavern in any small town along the Mediterranean, and you'll probably encounter older gentlemen in their daily ritual of sipping *pastis* (in France), or *ouzo* (in Greece), or *raki* (in Turkey).

These drinks are *digestifs*—after-dinner drinks flavored with the distinctive licorice-like taste of aniseed (also called anise), a spice traditionally used to soothe the stomach and ease digestion.

Scientists have discovered that the gut-calming compound in aniseed is *anethole*, and that it is yet another factor that makes the Mediterranean diet one of the healthiest in the world.

Relaxation from the Inside Out

Watching the men in their midday ritual, it's obvious that they're relaxed and content, enjoying each other's company. But that relaxation is also taking place *inside* the body. Research shows that anethole relaxes the parasympathetic nervous system, which controls the muscles of the digestive tract. In fact, when scientists first discovered the body-calming power of aniseed, they declared: "The relaxant effect justifies [the use of aniseed] in folk medicine."

ANISE FLAVORS DIGESTIFS
POPULAR IN TAVERNS ALONG
THE MEDITERRANEAN.

It also justifies its use in modern medicine. The use of aniseed for digestive ills has been endorsed by the German *Commission E Monographs*, which help guide health professionals in that country in the medicinal use of herbs. Commission E reports that aniseed can help alleviate:

- Bad breath
- Colic
- Constipation
- Flatulence
- Indigestion
- Stomach cramps

Aniseed also relaxes the muscles of the respiratory tract, and Commission E reports the seed can ease the bronchial spasms that cause the symptoms of asthma.

In an experiment in the Middle East, scientists found anethole works to reduce digestive spasms in the same way as the prescription drug atropine (Sal-Tropine), which is used to treat stomach and intestinal spasms. Aniseed extract also showed effects similar to the asthma drug theophylline, which relaxes the muscles of the respiratory tract. Writing in the *Journal of Ethnopharmacology*, the researchers also noted that anethole has anti-inflammatory properties that might help calm asthma.

In another study, scientists in Saudi Arabia found that aniseed extract "completely inhibited ulcer formation" in animals with damaged stomachs. They noted that aniseed stopped the formation of ulcers through at least four different mechanisms, including reducing the acid secretions that can irritate the stomach lining.

In Lebanon, a traditional remedy for constipation is drinking a glass of water in which aniseeds have been soaked—and when scientists there tested the remedy, they found it was effective. The same researchers also found aniseeds helped conserve body fluids during hot weather, preventing dehydration.

Getting to Know Aniseed

The ancient Romans were renowned for gluttony. A typical feast might include camel, giraffe, wild boar, ostrich, lobster, sea scorpions, and songbirds. Afterward, to help digest it all, they would always eat a piece of aniseed-studded cake called *mustaceus*. Today, Romans (as well as other Europeans) achieve the same effect after far more modest meals by chewing on roasted aniseeds.

Aniseed has been anciently popular both as flavoring and medicine. By the 14th century, it was in such great demand that King Edward I of England saw it as revenue-building opportunity and declared it a taxable drug. He used the money to help pay for the repair and maintenance of London Bridge.

Ounce for ounce, aniseed is 13 times sweeter than sugar, making it a natural for dessert—whether dessert is a handful of roasted seeds, an anise cake, or an after-dinner digestif. And almost every European country seems to have an anise liqueur. In addition to pastis, the French also have *anisette* and *pernod*. Italy's anise-flavored liqueurs are *strega* and *sambucca*. In Spain, it is *ojen*, in Egypt *kibib*, in Latin America *aguardiente*, and in the Middle East it's *arrak*.

Of course, there are non-alcoholic ways to end your dinner with aniseed. The Portuguese, Germans, and Scandinavians all have specialty cakes and confections made with anise. Anise cookies are a Christmas tradition in Germany and Italy.

Aniseed is popular in Asian cooking, especially Chinese, but it's used more in savory than in sweet dishes. Scandinavians also favor it in savory dishes, and put it in rye bread and a wide range of processed meats. In India, fennel seed (another licorice-tasting spice) is favored over aniseed.

You might also recognize the taste of anise in cough syrups and lozenges, where—as usual—it's used both as flavoring and medicine.

How to Buy Aniseed

The majority of aniseeds—oval-shaped, and yellow to green in color—are imported into the US from Turkey. They are sold whole, cracked, or ground. However, the seeds are so small that grinding isn't necessary—they're best used whole. In fact, ground aniseed starts to lose its pungency fairly quickly, so if you purchase it ground, use it within a few months. (If you have

Aniseed may help prevent and/or treat:

Asthma	Flatulence
Bad breath	Indigestion
Colic	Stomachache
Constipation	Ulcer
Dehydration	

Aniseed pairs well with these spices:

Allspice	Coriander	Nutmeg
Cinnamon	Cumin	Star anise
Clove	Fennel seed	

and complements recipes featuring:

Breads and biscuits	Pork
Cookies	Shellfish stews
Cheese	Tomato sauces
Chicken	Vegetable dishes
Pasta	

Other recipes containing aniseed:

Chaat Masala (p. 265)

ground aniseeds that have been sitting around for a long time, throw them away.) The whole seeds will keep in an airtight container in a dark place for about three years.

The anise plant—an annual with white flowers—grows almost everywhere the weather is warm, including Greece, North Africa, Spain, Italy, Malta, Central America, and Turkey. (Be careful if you see fresh anise for sale. Quite often, fresh fennel is mislabeled as anise.)

In the Kitchen with Aniseed

Aniseed's unmistakable licorice flavor is similar to the taste of fennel seed, but it's more delicate and doesn't have an aftertaste.

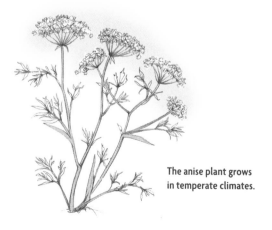

The anise plant grows in temperate climates.

Anise Kisses

Similar to the popular anise drops found in Germany, these little cookies are a pleasant way to freshen your breath and help digestion after a meal.

3 eggs
1 cup sugar
2 cups all-purpose flour
½ teaspoon baking powder
½ teaspoon cream of tartar
1½ tablespoons aniseed, slightly crushed

1. Beat the eggs and sugar with an electric mixer for 15 minutes. The mixture should look almost white and be thick enough to ribbon. Stir in the flour, baking powder, cream of tartar, and 1 tablespoon of the aniseed.

2. Grease two baking sheets or spray them with non-stick spray. Drop heaping teaspoons of the dough on the cookie sheet, separating them by an inch. Sprinkle the remaining aniseed on top. Bake in a preheated 350°F oven for 20 minutes or until the cookies are lightly browned. Remove them to a clean tea towel to cool.

Makes about 80 cookies.

Aniseed is popular in the United States in sweets, but it can also be used in savory dishes. You can roast and sauté it with other spices to enhance roasts, curries, tomato sauces, and stewed vegetables. You can use it to flavor cakes, relishes, marinades, salad dressings, and sausages.

Here are a few other ways to enjoy anise:

- Add a few crushed seeds to help balance rich sauces and gravies.

- When baking, slightly crush the seeds before adding to batter.
- Add a pinch or two of aniseed to vegetable soup, chicken potpie, and shellfish stews.
- Sprinkle the seeds on top of bread batters, sweet rolls, or into pancake batters.
- Put a small bowl of aniseed as a condiment on cheese trays.

ASAFOETIDA   *Fabled Flu-Fighter*

To say that asafoetida is an acquired taste is putting it mildly—or pungently. In fact, its sulfur-powered smell (think garlic and onions on steroids) is so intense that just cracking open a jar of asafoetida powder leaves an acrid odor in the air for hours. (Fortunately, asafoetida mellows in cooking.)

But that same smell (*foetida* is Latin for *stinky*) also allowed asafoetida to play a storied role in the US during the influenza pandemic of 1918. The Spanish flu, or La Grippe, as it was called, ravaged

the world for 20 months, killing close to 100 million people, with 10,000 Americans dying every week. During that time, thousands of people walked city streets in the US with a small bag of super-smelly asafoetida tied around their necks, trying to stave off the infection (and infected strangers). At the time, the US Pharmacopeia—an organization that sets standards for medications—sanctioned the spice as a flu remedy.

Fast forward to 2009 and laboratories in Egypt and Taiwan . . .

Facing Down the Flu

The Spanish flu infected the globe nearly a century ago, but descriptions of its devastation once again dominated the media in the spring of 2009, when a new flu pandemic—the swine flu—broke out in Mexico and speedily spread around the world.

As this book is written, the rate of infection and death from swine flu have been miniscule compared to the Spanish flu. But the two share some characteristics: both threaten young adults more than older people; and both are a type A influenza (denoting degree of severity, with "A" being the worst), with an H1N1 subtype (denoting the type of virus).

Asafoetida to the rescue?

Researchers in Egypt and Taiwan quickly tested the smelly spice to find out if it was a match for swine flu. And it was—at least in the laboratory, where asafoetida killed the swine flu virus more effectively than did amantadine (Symadine), one of the antiviral drugs prescribed for treating swine flu. Compounds in asafoetida "may serve as promising lead components for new drug development" against the swine flu, said the Taiwanese researchers in the American Chemical Society's *Journal of Natural Products*.

Corralling Cancer

Asafoetida announces itself to your nose through an abundance of sulfur compounds. However, scientists—pursuing the lead of asafoetida's traditional use as a medicine in many parts of the

DURING THE 1918 FLU PANDEMIC, ASAFOETIDA WAS USED TO WARD OFF INFECTION.

world—have isolated *hundreds* of active compounds in asafoetida, and are figuring out which ones have preventive and curative power. But whatever the active ingredients of asafoetida, they're definitely active against cancer.

One of the team of researchers who pitted asafoetida against swine flu also conducted a study on the spice's ability to battle cancer. Mixing the spice with lung, breast, liver, and oral cancer cells

One Doctor's Anti-Smoking Campaign

The acrid smell of the asafoetida necklace he wore for the duration of the Spanish flu epidemic was still in the memory of a Philadelphia ear, nose, and throat specialist when, in 1975, he came up with a novel way to help people stop smoking: by tainting cigarettes with the taste of asafoetida.

He based his hypothesis on Pavlov's method of conditioned reflex: if cigarettes tasted like asafoetida instead of tobacco, people would start to hate the taste of cigarettes. And they did!

For his experiment, he recruited 21 smokers between the ages of 23 and 60 who had been smoking about a pack a day for an average of 36 years. The instructions were simple: just before lighting up, they were to put an asafoetida lozenge under the tongue and keep it there while they smoked. Each person got 100 lozenges to get them through five packs of cigarettes. Within a week, 82 percent of the smokers had quit. Just putting a cigarette to the lips "gives a feeling of nausea and [the patient] doesn't even light the cigarette," explained Albert P. Seltzer, MD, in the *Journal of the National Medical Association*.

Four years later all the ex-smokers were still cigarette-free.

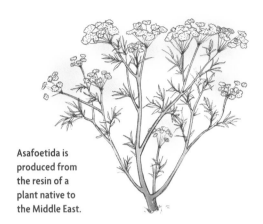

Asafoetida is produced from the resin of a plant native to the Middle East.

Asafoetida may help prevent and/or treat:

Cancer	Irritable bowel syndrome
Flatulence	
Flu	

Asafoetida pairs well with these spices:

Ajowan	Ginger
Black pepper	Mustard seed
Cardamom	Tamarind
Coriander	Turmeric
Fennel seed	

and complements recipes featuring:

Beans	Lentils
Cabbage	Nuts
Cauliflower	Pickles
Chutney	Red meat
Curries	

Other recipes containing asafoetida:

Brussels Sprouts Kulambu (p. 123)	Onion and Tomato Chutney (p. 113)
Chaat Masala (p. 265)	Sambaar Masala (p. 265)

cut cancer activity by 50 percent. Polyphenols—powerful antioxidants in asafoetida similar to those in green tea, red wine, and dark chocolate—may be the factors that corral cancer, said the researchers.

Researchers in India also tested the spice against cancer, and found that it slowed the formation of skin cancer in laboratory animals. It also boosted blood levels of cancer-fighting antioxidants.

And in a study on breast cancer, scientists in India found that feeding laboratory animals with asafoetida "resulted in a significant reduction" in the number and size of breast cancers induced by treatment with a toxic chemical. "These findings indicate the [cancer-preventing] potential of asafoetida," they concluded in *Breast Cancer Research and Treatment*.

Aiding Digestion

Asafoetida is a staple of Indian cuisine—and one reason why lentils, beans, and other gas-producing foods in India's diet are tolerated so well. In a study in the *Journal of Ethnopharmacology*, scientists in the Middle East reported the spice relaxes the muscles of the gastrointestinal tract. Two other studies found that regular ingestion of the spice can help relieve the symptoms of irritable bowel syndrome, including intestinal cramping, bloating, and gas.

Getting to Know Asafoetida

The world is a little schizophrenic about asafoetida, a spice produced from the resin (sap) of a plant native to Iran and Afghanistan—its common names include both *devil's dung* and *food of the gods*! That's because asafoetida is stinky when raw but smoothly flavorful when cooked, with a scent similar to cooked onions or garlic.

And that scent is a daily presence in kitchens throughout India, Nepal, and parts of the Middle East. A piece of asafoetida resin the size of a marble is almost always found under the lids of cooking pots filled with lentils,

Spiced Vegetable Fritters

Called bhajis, *these vegetable fritters are served warm as a snack with a chutney dipping sauce in India. This recipe comes from Alamelu Vairavan, an exceptional cook and author of* Healthy South Indian Cooking *(Hippocrene Books). I recommend serving these fritters with Onion and Tomato Chutney (p. 113), another recipe from Alamelu that also features asafoetida. Besan (chickpea flour) is available in Indian markets. If you cannot find it, you can use instant pakora mix in place of the flour, salt, and baking soda. The mix is available in Indian markets and some supermarkets that carry ethnic ingredients.*

1 cup besan (chickpea flour)
¼ cup rice flour
1 teaspoon salt
¼ teaspoon baking powder
½ teaspoon cayenne
½ teaspoon asafoetida powder
¼ teaspoon turmeric
30 thin slices eggplant, potato, or white onion
Canola oil for frying

1. Mix all the dry ingredients together by hand in a medium bowl.

2. Add approximately 1 cup of water to the dry ingredients, stirring until it makes a smooth, thick batter. Set aside for 30 minutes.

3. Heat enough oil in a deep skillet or wok for deep-frying. One by one, coat each vegetable with the batter and add to the frying oil. Fry a few slices at a time until golden brown on both sides, about two to three minutes. Drain the vegetables on paper towels. Repeat until all are fried.

Makes 6 servings.

---

cabbage, cauliflower, brussels sprouts, or other foods with a reputation for producing flatulence. Asafoetida is also a frequent flavoring in Indian curries, Indian ground meatballs called *koftas*, and fried bread called *papadum*. It's also a key ingredient in the Indian spice mix *chaat masala*, which is used in side dishes and snack foods.

Iranians rub asafoetida on warmed plates used to serve meat. In Afghanistan, cooks sprinkle asafoetida and salt on meat as a tenderizer.

Though it is virtually unheard of in Western culinary arts, chances are you might have some in your kitchen cupboard: rumor has it that it's a secret, unlisted spice in the popular American staple, Worcestershire sauce.

How to Buy Asafoetida

Asafoetida is sold in several forms, including solid resin, paste, and powder. I strongly suggest buying the powdered form. For the uninitiated,

the solid can be difficult to handle, as can the paste. (Even the powder requires judicious handling, as I'll discuss in a moment.)

The powder comes in two colors: light brown and yellow. The yellow is slightly milder because it's colored with turmeric, a golden-yellow spice. Yellow asafoetida blends more easily with other ingredients.

The resin ranges in shades from dark red to brown. Stay away from those that are almost black in appearance, which is a sign of age.

There are two varieties of asafoetida: hing and hingra. Hing is considered the superior of the two, because of its richer odor.

As you'll quickly discover, the biggest challenge isn't *purchasing* asafoetida but *storing* it. If the spice isn't stored properly, the acrid odor of raw asafoetida powder can overpower your spice cupboard and contaminate other ingredients. One way to keep the odor contained is to double wrap the spice. Keep the container tightly closed and place it in *another* airtight container or plastic ziplock bag. Or keep it in the garage!

In the Kitchen with Asafoetida

As I've pointed out, for all the ridicule asafoetida receives because of its overpowering stench *outside* the pot, it mellows *in* the pot, imparting a mild, sweet taste to food. Be forewarned, however, that it takes only a very little to get this effect. A pinch is all you need, even if you're making a large pot of curry or stew for company.

The best way to use the powder is to fry it in oil at the beginning of cooking. That will dispel the odor before you add other ingredients.

BASIL   *The Garden of Youth*

Basil has a lot more to boast about than the burst of succulent flavor that comes from biting into its summer-fresh leaves. For starters, it may help keep you young!

In a study on basil and aging, Indian researchers found that compounds in this culinary favorite neuter dangerous molecules called *free radicals*. These molecules roam through the body and create oxidative damage (a kind of internal rust)—corroding arteries, decaying neurons, and eroding DNA (a possible trigger for cancer).

"The study validates the traditional use of basil as a youth-promoting substance in the Ayurvedic system of medicine," reported Dr. Vaibhav Shinde, at the annual British Pharmaceutical Conference in London. (Ayurvedic medicine is the ancient Indian system of health maintenance and natural healing, in which basil was used not only to delay aging, but also as a remedy for diabetes, digestive disorders, skin problems, infections, and even snake bite.)

The researchers studied *holy basil*, a variety of the spice native to India. But all of the more than 30 varieties of basil contain the same uniquely health-giving phytonutrients, including the antioxidants *orientin* and *vicenin*, and the volatile oils (concentrated compounds that give a plant its distinctive smell) *eugenol* and *apigemen*. Studies show that these and other compounds in basil may help prevent or treat a wide variety of health conditions.

The Stress-Busting Spice

When you're under stress—stuck in a traffic jam, worried about your bank account, being chewed out by your boss—the adrenal gland generates *stress hormones*, such as cortisol and adrenaline. Short-term, they charge up your system, helping you cope. Long-term, however, they *weaken* the body, setting you up for conditions as commonplace as a cold or as life-threatening as heart disease. (In fact, studies show that unrelenting stress can cause or complicate nearly *every* health problem.)

But researchers in India found that several compounds in basil extract had "anti-stress effects" in stressed laboratory animals. Basil normalized levels of cortisol, lowered blood sugar (which spikes when you're under stress), decreased *creatine kinase* (an enzyme generated when the body is under severe stress, such as during a heart attack), and stopped "adrenal hypertrophy" (a sign of overworked adrenal glands). In a similar study, another team of Indian researchers exposed animals to the stress of constant noise—and found that those given basil had much lower cortisol levels.

Help for Damaged Hearts

Researchers in India studied animals with induced heart attacks—and found that basil extract protected their hearts by "improving the body's antioxidant defense mechanism and by diminishing free radical production."

Basil "may provide potential therapeutic value in the treatment of heart attack," concluded the researchers in *Molecular and Cellular Biochemistry*. Other laboratory studies show that basil extract can reduce heart-harming blood fats, including total cholesterol, LDL cholesterol, and triglycerides.

A Bounty of Healing

Other conditions that basil may help prevent or treat include:

Acne. Basil can kill the bacteria that cause acne, according to a study in the *International Journal of Cosmetic Science*. "These findings indicate the possibility to use Thai, sweet, and holy basil in suitable formulations for acne skin care," the researchers concluded.

Cancer. Laboratory studies in India found that the antioxidant activity in basil has "the potential to block or suppress" liver, stomach, and lung cancer.

Diabetes. Extract from basil leaves "significantly lowered the blood glucose [blood sugar]" in laboratory animals with and without diabetes, reported a study in the *Journal of Ethnopharmacology*.

Eye problems. Eye drops containing basil and several other natural compounds helped relieve eye problems in more than 90 percent of those using the over-the-counter medication, according to a study in *Phytotherapy Research*. The drops were used for dry eyes, conjunctivitis (pink eye), dacryocystitis (an infection of the lower eyelid), and recovery from cataract surgery. (The product is Ophthcare, an Ayurvedic formulation.)

Pain relief. Take a whiff of fresh or dried basil—especially the variety known as *sweet basil*—and you'll detect a slight scent of clove. The source of this aroma is eugenol, the same compound that makes oil of clove an effective painkiller. Eugenol works by blocking *cyclooxygenase* (COX), the pain-triggering enzymes also blocked by nonsteroidal anti-inflammatory drugs (NSAID) such as aspirin, ibuprofen, and naproxen.

Wound healing. Indian researchers found that basil leaf extract speeds wound healing. Basil

---

Basil may help prevent and/or treat:

Acne	Eye infection,
Cancer	dacryocystitis
Cholesterol problems (high total cholesterol, high "bad" LDL cholesterol)	Gout
	Heart attack
	Malaria
	Pain
Conjunctivitis (pink eye)	Stress
	Triglycerides, high
Diabetes, type 2	Ulcer
Dry eye syndrome	Wounds

"could be a fairly economic therapeutic agent for wound management," they concluded in the *Indian Journal of Experimental Biology*.

Gout. In animal research, scientists in India reported that basil reduced levels of uric acid—the substance that causes the pain and inflammation of gout.

Ulcers. Holy basil inhibited the formation of stress- and NSAID-induced stomach ulcers in laboratory animals.

Malaria. An Ayurvedic preparation containing fresh holy basil leaves and black pepper relieved malarial symptoms.

Getting to Know Basil

Basil is one of the most recognized and versatile seasonings. But it didn't become popular in American kitchens until the 1970s, when the populace as a whole started patronizing Italian restaurants—and found out that pasta sauce doesn't have to be red. These days, green pesto sauce—made from sweet basil (the kind most often used in American kitchens), olive oil, pine nuts, and garlic—is as common as red marinara sauce.

Many people think basil has an Italian heritage, because it's so often teamed with the tomato. And it does grow profusely along the

Mediterranean. But it's actually native to India, Southeast Asia, and North Africa.

In days gone by, basil had a checkered reputation. To the Italians, it was the symbol of love—a pot of basil on the windowsill was a sign that a courting beau was welcome. When a Romanian man accepted a sprig of basil from a woman, they were considered engaged. But

---

BASIL IS A REVERED

PLANT IN INDIA, WHERE THE

ROOT IS CARVED INTO PRAYER

BEADS (TULSI BEADS).

---

ancient Greeks viewed basil with suspicion, naming it after the *basilisk*, a deadly mythological creature.

In culinary history, basil was most widely used in Italy's Liguria region, which includes Genoa, where pesto was invented. Not too far away, in the Provence region of France, cooks made a similar basil sauce called *pistou*. It includes garlic and sometimes tomatoes, but never pine nuts, and is added to soup instead of pasta. Nowadays, basil is also an ingredient in the liver-based pates and terrines of France; the volatile oils counteract the richness. And throughout the Mediterranean, basil is favored with fish and in fish sauces.

Holy basil and Thai basil are commonly used in Oriental cooking. Basil is a popular flavoring in the cuisines of Southeast Asia, especially in Vietnam, where it is used in just about everything—soups, salads, stir-fries, stews, curries,

and condiments. The Japanese cultivate a basil called green shiso, which is put in sushi rolls and salads. It is also fried in tempura batter.

Basil is a revered plant in India, where it was traditionally planted around temples and used in religious ceremonies (the root was even carved into prayer beads)—hence the name holy basil, or *tulsi*. In some weddings, parents give the bride away with a present of basil leaf. In winter, Indians make a basil tea called *tulsi ki chah*, which is brewed with holy basil leaves, shredded ginger, and honey.

Basil seeds become gelatinous when mixed in water, making for culinary adventures. In Thailand basil seeds are used in a popular milk-based dessert called *mang nak lam ka-ti*. In Iran and Afghanistan the seeds are used in a sherbet-like beverage.

How to Buy Basil

Basil is a beautiful, lush (and popular!) plant, with full, dark green leaves—freshly picked it can perfume a room like a bouquet of flowers. It grows profusely as long as you keep it warm and watered, and nip it back so it doesn't flower and go to seed. It loves warmth and wilts at the first sign of cold.

Basil comes fresh, dried, or as a paste in oil. Though sweet basil is the most popular variety, you can purchase fresh basil plants in other varieties. Check with your local nursery.

The fresh basil available at the supermarket is sweet basil. Avoid buying leaves that are wilted or have black marks. Store fresh basil in the refrigerator, wrapped in a slightly damp paper towel. However, it doesn't take well to being refrigerated, and starts to wilt after a few days.

You can freeze fresh basil, but it's a little tricky. A clever technique: gather the fresh leaves in a loose bundle and place them in a clear plastic bag. Blow air in the bag and tie it tightly. Place the bag on a freezer shelf where the leaves won't be disturbed, and take them out one by one, as needed. You can also cut a full sprig from your garden and freeze it the same way.

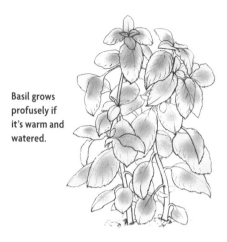

Basil grows profusely if it's warm and watered.

Dried basil doesn't have the lush fragrance of fresh, but the dehydrated leaves have a large concentration of the health-giving volatile oils—a fact that quickly becomes apparent when you open the jar! Dried basil is also the best for long-simmering recipes. Look for dried basil that is uniformly dark green in color.

Dried basil will keep for six months in an airtight container stored in a dry place away from direct light.

Varieties other than sweet basil are difficult to find, even dried. Check the "Buyer's Guide" on page 309 for specialty spice retailers.

Holy basil is also available as a nutritional supplement.

Caution: Animal studies indicate that basil extract in very large amounts may have anti-fertility effects in both males and females. The supplement should not be taken by any individual or couple intending a pregnancy, or by a woman during pregnancy. As with all supplements discussed in this book, use only with the approval and supervision of a qualified health practitioner.

In the Kitchen with Basil

Even if you grow your own basil, you should always have a jar of dried basil in the pantry. Fresh basil is wonderful raw but it doesn't take well to cooking, especially long cooking, as its flavor dissipates easily. It's also finicky about

Basil pairs well with these spices:

Allspice	Lemongrass	Sage
Ajowan	Juniper berry	Saffron
Black pepper	Marjoram	Sun-dried
Celery seed	Mint	tomato
Galangal	Oregano	Thyme
Garlic	Parsley	
Ginger	Rosemary	

and complements recipes featuring:

Beans	Pasta
Bread	Poultry
Cheese, hard and pungent	Salads
Corn	Squash
Eggplant	Stuffings
Lamb	Tomatoes and tomato sauces
Nuts	Zucchini
Olives and olive oil	

Other recipes containing basil:

All-American Chili con Carne (p. 110)	Shellfish in Saffron Broth (p. 211)
Pizza Spice Blend (p. 272)	Thai Red Curry Paste (p. 286)

being handled, and can turn black if bruised or cut with a knife. Only use fresh basil in the last few minutes of cooking. If a recipe calls for chopped fresh basil, tear it with your hands.

Two of the best ways to enjoy fresh basil: take a handful of whole leaves and toss them into hot pasta and dress with extra-virgin olive oil; or layer fresh basil leaves between slices of fresh vine-ripened summer tomatoes and fresh mozzarella cheese, sprinkle with freshly ground black pepper, and drizzle with extra-virgin olive oil.

Dried basil has a strong scent. But it isn't as penetrating in the pot as its aroma suggests, so you can use it liberally. It is a natural for intense, full-flavored sauces.

Basil has a natural affinity with tomato. Its assertive flavor goes well with other equally assertive flavors, such as dry-roasted tomatoes, roasted peppers, and olive oil.

Ian Hemphill, an herb and spice expert from Australia, offers this suggestion on how to make dried basil taste closer to fresh: Mix ½ teaspoon of basil with ½ teaspoon of lemon juice, ½ teaspoon water, ½ teaspoon oil, and a pinch of ground cloves. Let it stand for a few minutes before using.

Here are some other ways to get more basil into your diet:

- Add basil leaves to Italian hoagies, grilled cheese and tomato sandwiches, and other sandwiches.
- Put fresh basil leaves in a bottle of white wine vinegar to mix with olive oil for salad dressings.
- Team fresh basil with mint and cilantro along with Bibb lettuce, bean sprouts, and chiles for a Vietnamese salad plate.
- Add basil leaves to stir-fries in the last moments of cooking.
- Make a healing tea by infusing chopped basil leaves in green or black tea.
- To make pesto, put 1 cup of fresh basil leaves, 1 cup of Parmesan cheese, ½ cup of pine nuts, and 5 cloves of garlic in a blender or food processor. Process while slowly adding olive oil (about ¼ cup), until it reaches a creamy consistency. Use pesto on pasta, grilled meat, or fish. Stir a tablespoon into soups at the last minute.
- Make a pistou as you would the above pesto, combining the basil leaves with 4 cloves of garlic and salt. Eliminate the cheese and the pine nuts. Spoon pistou over cold or hot salmon, broiled or grilled steak, sliced tomatoes, or bruschetta.

Meet the Basils

Basil is not one but a huge variety of plants, all of which botanically belong to the genus *Ocimum*—but only a handful are used as a culinary spice. These are the basils you might come across in culinary specialty markets:

- *Sweet basil* is the basil popular throughout the United States and Europe, and it's by far the most popular for culinary use. It has a full-flavored, sweet, mint-like taste, with a hint of anise and clove. The color is brilliant green.

- In recent years sweet basil has been hybridized into other varieties, with subtle flavors reflected in their names, such as *cinnamon basil, lemon basil,* and *anise basil.*

- *Thai basil*, also called *hairy basil* or *anise basil,* is similar in appearance to sweet basil, but with purplish stems and veins. Many gourmet cooks like to use it for its stronger anise-like notes and a spiciness that is not found in sweet basil.

- *Holy basil*, also called *tulsi,* is grown in India, where it's considered a holy plant and is infrequently used as a culinary spice. It contains more eugenol than other basil, hence its pungent, clove-like fragrance. (Clove also contains a lot of eugenol.) It's smaller than sweet basil, with tinges of purple, and produces mauve-pink flowers when it goes to seed. Among basils, it's the only perennial.

- *East Indian basil* is now cultivated in many parts of the world. It's grown both as a spice and to keep away mosquitoes. It also has a clove-like fragrance.

- Tea-bush basil is grown and used in West Africa. It's the least aromatic of all the edible basils.

- Purple basil comes in two varieties, *Purple Ruffle* and *Dark Opal,* which you might spot in your salad at a gourmet restaurant. It's milder than sweet basil.

Spaghettini with Basil-Tomato Sauce

This tomato sauce couldn't be easier to make. It has the rich taste and texture of homemade that can't be found in commercial varieties. It can also be used as a pizza topping; just continue to cook until it thickens to the desired consistency. The sauce can be frozen for up to three months.

2 tablespoons extra-virgin olive oil
2 cups diced onions
3 cloves garlic, minced
1 twenty-eight-ounce can crushed tomatoes with their juices
1 tablespoon dried basil
¼ teaspoon dried rosemary
¼ teaspoon celery seed
Bouquet garni (p. 271) including fresh celery leaves
Salt to taste
1 pound spaghettini

1. Heat the oil in a medium-sized Dutch oven over medium-high heat. Add the onions and sauté for five minutes, stirring frequently. Add the garlic and continue to sauté until the garlic releases its aroma, about two to three minutes.
2. Add the canned tomatoes, basil, rosemary, celery seed, bouquet garni, and salt and simmer, uncovered, until sauce begins to thicken, about 20 minutes. Meanwhile, make pasta according to package directions. Ladle the sauce over the pasta.

Makes about 3 cups of sauce.

- Make a basil vinaigrette for a rack of lamb or lamb roast by combining ¼ cup of the juices from the bottom of the roasting pan and putting it in a blender with ½ cup of packed basil leaves and 3 tablespoons of white wine vinegar. Blend while slowly adding 2 tablespoons of olive oil. Just before serving, whisk in 2 tablespoons of extra-virgin olive oil, and salt and pepper to taste.
- Make a basil marinade for chicken by putting a big handful of fresh basil or a table-spoon of dried basil, salt, and chopped garlic in equal parts of extra-virgin olive oil, lemon juice, and water.
- Wrap shrimp in a basil leaf fastened with a toothpick and serve with traditional red cocktail sauce.
- Help keep salad greens and other raw food fresh from contamination, especially during warm weather, by adding fresh basil to the mix or adding dried basil to your basic vinaigrette dressings.

BAY LEAF *An Infusion of Antioxidants*

Who would have guessed that so much healing could come from one small dried leaf! But that's bay leaf—infusing your body with antioxidant protection as easily as it infuses flavor into poached fish.

While cooking, the aroma of bay leaf intensifies as it releases its *volatile oils*—its scent-giving plant compounds that are also among the most powerful antioxidants in existence.

In fact, when researchers in Korea tested 120 spices, herbs, and vegetables for their antioxidant power—their power to reduce *oxidation*, the internal rust that can erode every cell of your body (and the precious DNA within cells)—they found bay leaf was at the top of the list. It was *stronger* than vitamin C, an A-1 antioxidant. It was *stronger* than BHA and BHT, synthetic antioxidants so powerful they're routinely used to preserve food. And it was equal to several anti-oxidant superstars, such as the resveratrol in red wine and the EGCG in green tea.

There are more than 80 active compounds in bay leaf, but the specific antioxidants that it uses to help keep disease at bay are the volatile oil *cineole* (also found in eucalyptus) and a class of compounds called *sesquiterpenes*. And they may be particularly effective against an epidemic blighting the health of more than 20 million Americans: type 2 diabetes, the disease of excess of blood sugar (glucose).

Taming the Sugar Disease

A team of researchers (led by Richard Anderson, PhD, a scientist at the Beltsville Human Nutrition Research Laboratory of the US Department of Agriculture, who is an expert in natural treatments for type 2 diabetes) studied 40 people with the disease, dividing them into four groups.

Three of the groups took bay leaf supplements—either one, two, or three grams a day. Another group took a placebo.

After one month, the bay leaf groups had big drops in blood sugar levels—up to 26 percent. But that's not all. They also had a 32 to 40 percent drop in "bad" artery-clogging LDL cholesterol, a 20 to 24 percent drop in total cholesterol, a 20 to 29 percent rise in "good" artery-cleaning HDL cholesterol, and a 25 to 34 percent drop in triglycerides, another heart-harming blood fat. Meanwhile, the placebo group had no changes in any of those parameters.

How did this spice produce such a powerful effect? Writing in the *Journal of Clinical Biochemistry and Nutrition*, the researchers speculate that the "bioactive compounds" in bay leaf might improve: insulin sensitivity (the ability of the hormone insulin to usher glucose out of the bloodstream and into cells), glucose uptake (the ability of the cells to deal with insulin once it arrives), antioxidant status (less oxidation translates into better control of glucose), inflammatory response (ditto for less chronic inflammation), and glucose emptying (the speed at which glucose is absorbed—with slower being better for balanced blood sugar).

Given the fact that type 2 diabetes increases the risk of heart disease six-fold, with 75 percent of people with diabetes dying from cardiovascular disease—those results are, well, heartening.

Healing by the Bay

But bay leaf doesn't stop at type 2 diabetes. Cellular and animal studies—the first scientific steps in proving the power of the spice to improve health in us humans—show that it might be natural medicine for:

Cancer. Several studies on cancer cells show that *parthenolide*—a compound in bay leaf—works several ways to foil cancer. And in a Russian study, an injection of bay leaf extract slowed the appearance and growth of breast tumors in mice with experimentally induced breast cancer. Other studies show that bay leaf inhibits leukemia and cervical cancer.

Arthritis. Bay leaf is a traditional remedy for the symptoms of arthritis. And in animal experiments, doctors in the Middle East found its volatile oils could alleviate the pain and swelling of the disease. Bay leaf possesses anti-inflammatory properties "comparable to those of analgesics [painkillers] and non-steroidal anti-inflammatory drugs [such as ibuprofen and naproxen]," they concluded in *Phytotherapy Research*.

Ulcers and poor digestion. Another traditional use of bay leaf: treating stomach problems. Recently, researchers in Turkey found bay leaf oil prevented stomach ulcers in rats. Other studies show it can aid digestion by stimulating the healthy secretion of stomach acids that break down food.

Bacterial infection. Bay leaf fights bacteria. Researchers in Morocco infected animals with 16 different strains of an infectious organism—but bay leaf helped keep the germs in check, showing a "strong inhibitory effect" on *E. coli*, *Salmonella*, and *Listeria* (all of which can cause food poisoning). In Pakistan, researchers found bay leaf was effective at controlling 176 different strains of bacteria.

SARS (severe acute respiratory syndrome). Bay leaf can beat back viruses, too. Research from laboratories around the world shows bay leaf oil can slow or kill the SARS virus—the cause of the highly contagious respiratory illness that, in 2003, infected 8,000 people and killed 800 before it was contained.

Wound healing. Researchers found that volatile oils in bay leaf helped speed wound healing in laboratory animals.

Mosquito bites. Essential oil from bay leaves is a traditional mosquito repellant, and a study in the *Journal of Ethnopharmacology* found it could repel mosquitoes for up to two hours.

Getting to Know Bay Leaf

The bay leaf is picked and dried from the bay laurel tree, a densely leafed evergreen that grows profusely along the Mediterranean Sea (although it's cultivated in many countries). And people have been picking it for thousands of years.

When physicians in ancient Greece completed their studies they were crowned with laurel

THE ANCIENT ROMANS

CROWNED THE WINNER OF

A CHARIOT RACE WITH A

WREATH OF BAY LAUREL.

branches—*baca* (branches) *lauris* (laurel), the origin of the word *baccalaureate*. Likewise, for the ancient Romans, bay laurel was a symbol of

victory and courage—with winners of chariot races crowned with leafy branches of bay laurel.

While people no longer wear it, we certainly cook with it. Bay leaf is one of the most popular and well-used spices in North American cooking. It's a rare kitchen that doesn't contain a jar of bay leaves—unless they've been used up! Bay leaf adds aroma to soups, stews, soups, beans, marinades, and fish boils. It's a key ingredient in San Francisco's famed *cioppino*, a fisherman's stew simmered in a rich tomato sauce. It's frequently used in pickling spices. And it's one of the spices used to cure corned beef—not an American original, but definitely an American favorite.

Bay leaf is generally used in savory dishes in both the US and Europe—though the British (ever the culinary oddballs!) like to add it to custards and puddings, too.

Bay leaf and French cooking are *bons amis*. It's the key spice in the *bouquet garni* that is enclosed in cheesecloth and added to long-simmering soups, stews, and stocks. It's also key to the simmering poaching liquid called *court boullion*. It's added to food made *en papillote*, a technique in which fish is wrapped in parchment to steam in its own juices. And it's used to aromatize the French fish stews *bouillabaisse* and *bourride*.

In fact, bay leaf is indispensable to *all* the cuisines in the Mediterranean basin—it's one of the ingredients that make the Mediterranean diet among the healthiest in the world. On the Greek island of Corfu, for example, fresh bay leaves are wrapped around *sikopsoma*, a flat cake made of dried, spiced figs.

How to Buy Bay Leaf

The only true bay leaf—and the one used in most scientific studies—comes from the bay laurel tree. But around the world, the term *bay leaf* is used to describe a variety of different leaves, none of which are bay laurel. If you encounter California bay, Mexican bay, Indian bay, Indonesian bay, or West Indian bay, be aware that they're *not* true

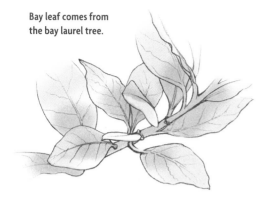

Bay leaf comes from the bay laurel tree.

bay leaf. In fact, they're an entirely different species. Indian bay, for example, is the dried leaf of the same tree that produces cinnamon, and West Indian bay comes from the bay rum tree. Most of these bay leaves have a stronger flavor than bay laurel.

Bay leaf is rarely sold fresh for culinary use, as its perfume is more pronounced and less bitter when dried. Dried leaves also infuse more flavor into food.

The majority of bay leaves produced and sold for export are from Turkey and Greece, with most bay leaf sold in the US from Turkey. It comes in two grades, but only one (usually referred to as "hand selected") is considered suitable—because it's not shipped with extraneous debris.

Look for leaves that are whole, uniform in size and color, and free of stems and bits of bark. The leaves should be clean and green. The darker the color and the larger the leaves, the better. Yellowing is a sign that they have been exposed to light for too long.

In the Kitchen with Bay Leaf

The woodsy, pungent aroma and flavor of bay leaf, with its slight hint of eucalyptus, is infused when it comes in contact with simmering liquid. The scent and flavor intensifies the longer it cooks, though if you leave bay leaf in the pot too long (more than a few hours) it starts to lose its aroma.

Bay leaf may help prevent and/or treat:

Arthritis (osteo- and rheumatoid)	Mosquito bites
	Severe acute respiratory syndrome (SARS)
Cancer	
Diabetes, type 2	Ulcer
Food poisoning	Wounds
Indigestion	

Bay leaf pairs well with these spices:

Amchur	Onion
Black cumin seed	Oregano
Black pepper	Parsley
Basil	Rosemary
Cinnamon	Sage
Cumin	Thyme
Garlic	

and complements recipes featuring:

Pot roast	Steamed food
Sauces	Stews
Soups	Tomato sauces
Seafood boil	

Caution: Bay leaves should always be removed and discarded before serving. Swallowing bay leaf can obstruct or even puncture the intestine.

Other recipes containing bay leaf:

Alsatian Pork and Sauerkraut (p. 148)	Penne and Sausage with Fennel Tomato Sauce (p. 117)
Boeuf Bourguignon (p. 240)	Spice de Provence (p. 271)
Bouquet Garni (p. 271)	
Chesapeake Bay Seafood Seasoning (p. 273)	

By-the-Bay Fisherman's Chowder

There are as many recipes for fisherman's stew as there are fishermen. This hearty meal-in-one is based on San Francisco's famed cioppino, which is characterized by a tomato-based broth and, of course, by bay leaf. This recipe makes good use of other healing spices, such as cumin and cinnamon. Substitute any fish or seafood of your liking.

2 tablespoons olive oil
2 cups chopped white onion
1 cup chopped celery
3 cloves garlic, minced
2 cups canned crushed tomatoes with puree
1 twenty-eight-ounce can diced tomatoes with juices
1 cup clam juice
2 cups fish or vegetable stock
1½ cups white wine
¼ tablespoon red wine vinegar
2 tablespoons Asian chili sauce
½ teaspoon dried oregano
1 teaspoon ground fennel
1 teaspoon celery seed
½ teaspoon chili powder
½ teaspoon black cumin seeds
½ teaspoon ground cumin
½ teaspoon ground cinnamon
½ teaspoon dried thyme
2 bay leaves
Salt and freshly ground black pepper to taste
½ pound sea scallops, cut in half

½ pound shrimp, peeled, deveined, and coarsely chopped
2 pounds firm white fish, such as sea bass
1 cup fresh parsley

1. Heat the oil in a large heavy pot over medium-high heat. Add the onions and celery and sauté until soft but not brown, about six minutes. Add garlic and cook one minute more. Lower the heat and add the crushed and diced tomatoes and their juices and simmer 10 minutes.

2. Add the clam juice, stock, wine, red wine vinegar, and Asian chili sauce. Combine the oregano, fennel, celery seeds, chili powder, black cumin, cumin, cinnamon, and thyme. Add the combined spices and bay leaves. Simmer, partially covered, for 30 minutes. Add the salt and pepper to taste.

3. Add the scallops, shrimp, and fish to the broth, cover and simmer until cooked through, about 10 minutes. Adjust seasoning and turn off the heat. Let the soup sit for about an hour. Reheat and serve, sprinkled with parsley.

Makes 6 servings.

Bay leaf goes with virtually any food simmered in liquid, especially roasting meat and boiled seafood. Steaming brings out even more of its natural flavor.

One or two medium-sized bay leaves are all that you need to flavor a dish for a family-size meal. Add it at the beginning of cooking.

Generally, bay leaf is used in savory dishes, but it will enhance sweets based in milk or cream sauces.

Bay leaves are used for flavoring only, as their infused oils permeate the ingredients in which they're cooked. Make sure you discard the leaves when cooking is complete. (The medical literature doesn't only contain research about bay leaf's many virtues—it's also filled with scary stories of digestive damage after a spiky bay leaf was mistakenly consumed.)

Here are ideas for getting more bay leaf in your life and your diet:

- Add a leaf or two to the water when boiling carrots, potatoes, or noodles.
- Add bay leaf to simmering tomato sauces,

even when you are heating up commercial pasta sauce.

- Steam shrimp in beer infused with bay leaf.
- Add more fragrance to rice by putting a bay leaf or two into your dried rice canister.
- Add a bay leaf to meat or to fish baked or grilled in foil.

- Make a French court bouillon for poaching fish, by combining two parts water to one part white wine, along with chopped carrots, onions, a pinch of thyme, and a bay leaf. Cover and simmer one hour before adding fish. Use enough liquid to immerse the fish completely.

BLACK CUMIN SEED *The "Amazing" Cure-All*

"It is a remedy for every disease, except death."

Religious pundits and scholars attribute that statement about the amazing therapeutic powers of black cumin seeds to the Prophet Muhammad, the founder of Islam.

The Bible weighs in too, describing it as "curative black cumin," in Isaiah 28:25.

And in this case, religion and science are in agreement. A team of researchers from the Medical University of South Carolina reviewed more than 160 scientific studies on the medical qualities of this jet-black spice, which is native to the Middle East and western Asia, and is formally known as *Nigella sativa*. "Among the promising medicinal plants," they said, black cumin is "amazing."

Studies show that black cumin seeds may help prevent and treat a wide range of chronic illnesses, including cancer, heart disease, and asthma, as well as many other conditions. The seeds' star component is a uniquely potent antioxidant called *thymoquinone* (TQ)—a compound yet to be detected in any other plant. Black cumin is also rich in many nutrients, including essential amino acids (the components of protein), essential fatty acids (the components of fat), the vitamin beta-carotene, and the minerals calcium, iron, and potassium. In all, more than 100 compounds important to health have been found in black cumin's volatile oils— and researchers believe many more are yet to be discovered.

But here's some of what researchers *already* have discovered about the therapeutic powers of black cumin . . .

Boosting Immunity

One of the "precious properties" of black cumin, noted the South Carolina researchers, is its ability to strengthen the immune system. "Studies . . . suggest that if it is used on an ongoing basis, *N. sativa* [black cumin] can enhance immune responses in humans," they wrote.

In one study, people treated with black cumin oil for four weeks had a 30 percent increase in the activity of *natural killer cells*, immune cells that slay viruses and thwart tumors.

Immunity declines with age, a condition scientists call *immunosenescence*. In fact, some experts believe aging is *caused* by the decline in immunity. But oil from black cumin seeds can improve the immune response even in the elderly, said the South Carolina researchers—probably because the spice provides a mixture of essential fatty acids (the molecular components of fat) that is highly nourishing to the immune system.

Protecting the Heart

Several studies show that extracts of black cumin seeds can help treat heart disease.

Researchers in Pakistan studied 123 people, dividing them into two groups—for 10 months, half took supplements of powdered black cumin seeds and half didn't. "Favorable impact" of the seeds "was noted on almost all" risk factors for heart disease—including blood pressure, blood fats such as cholesterol, weight, blood sugar levels (75 percent of those with diabetes die of cardiovascular disease), and waist-hip ratio (the more belly fat, the higher the risk). The study was published in the *Journal of Alternative and Complementary Medicine*.

Researchers in the Middle East studied people with high blood pressure, dividing them into three groups. One received 200 milligrams (mg) a day of black cumin seed extract, one received 100 mg, and one received a placebo. After two months, those receiving the spice had a significant reduction in blood pressure, compared to the placebo group. The spice also lowered "bad" LDL cholesterol. "The daily use of *Nigella sativa* seed extract for 2 months may have a blood pressure-lowering effect in patients with mild hypertension," concluded the researchers in *Fundamentals of Clinical Pharmacology*.

Battling Cancer

Numerous animal and test tube studies show that both TQ and black cumin seeds can fight cancer—including research conducted by my colleagues and I, both at the University of Texas M.D. Anderson Cancer Center and at the Center for Cancer and Stem Cell Biology at the Texas A&M University System Health Science Center. Our studies, and those from other laboratories, shows that TQ can fight cancer in many different ways. It can stop *proliferation*—cancer cells dividing and multiplying. It can stop *metastases*—cancer cells moving from the initial tumor to other areas of the body. It can stop *angiogenesis*, the formation of a new blood supply to a tumor. It can trigger *apoptosis*—the death of cancer cells. And it can enhance the effectiveness of chemotherapeutic drugs.

One or more of these cancer-fighting actions have been demonstrated for more than a dozen kinds of cancer, including breast, colon, prostate, lung, skin, esophageal, pancreatic, ovarian, and blood.

Black cumin seed may help prevent and/or treat:

Age-related immune decline	Dermatitis, contact
Allergies	Eczema (atopic dermatitis)
Asthma	Epilepsy
Cancer	Heart disease
Cholesterol problems (high "bad" LDL cholesterol)	High blood pressure (hypertension)
	Multiple sclerosis
Colitis (inflammatory bowel disease)	Pain
	Ulcer

For example, we tested TQ on human leukemia cells. The compound worked on the genetic level, by stopping the disordered regulation of proteins that control DNA—and mutations in DNA are *the* pathway to cancer. We also found that pretreatment with TQ enhanced the effectiveness and reduced the toxicity of two drugs used to treat pancreatic cancer—a crucial finding for the 50 percent of cancer patients who don't respond to cancer drugs or relapse after a positive response.

Recent studies from other laboratories have produced similarly exciting findings:

Researchers at the Institute of Genetics and Hospital for Genetic Diseases in Hyderabad, India, tested an extract from the powder of black cumin seeds against cervical cancer cells—and it killed them. The spice is a "potential therapeutic against cervical cancer," they concluded in *Cancer Cell International*.

Researchers at the Barbara Ann Karmanos Cancer Institute, at Wayne State University School of Medicine, in Detroit, Michigan, studied TQ. They found it sensitized pancreatic tumors in laboratory animals to treatment with chemotherapeutic drugs, resulting in 60 to 80 percent "tumor inhibition" with TQ, compared to 15 to 25 percent when the drugs were used alone. They found that TQ worked by "down-regulating" (reducing the activity of) two genes linked to the survival of cancer cells. They reported their results in *Cancer Research*.

Researchers in the Department of Hematology/Oncology at Henry Ford Hospital in Michigan studied prostate cancer cells. They found that TQ blocked cellular receptors for androgen, the hormone that powers the growth of prostate tumors. "We conclude that thymoquinone, a naturally occurring herbal product, may prove to be effective in treating . . . prostate cancer," wrote the researchers in *Cancer Research*. "Furthermore," they continued, "because of its selective effect on cancer cells, we believe that thymoquinone can also be used safely to help prevent the development of prostate cancer."

Because TQ is so powerfully anti-cancer, my colleagues and I declared, in a scientific paper in the journal *Molecular Cancer Therapeutics*, that it "could be used as a potential drug candidate for cancer therapy."

Calming Asthma and Allergies
Because it's a powerful antioxidant and anti-inflammatory, black cumin can also quiet down the symptoms of asthma and allergies, two inflammatory conditions.

Researchers in the Middle East studied 29

A Case of Mistaken Identity

In the US, this spice is most commonly called *black cumin*. As a result, it's often confused with the spice *cumin*. Even some supposedly accurate reference books on spices link black cumin and cumin, giving the impression that they're similar or even botanically related.

Well, black cumin and cumin do have a few things in common. They are both spices, they're both grown in India, and they're both common in Indian cooking. But they don't look alike or taste alike. And they aren't from the same botanical family.

people with asthma, dividing them into two groups. One group took an extract of black cumin seeds daily and the other didn't. After six weeks, those taking the spice showed significant improvements in their condition—*fewer* asthma symptoms, less *frequent* symptoms, and fewer occasions of *severe* asthma. They also had better overall lung function and took less asthma medications. There was little or no change in those not taking the extract. The results, said the researchers, show that black cumin seed extract has a protective effect against asthma.

German researchers conducted four studies on black cumin seed extract and asthma, hay fever (allergic rhinitis), and eczema (an allergic condition that results in skin rashes and other symptoms), involving 152 patients. They found that supplements of oil from black cumin seeds reduced the "subjective severity" of the diseases—that is, the people who took the spice said their symptoms were reduced. "Black seed oil proved to be an effective adjuvant [addition] for the treatment of allergic diseases," they concluded in *Phytotherapy Research*.

Health in the Black
Black cumin may influence many other conditions, including:

Ulcers. Egyptian researchers found that animals pretreated with black cumin had a 54 percent lower rate of developing stomach ulcers. Another animal study found that black cumin seeds reduced the rate of aspirin-induced stomach ulcers by 36 percent.

Ulcerative colitis. Researchers found that TQ offered "complete protection" against flare-ups in lab animals with this inflammatory digestive disease.

Pain. In animal research, black cumin was as effective as medications in reducing pain and inflammation.

Multiple sclerosis. Two studies found that TQ slowed the progression of multiple sclerosis in animals. "These data reveal the therapeutic potential of TQ . . . in treatment of multiple sclerosis in humans," said the South Carolina researchers.

Dermatitis (skin allergy). An ointment containing black cumin seed oil was as effective as commercial products in treating contact dermatitis in animals.

Epilepsy. Doctors in the Middle East added 120 mg a day of black cumin extract to the treatment regimen of 20 children with epilepsy who weren't responding well to seizure-preventing anticonvulsant medication. The frequency of seizures "decreased significantly during treatment with the extract," concluded the researchers in *Medical Science Monitor.*

Getting to Know Black Cumin Seed

Maybe you've been to one of the famous, world-touring exhibits of objects from the tomb of the Egyptian Pharoah Tutankhamen. Well, black cumin seeds were also found in King Tut's tomb.

The foot-tall flowering plant that supplies the seeds is found in the Middle East and in India,

> BLACK CUMIN SEEDS WERE
> FOUND IN KING TUT'S TOMB,
> AN ACCOMPANIMENT
> TO THE AFTERLIFE.

Pakistan, and Afghanistan. Hippocrates referred to black cumin as *melanthion.* In old Latin, the spice was called *panacea,* or cure-all. In Arabic, it was known as *habbat el baraka,* or seeds of blessing. In India it is called *kolonji*; in China, *hak jung chou.*

Black cumin seed pairs well with these spices:

Cardamom	Ginger
Chile	Kokum
Cinnamon	Nutmeg
Cocoa	Pumpkin seed
Coconut	Turmeric
Clove	Vanilla

and complements recipes featuring:

Breads and biscuits	Mango
Chocolate	Potatoes
Chutney	Rice
Lamb	

Other recipes containing black cumin seed:

Baharat (p. 268)	Garbanzo Beans with Mushrooms and Toasted Almonds (p. 29)
By-the-Bay Fisherman's Chowder (p. 46)	
	Panch Phoron (p. 266)

The spice was used like pepper in the countries where it grows, and it was brought to the Americas by early settlers for the same use. Today, it's a stranger to most Americans, though you've tasted it if you've eaten Indian *naan* bread or Armenian string cheese. But black cumin is a staple in the cooking of India and the Middle East.

In India, it's used whole and roasted in chutneys, curries, rice, and yogurt dishes. It is an ingredient in the whole-seed spice mix *panch phoron.* It's an essential ingredient in Kashmiri cuisine, where it's used to spice meats and in rich creamy sauces.

In the Middle East, it's a key spice in *kibbeh,* a hot dog-shaped fried croquette made with bulgur and lamb. It is often added to the Middle

Eastern spice mix *baharat*, which you can find on page 268. Its nutty flavor also makes it popular in breads and sweets—in fact, it's often mixed with honey as a sweet.

In Ethiopia, it's used as a spice in alcoholic beverages, much like Americans add celery seed to Bloody Marys.

Black cumin is also grown in Russia and is the topping on Russian rye bread.

How to Buy Black Cumin Seed

You won't find black cumin (though you will find cumin) in your typical supermarket, but you can find it in Indian markets or specialty spice shops. You may not, however, find it under the name black cumin. Your best bet is to look for *kolonji* or *nigella*, the Indian names for the spice.

You might find it on the Internet under *black cumin, kolonji, nigella, black caraway, blackseed, fennel flower, Roman coriander*, or *black onion seeds*. (Even though it has no relationship whatsoever to caraway, fennel, coriander, or onion.) But you could also end up with caraway seeds or onion seeds. To be certain you're getting the

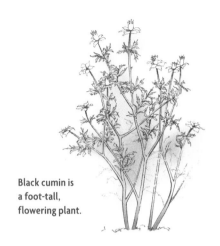

Black cumin is a foot-tall, flowering plant.

real thing, ask for black cumin seed by its botanical name, *Nigella sativa*. You're also certain to get what you want by *looking* at it. The shiny, smooth black seeds are unmistakable.

The seeds are always sold whole, as that's the way they're usually used. And they're not expensive—a three-ounce jar of seeds goes for about three dollars at an Indian market. They will keep in a dry, cool place for up to three years.

Black Mango Chutney

Mango chutney is a popular Indian chutney and black cumin is one of the reasons for its special taste. Serve this as an accompaniment to fish, poultry, or risotto, or put it on top of baked Brie. This chutney will keep refrigerated for about a week.

2 tablespoons vegetable or canola oil
1 teaspoon *panch phoron* (p. 266)
3 dried red chiles, seeds removed and diced
1 teaspoon black cumin seeds
2 tablespoons sugar
1 cup water
2 ripe mangoes, peeled, cored, and diced
¼ cup shredded, sweetened coconut
½ teaspoon salt
¼ cup cilantro

1. Heat the oil in a medium saucepan over medium-high heat. When hot, add the panch phoron, chiles, and black cumin seeds and fry until the seeds start to pop and the chiles are browned. Be careful not to burn.

2. Add the black cumin and stir one minute. Add the sugar and water and stir until the sugar is dissolved. Add the mangoes, coconut, and salt, and bring to a boil. Lower the heat and simmer until the mixture softens, melds, and thickens slightly, about 15–20 minutes.

3. Remove from heat and cool. Stir in the cilantro. Serve hot or room temperature.

Makes about 2 cups.

Black cumin seed oil, or TQ, is also available as a dietary supplement. Because of its potential in cancer prevention and its positive effects on the immune system, I recommend it as a daily supplement for general health. No side effects have been found from taking supplements, but pregnant women should not take them, as they can cause uterine contractions.

In the Kitchen with Black Cumin Seed

There's confusion around the *name* of black cumin—and there's controversy around the *taste*. Some say the seeds are pungent. Others describe them as slightly peppery. I agree with the latter. Some say they detect an aftertaste of lemon. Some claim the aftertaste is akin to strawberry. I agree with the former. There is no question as to their nutty flavor, though, which is why you'll find black cumin is quite versatile in the kitchen.

The seeds can be used as is, but dry roasting brings out more aroma. You should roast them if you plan on grinding them.

Here are some suggestions on ways to use black cumin:

- They're a classic addition to Indian chutneys—add a pinch to your favorite recipes.
- Black cumin will enhance meat dishes, especially stews made with lamb.
- Use the seeds to flavor rice pilafs or put them in mashed potatoes.
- Sprinkle them on homemade cookies and breads.
- Add them to spice blends.
- Put them in hot pepper sauces.

BLACK PEPPER *The King of Spices*

This common condiment has a royal pedigree.

During the Middle Ages, black pepper was considered the "King of Spices"—and it was more valuable than gold. Only the wealthy could afford it, and social status was measured by how much black pepper you had stored away.

To increase its mystery and desirability, Arab traders kept its origins a closely guarded secret, inventing wild tales of perilous searches for the spice in make-believe lands.

And when the Spice Wars—the conflict between nations to dominate the spice trade—intensified during the 15th century, tariffs and taxes drove the price of pepper up 30-fold. That sent Christopher Columbus westward from Spain to discover the land of pepper—and riches for the Queen of Spain.

But Columbus was off course by about 8,000 miles. The "secret" land of pepper was India's Malabar Coast, where the best-tasting pepper in the world is still grown today.

Pepper, Healer for Millennia

Indian black pepper is considered superior because it's particularly rich in *piperine*, the compound that zaps your taste buds and triggers a sneeze when it hits the nerve endings inside your nose.

The Ayurvedic physicians of India—the practitioners of the millennia-old science and art of natural healing native to that country—may not have known about piperine, but they did know about pepper's curative power. They prescribed black pepper for a variety of everyday and serious conditions, including constipation, diarrhea, insect bites, tooth decay, sunburn, arthritis, heart disease, and lung disease.

When pepper reached China, the spice was incorporated into traditional Chinese medicine—another millennia-old medical tradition—where one text described it as able to "warm the middle, disperse cold . . . while dispelling phlegm . . . and relieving diarrhea." One Chinese herbal remedy still in use today consists of a dried powder made from one radish—and 99 peppercorns!

In ancient Rome, pepper was more valued for its culinary impact—the Romans loved to season their food with pepper, and they buried meat and other perishable foods under piles of pepper to keep it from spoiling. (That was the first clue that the spice had potent antibacterial powers. Scientist now know that piperine can even inhibit the deadly bacteria that cause botulism.)

When in Rome—or anywhere else in the world—pepper as the Romans peppered. Because pepper is very good for you. Starting the moment you eat it.

Jumpstarting Digestion

Piperine stimulates the taste buds, triggering the pancreas to start producing digestive enzymes. It also tones the lining of the intestines. That boost in digestive power and speed is very helpful:

Speeding up transit time. In a study in the *Journal of the American College of Nutrition*, gastroenterologists found that 1.5 grams of black pepper (about 1/20 of an ounce) sped up "transit time"—the time it takes for food to move all the way through the digestive tract. Slow transit time has been linked to many GI problems, from constipation to colon cancer. The researchers noted that black pepper "is of clinical importance in the management of various gastrointestinal disorders."

Enhancing the effectiveness of medications. Pepper helps you digest food better—and metabolize medications faster. In studies on animals and people, researchers have found that piperine can increase the bioavailability of a range of drugs, including antibiotics, beta blockers for high blood pressure, calcium channel blockers for heart disease, cough medicines, and also drugs used to treat arthritis, epilepsy, respiratory problems, tuberculosis, and HIV/AIDS. It works by influencing enzymes in the liver that are active in the metabolism of drugs. "Piperine is exceptional in its influence on the liver drug-metabolizing enzyme system," concluded a team

of Indian researchers in the *Canadian Journal of Physiology and Pharmacology*.

Fighting Cancer

Laboratory studies on animals and on human cells show that piperine may play a role in preventing or treating cancer.

Colon cancer. In the laboratory, researchers in the US found that adding black pepper to a culture of human colon cancer cells produced "significant inhibition" of growth. Regular intake of low doses of black pepper may "offer preventive effects against colon cancer," concluded the researchers in *Annals of Clinical and Laboratory Science.*

Lung cancer. "Black pepper has been used widely in various systems of traditional medicines," wrote a team of Indian researchers in *Molecular and Cellular Biochemistry*—which led them to test the power of pepper against lung cancer. In their animal study, they found that treating lung cancer with piperine changed the level of several enzymes, "which indicated an anti-tumor and anti-cancer effect."

Breast cancer. A team of Indian researchers found that adding black pepper extracts to the diet of mice with breast cancer increased their lifespan by 65 percent. The findings were in *Cancer Letters.*

Pepper Your Health

Scientists around the world have discovered many other ways that black pepper may enhance health.

Easing arthritis. Korean researchers tested piperine against arthritis in two ways: they added the black pepper extract to a culture of human rheumatoid arthritis cells, and they fed it to animals with experimentally induced arthritis. In the human cells, piperine reduced compounds known to worsen inflammation, the hallmark of rheumatoid arthritis. In animals, piperine reduced inflammation and other arthritis symptoms. Piperine may have a role as a "dietary supplement for the treatment of arthritis," the researchers concluded in *Arthritis Research & Therapy.*

Preventing Alzheimer's. Researchers in Thailand tested piperine in animals with Alzheimer's-like brain changes and found the extract "significantly improved memory impairment and neurodegeneration [the destruction of brain cells]."

Better brains. In another study, the same team of researchers found that piperine had "antidepression-like activity and cognitive-enhancing effect" when fed to laboratory animals. Piperine may "improve brain function," they concluded.

Helping seniors stand up. Researchers in Japan found that sniffing black pepper oil stabilized the ability to stand (and therefore lowered the risk of falling) in 17 people aged 78 and older. "Olfactory stimulation" with black pepper "may improve postural stability in older adults," they concluded in the journal *Gait and Posture.*

Helping with post-stroke swallowing. After a stroke, many people suffer from *dysphagia*—difficulty swallowing. The same team of Japanese researchers found that sniffing black pepper oil for one minute helped improve the ability to swallow in more than 100 people who had suffered a stroke. "Inhalation of black pepper oil . . . might benefit older post-stroke patients with dysphagia, regardless of their level of consciousness or physical or mental status," concluded the researchers in the *Journal of the American Geriatric Society.*

Helping brain-damaged children on feeding tubes. In a third study, the Japanese researchers found that sniffing black pepper oil could stimulate the appetite of neurologically damaged children on feeding tubes, helping them eat more solid foods.

Quitting smoking. Scientists at the Nicotine Research Laboratory in Durham, North Carolina, found that the craving for cigarettes decreased after smokers puffed on a vapor containing black pepper essential oil. "Cigarette substitutes delivering pepper constituents may prove useful in smoking cessation treatment," they concluded in the journal *Drug and Alcohol Dependency.*

Lowering high blood pressure. A study by Pakistani researchers in the *Journal of Cardiovascular Pharmacology* showed that piperine lowered blood pressure in laboratory animals.

Preventing heart disease. High-fat diets and heart disease go hand in hand. Researchers in India found that laboratory animals fed a high-fat diet *and* black pepper or piperine had much less *oxidation*—a crucial step in the process that turns dietary cholesterol into artery-clogging plaque. "Supplementation with black pepper or piperine can reduce high-fat diet induced oxidative stress to the cells," concluded the researchers.

Healing hyperthyroidism. Indian researchers found that piperine worked as effectively as thyroid medication in treating overactive thyroid in animals.

Protecting hearing. Korean researchers found that piperine protected cells in the cochlea (the sensory organ of hearing in the ear) from chemical damage. Cochlear damage leads to hearing loss.

Reversing vitiligo. In the skin disease *vitiligo*, a malfunction in pigment-producing cells called *melanocytes* leads to irregular patches of pale skin. Researchers in the UK found that piperine promotes the growth of melanocytes. "This finding supports the traditional use of [black pepper] in vitiligo," concluded the researchers in the *Journal of Pharmacy and Pharmacology.*

Getting to Know Black Pepper

Like grapes, black pepper grows on perennial vines. But pepper vines soar to a height of 30 feet or more—you can see them trellising swaying palm trees in the state of Kerala on India's Malabar coast, where black pepper is big business and pepper vines are everywhere.

The vines have large, shiny leaves with spiky extensions called *catkins* that fill with peppercorns, the fruit of the pepper vine. A catkin full of peppercorns is a twisty stalk densely packed with what looks like shiny beads.

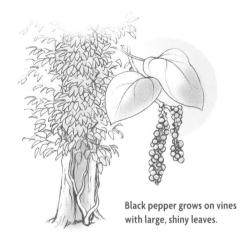

Black pepper grows on vines with large, shiny leaves.

After peppercorns bud, they gradually turn dark green—the sign that they're ready to be picked and dried.

As peppercorns dry, the peppercorn's outer layer (called the *pericarp*) turns thick, rough, oily, and black. At this point, the peppercorn is *pepper*—warm, penetrating, full-bodied, with lingering heat.

But not all peppercorns that you find in the market are black.

Green peppercorns (which became all the rage in the 1970s, with the popularity of French *nouvelle cuisine*) are unripe black peppercorns that have been plunged into boiling water, which inactivates the ripening enzymes and stops them from turning black. They have a fresh, hot bite but are much more subtle than the black. You can eat them whole and still smile!

White peppercorns—also known as white pepper—are black peppercorns with the pericarp removed, revealing a smooth, creamy white center, called the heart. Removing the pericarp is arduous, which is why white peppercorns are considered a gourmet spice, and are more expensive than black. White peppercorn is hotter and sharper than black, but slightly sweet.

Pink peppercorns have been left on the vine, turning from green to yellow to ripened red. Then they're picked and sold as so-called pink peppercorns. Like white, they're considered a gourmet spice. They're aromatic, with a benign and subtle flavor.

Piperine is found in all the peppercorns, but it's most abundant in black pepper. And there's a lot of black pepper out there.

Next to salt, pepper is the world's most frequently used spice. It is an ingredient in about 95 percent of recipes, and you can find it on almost every table in America. And no wonder—it offers a "bite" not found in any other spice. Even restaurants that consider salt an insult to the chef will offer pepper, usually freshly ground at tableside.

Indian cuisine makes elaborate use of black peppercorns, but eschews the other colors. Black pepper is a principal ingredient in many of India's most beloved spice blends, including *garam masala* and *sambaar masala*. Black peppercorn is also the key ingredient in *baharat*, a spice mix used throughout the Middle East.

The French are fond of white pepper, which blends nicely with the many cream-based sauces in their cuisine. They also grind white and black pepper into a blend called *mignonette*. White pepper is one of the four ingredients in the spice blend *quatre épices*. But black peppercorns aren't totally *disgracié*—they're often bundled in the *bouquet garni* found in many kitchens.

In America, black peppercorns are key to fiery Cajun and Creole cooking.

Peppercorns require a warm climate, and most of the black pepper imported into the US comes from Indonesia or Brazil. Other pepper-growing countries include Malaysia, Madagascar, Tasmania, and Vietnam, which recently surpassed India as the world's largest producer of peppercorn.

How to Buy Black Pepper

While India is no longer the world's largest supplier, it still produces the finest quality—90 percent of which is harvested on the Malabar coast, a variety prized for its high content of piperine and other volatile oils.

There are two varieties from this region: Malabar peppercorns (formerly called Alleppy peppercorns) and Tellicherry peppercorns. Of the two, Tellicherry is the superior. The best Tellicherry is labeled TGSEB, which stands for: Tellicherry (place of origin), Garbled (free of grit and inferior berries), Special (the finest quality), and Extra Bold (largest in size). Malabar Garbled No. 1 (MG1) indicates top-grade, cleaned peppercorn.

The American Spice Trade Association (ASTA) also applies its standards to peppercorn. ASTA on a label means that the pepper meets standards of cleanliness, volatile oil content, moisture level, and other technical specifications.

Black pepper comes whole, cracked, or ground.

Your best strategy: buy whole peppercorns and grind them *as needed*, for the best taste and maximum health benefit. Once pepper is ground, it begins to lose its piperine and other

Other recipes containing black pepper:

Adobo (p. 270)

Alamelu's Salt Substitute (p. 289)

All-American Chili con Carne (p. 110)

Baharat (p. 268)

Basic Barbecue Rub (p. 272)

Berbere (p. 267)

Bloody Mary Soup with Jumbo Lump Crabmeat (p. 70)

Boeuf Bourguignon (p. 240)

Caribbean Curry Paste (p. 287)

Chaat Masala (p. 256)

Chesapeake Bay Seafood Seasoning (p. 273)

Chicken Oreganata (p. 186)

Chimichurri Sauce (p. 190)

Cocoa Rub (p. 270)

Coconut Meatballs with Peanut Sauce (p. 101)

Colombo Powder (p. 270)

Dukkah (p. 268)

Garam Masala (p. 264)

Grilled Pork Chile Adobo (p. 78)

Hot Curry Powder (p. 284)

Jamaican Jerk Marinade (p. 269)

La Kama (p. 266)

Madras Curry Paste (p. 286)

Madras Curry Powder (p. 284)

Malaysian Curry Paste (p. 287)

Pickling Spice (p. 272)

Potato Cauliflower Curry (p. 252)

Prawns with Almond Hot Pepper Sauce (p. 26)

Quatre Épices (p. 271)

Roast Chicken with 40 Cloves of Garlic (p. 134)

Rosemary Barbecue Rub (p. 272)

Sambaar Masala (p. 265)

Spiced Milk Tea (p. 66)

Vindaloo Curry Paste (p. 286)

Yucatan Pickled Red Onions (p. 21)

volatile oils. It retains its bite, but loses flavor.

The best black peppercorns are large, with dark brown to jet black rough skin, and a dull patina. A shiny patina indicates inferior quality.

Ground pepper is available as coarse or fine. There's also an indication of inferior quality in ground pepper—it's too black. Here's why:

When peppercorns are harvested and dried, there's always a percentage that are hollow inside, lacking white hearts. They are referred to as *light berries*. There's typically a government-mandated specification that limits the percentage of light berries permitted in a crop, but growers sometimes circumvent the rules. The best ground black pepper is gray, because the entire berry—black pericarp and white core—was ground. Pepper that is too black is an indication that too many light berries were part of the grinding.

White peppercorns are sold whole. The best quality is Montok.

You can purchase green and pink peppercorns either dried or in brine.

The best dried green peppercorns—called *late-picked* berries—are freeze-dried. They should look full, plump, and bright green. They're excellent for cooking but shouldn't be put in a peppermill, as they're too soft and can clog the mechanism.

Pink peppercorns are the least popular because they have the least flavor. They're also too soft for a peppermill.

There is also a pink "peppercorn" from Brazil that belongs to the cashew family. It has no relationship to true peppercorns, and isn't considered particularly useful in cooking. They were banned from the US several years ago because of concern about toxicity, but shipments sometimes make it to store shelves. Be sure the pink peppercorns you buy are *Piper nigrum*.

Both whole and ground pepper will keep indefinitely, although old ground pepper won't have much flavor.

Both green and pink peppercorns purchased in brine should be used within two weeks of opening.

There are numerous varieties of black pepper, including popular Chinese Szechwan peppercorns, but they aren't true pepper. Szechwan pepper has no resemblance in taste to black

Black Pepper Rice with Almonds

Rice is a staple in Indian cooking, but you'll never find it plain. The combinations of spices that complement rice are huge. This pepper-rich recipe, compliment of Alamelu Vairavan, author of Healthy South Indian Cooking, *is one of my favorites.*

1 cup basmati or extra long-grain rice
1 tablespoon canola oil
3 curry leaves (optional)
1 small dried red chile
1 teaspoon black mustard seeds
1 teaspoon cumin seed
1 cup chopped onions
1½ teaspoons freshly ground black pepper
½ teaspoon ground cumin
1 teaspoon salt
¼ cup sliced almonds

1. Cook rice according to package directions, but omit using salt or oil. Cool rice for about an hour. Stir so the grains do not stick together.
2. Heat the oil in a wok or large skillet over medium-high heat. When the oil is hot, but not smoking, add the curry leaves and red chile. Add the mustard and cumin seeds. Cover and heat until the mustard seeds pop, about 30 seconds.
3. Add the onions and cook for one minute. Add the cooked rice and stir well. Add black pepper, ground cumin, and salt and mix well. Stir in the almonds and serve.

Makes 4 servings.

pepper. Neither makes a satisfactory substitute for the other.

In the Kitchen with Black Pepper

Black pepper is the most useful and indispensable of all culinary spices. When faced with a plate of uninspiring food, the judicious grind of a peppermill can salvage a meal.

The robust flavor of black pepper is most closely associated with strong-flavored food. Apply it liberally to red meat, game, seafood, beans, and lentils. Use it lightly on more delicate food.

But you *can* put black pepper on anything, even fruit. Berries, apples, pears, and even cheese take well to a grind of fresh black pepper. Use black pepper to flavor soups, stews, fish, and poultry.

Keep white peppercorns on hand for those times you want to give a dish a pepper bite without an overpowering pepper fragrance.

And you should always add pepper to liquids and sauces at the last minute. If added early in cooking, it loses its aromatic fragrance and can leave a bitterness that is hard to erase.

Keep black peppercorns in a metal, plastic, or glass peppermill, not wood. Wood will leach pepper of its volatile oils.

Here are a few ways to get more black pepper into your diet:

- Rub coarsely ground peppercorns into red meats before grilling, roasting, or braising. Don't be timid. It can take a lot.
- Add whole peppercorns to marinades, stocks, and dishes being pickled.
- Slice strawberries over watercress and sprinkle generously with black pepper. Dress lightly with a balsamic vinaigrette.
- Add cracked pepper to homemade salad dressing.
- Keep a peppermill, rather than a shaker of already ground pepper, on your table.

CARAWAY *After-Dinner Relief*

When Alice of Wonderland fell down the rabbit hole, she didn't have a toothbrush with her—but she did have a box of *comfits* in her pocket. These little cakes coated in caraway seeds were a popular confection in Victorian England, when caraway seeds were highly regarded for keeping the breath fresh and the digestive system running smoothly.

Rural Victorians celebrated a successful spring sowing of wheat with ale and *wiggs*, another caraway cake. The superstitious among the Victorians believed that anything caraway touched couldn't be stolen, and women put caraway seeds in their husbands' pockets in the belief that it would keep them from straying. The spice was also bottled as a love potion and became known as "kissing caraway."

But caraway's popularity among the English went the way of chimney sweeps and "pantalettes" for covering piano legs. Perhaps it's time for a revival of the spice—in the UK *and* the US, where post-meal tummy troubles such as burning, bloating, belching, cramping, and nausea plague an estimated 40 percent of the population. New scientific studies show what Alice and her contemporaries on this side of the looking glass knew from firsthand experience: caraway is one of the most powerful digestive aids around.

Better than Antacids

Researchers in the UK reviewed 53 studies on antacids and found they provided "little relief" for digestive woes. Then they looked at 17 studies on herbal remedies, including a combination of peppermint and caraway oil, both of which contain *carvone*, a component of some essential oils that relaxes spasms in the digestive tract. The herbal combo effectively reduced stomachache and other post-meal problems anywhere from 60 to 95 percent of the time. In one study, people who used the combo for four weeks had an average 45 percent reduction in gastrointestinal pain.

A Folk Remedy for Diabetes

The English aren't the only traditional fans of caraway. Ancient Greeks, Romans, and Egyptians considered the spice both food and medicine, baking it into bread, cakes, and fruit dishes to stimulate digestion and fight colds and bronchitis.

Caraway continues to be a popular folk remedy in Morocco, where many of the populace chews on lightly roasted seeds after dinner. It's also considered a way to prevent and control blood sugar problems. In fact, in 2004, Moroccan researchers tested the remedy on rats with drug-induced diabetes—and found that the daily administration of the remedy for two weeks completely normalized the ailing animals' blood sugar levels. The finding "represents an experimental confirmation of the Moroccan traditional use" of caraway seeds for the control of type 2 diabetes, said the researchers in the *Journal of Ethnopharmacology*.

Way More to Caraway

In fact, caraway seeds contain more than *50* healing compounds, which studies show can fight all kinds of health problems. Those include:

Cancer. Caraway seeds are loaded with *limonene*, a compound with known anti-cancer activity. Animal studies show that limonene can stop the growth of breast, liver, lung, and stomach cancer. Some animal studies show that limonene and carvone combined reduce the risk of colon cancer.

Food poisoning. *E. coli* is the germ behind most cases of food poisoning, an infection that strikes

76 million Americans a year. (That's 21,000 per *day*.) Chicken is a favorite hangout of *E. coli*—but researchers who contaminated a pot of chicken soup with the bacteria found that carvone prevented it from multiplying.

Cholesterol and triglycerides. Moroccan researchers found caraway reduced levels of these two blood fats in both normal and diabetic laboratory animals. The spice has "potent lipid [fat] lowering activity," the researchers concluded.

Constipation. In Bulgaria, doctors treated 32 people with chronic constipation with a laxative containing caraway—and 29 of them started having regular daily bowel movements.

Tuberculosis. In India, where tuberculosis is the leading cause of death from infectious disease, researchers found that dietary caraway enhanced the absorption of three anti-tuberculosis drugs.

Getting to Know Caraway

Unlike most healing spices, caraway thrives in a moderate (rather than tropical) climate, and is grown in many parts of the world, including Europe, Central Asia, North Africa, and the United States. Americans haven't adopted a fondness for caraway in the same way as other nations, however. We're most familiar with caraway as the seed on the crust of German and Jewish rye breads.

Real caraway country is in Europe. The intense anise-like flavor is particularly characteristic of German cuisine, where chefs discovered it balances the starches and fats in the traditional meat-and-potato diet. Germans put it in all kinds of dishes—soups, meat stews, sausages, potato casseroles, and cakes. It's always added to sauerkraut and boiled cabbage, to banish the lingering sulfuric odor—and flatulence—that cooked cabbage leaves behind. And it's used to flavor the German liquors *kummel* (a word for caraway) and schnapps.

Caraway also defines the flavor of aquavit, Scandinavia's national liquor. It gives a savory

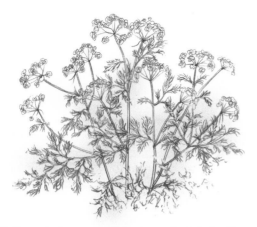

Unlike most spices, caraway thrives in a moderate (rather than tropical) climate, and grows in many parts of the world.

Caraway may help prevent and/or treat:

Cancer	Heartburn
Cholesterol problems	(gastroesophageal
(high total cholesterol)	reflux disease, or
Constipation	GERD)
Diabetes, type 2	Indigestion
Food poisoning	Triglycerides, high
	Tuberculosis

Caraway pairs well with these spices:

Allspice	Coriander
Almond	Fennel seed
Cardamom	Juniper berry
Chile	Onion
Cinnamon	

and complements recipes featuring:

Apples	Pork
Cabbage	Sausages
Cheese	Sauerkraut
Pears	

Other recipes containing caraway:

Alsatian Pork and	Ras-el-hanout (p. 266)
Sauerkraut (p. 148)	Tabil (p. 267)
Garam Masala (p. 264)	

sweetness to Hungarian goulash. In Russia, it's put in borscht. In France, it's used as a preservative in *choucroute*.

Lightly roasted caraway seeds often accompany a cheese plate in central Europe: people in the Alsace-Lorraine region of France eat caraway with Muenster cheese; the Dutch eat it with Tilsiter cheese; and in Hungary it's served with Liptauer cheese along with mustard, butter, and chopped chives.

Caraway is a key ingredient in Tunisia's famous fiery *harissa*, one of the hottest condiments on earth. In Nigeria, it's the spice on the sweet deep-fried wafer *chin-chin*. In India, caraway is often found in snacks.

How to Buy Caraway

There are two types of caraway: one is from an annual plant native to Europe, the other is from a biennial native to the Middle East. Caraway connoisseurs say the best is grown in Holland. But none of these facts are particularly relevant unless you buy your spices at a specialty shop.

The most important fact: always buy caraway seeds *whole*. Grinding releases the spice's volatile oils, dissipating the flavor. When stored in an airtight container in a cool place and out of the sunlight, the whole seeds will keep for two years or longer.

Raw caraway will have a slight aroma, but the full flavor doesn't come out until the seed is cooked.

In the Kitchen with Caraway

The taste of caraway (which some feel is an *acquired* taste) is earthy, similar to fennel and anise, with a nutty aftertaste. Even if you buy ground seeds, you will get the best flavor out of caraway by dry roasting. Roast until you detect

Hungarian Goulash

Paprika doesn't overpower this national dish because caraway helps balance it—together, they create the unique flavor that defines Hungarian goulash. Use Hungarian paprika, if possible—it makes a difference. Serve over egg noodles.

2 strips bacon
2 pounds veal or beef cubes
¼ cup flour
2 cups sliced onion
3 cloves garlic, chopped
1½ teaspoons caraway seeds
1 teaspoon lemon zest
⅓ cup Hungarian paprika
1 cup peeled and cubed potatoes
1 cup sliced carrots
¼ teaspoon dried thyme
¼ teaspoon dried marjoram
¼ teaspoon dried rosemary
2 cups beef stock
1 cup strong beer
2 tablespoons tomato paste
1 cup low-fat sour cream

1. Cook the bacon over medium-high heat in a large Dutch oven until crisp. Remove. Dredge veal cubes in the flour and brown in the bacon fat. Remove from pot with a slotted spoon and set aside. Season with salt and pepper, if desired.

2. Add the onions and cook until soft but not browned. Add the garlic, caraway seeds, and lemon zest and cook one minute. Stir in the paprika and stir to coat well. Return the meat to the pot and stir again. Add the potatoes, carrots, thyme, marjoram, rosemary, stock, and beer. Stir in the tomato paste. Bring to a simmer, reduce the heat, cover, and cook for 1½ hours.

3. Turn off the heat and remove the meat and vegetables with a slotted spoon and keep warm. Let the liquid cool slightly. Skim off the fat. Stir in the sour cream. Whip the mixture into the sauce and simmer until the sauce thickens. Return meat and vegetables to the sauce and heat through.

Makes 6 servings.

the release of the volatile oils (your nose will know), then stop immediately. If cooked too long, the seeds turn bitter.

Caraway's flavor is strong and tends to dominate other flavors. Unless you want to feature its flavor, use less caraway than other spices in your recipes. Here are some ideas for adding more caraway to your diet:

- Caraway goes naturally with pork. Sprinkle it on or around a roast or chops in the last 15 minutes of baking.
- Caraway goes well with apples. Add it to your favorite spiced-apple recipe.
- Add a pinch of caraway to an onion tart recipe.
- Serve apples and caraway on a cheese tray. In addition to the cheeses already mentioned, caraway goes well with Gouda and Gorgonzola.
- Mix toasted seeds into cottage cheese or yogurt.
- Make this popular German potato dish: Halve unpeeled potatoes lengthwise. Dip the flesh side in melted butter, then in a plate of caraway seeds. Bake, cut side down, at 400°F for 30 minutes or until soft.

CARDAMOM   *The Stomach Sentinel*

As old as civilization itself, cardamom always has been and still is one of the world's most expensive spices. During the end of the Middle Ages, in the late 16th century, when the price of all spices was sky high, cardamom was among the costliest. A handful of cardamom pods cost the equivalent of a poor man's yearly salary—and prosperous Europeans paid it gladly, because of cardamom's special medicinal and culinary value. No wonder it's known as the "Queen of Spices." (Pepper is King.)

Cardamom's delicately pleasant, one-of-a-kind aroma and flavor is derived from its rich and varied content of more than 25 *volatile oils*, plant compounds that impart fragrance. And the most medicinally active of the oils is the antioxidant *cineole* (which is also found in bay leaf).

In the traditional medicines of the East, cardamom has been used to treat an impressive variety of health problems, including heart disease, respiratory ailments such as asthma, bronchitis, colds, and flu, and all forms of digestive problems, from bad breath and colic to constipation and diarrhea.

After centuries of use in traditional medicine, the 20th century saw the first scientific research into the health benefits of cardamom. In 1978, the Indian Cardamom Research Institute was established, which later became the Indian Institute of Spices Research.

Today, medical research on cardamom and cineole is conducted worldwide, although the majority of studies are still from India. Here's the best of what researchers are discovering:

Digestive Relief

Cardamom's stomach-soothing ability is legendary. But it wasn't until recently that studies started to show *why* it works. In the last 20 years, dozens of studies have shown that the volatile oils in cardamom are powerful anti-inflammatory and anti-spasmodic agents that can work together to improve digestion.

Calming the gut. For example, a study by a team of researchers in Saudi Arabia showed that volatile oils in cardamom may calm the gut by blocking receptors on cells that regulate muscle contraction. And a team of Indian researchers discovered that cardamom acted like cholinergic and calcium antagonist drugs: cholinergic drugs stimulate the parasympathetic nervous system, which is responsible for salivation, digestion, and muscle relaxation; calcium antagonist drugs also relax muscles, by affecting the movement of calcium into and out of muscle cells.

Beating bad breath. Cineole is an antiseptic that kills bacteria that can cause bad breath.

Stopping ulcers. Several studies show cineole can slow or stop the development of aspirin-induced and alcohol-induced stomach ulcers in laboratory animals.

Preventing colon cancer. Animal research in India shows that cardamom can fight colon cancer cells several ways—reducing the inflammation that fuels cancer growth, stopping cancer cells from dividing, and killing cancer cells.

Cardamom for Cardiac Ills

Several studies show that cineole helps protect the cardiovascular system by:

Lowering blood pressure. In a study reported in the *Journal of Ethnopharmacology*, cardamom lowered blood pressure in laboratory animals—the greater the dose, the greater the drop. The same study showed cardamom worked like a diuretic, a type of drug used to treat hypertension.

Preventing blood clots. Heart attacks and strokes are often caused by blood clots that block an artery. Indian researchers tested cardamom extract on human *platelets*, the structures in blood that stick together and form clots. The spice decreased *platelet aggregation*, the platelets' ability to adhere to one another to create a clot.

Cardamom may help prevent and/or treat:

Asthma	Heart disease
Bad breath	High blood pressure (hypertension)
Blood clots	
Colic	Indigestion
Colon cancer	Sinusitis
Constipation	Stomachache
Diarrhea	Ulcer

Breathing Easier

Just as cardamom can relax the gut, it can also relax the airways, restoring breathing in people with respiratory ills.

Easing severe asthma. German researchers studied 32 people with severe asthma who were dependent on anti-inflammatory steroid drugs, dividing them into two groups. One group added a supplement of cineole to their drug regimen; the other group didn't. After two months, those taking cineole reduced their need for steroids by 36 percent, compared to 7 percent for the non-cineole group. "Long-term therapy with cineole has a significant steroid-saving effect in steroid-dependent asthma," concluded the researchers in *Respiratory Medicine*.

Clearing up a sinus infection. Two German studies have found that cineole offers relief for sinus infection. In one, 152 people with acute sinus infections were asked to take either cineole (two 100-milligram capsules, three times a day) or a placebo. After just four days, those taking cineole had fewer headaches, less sinus pain, and less nasal secretion and obstruction. "Timely treatment with cineole is effective and safe," concluded the researchers in *Laryngoscope*. In fact, they recommend those with an acute sinus infection take a supplement of the spice extract *before* trying antibiotics.

In a similar study involving 150 people with acute sinus infections, researchers once again found that treatment with cineole relieved sinus headache, eased tender sinuses, reduced nasal secretions, and decreased nasal obstruction. Treatment with the spice extract is "clinically relevant," concluded the researchers.

Getting to Know Cardamom

India is the land of cardamom—for millennia, spice traders searched the mountainous rainforests of the Cardamom Hills in southern India, looking for precious pods growing wild on the roots of cardamom bushes.

The early Romans loved the Indian spice and imported it in vast quantities. They used it as many people in India still use it today—as Mother Nature's toothbrush. Cardamom cleans the teeth and freshens the breath. In fact, it is one of the few substances that will help you dissipate "garlic breath" after eating a heavily spiced meal.

Today, cardamom is most popular in the cooking of India, Iran, Morocco, and the Arab nations. In Arabian cooking, it imparts a sweet aroma to savory curries and other dishes. It is a key ingredient in the Moroccan spice mix *ras-el-hanout* and the well-known Indian mix *garam masala*. It is also used in Indian sweets called *halva*, and in puddings, yogurt, custards, and ice

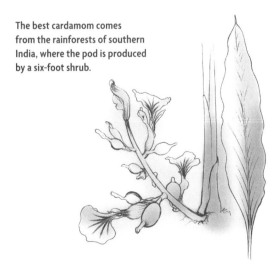

The best cardamom comes from the rainforests of southern India, where the pod is produced by a six-foot shrub.

True Cardamom and False Cardamom

There is Chinese brown cardamom. Thai green cardamom. Nepal or large cardamom. Java cardamom . . . and on and on. But they are all "false" cardamom. There is only one true cardamom—green cardamom, the Queen of Spices, the culinary spice universally referred to simply as cardamom.

India, however, has a second cardamom that's somewhere between true and false—brown (or black), disparagingly called "bastard" cardamom. It is an integral spice in some of India's most famous dishes, including those that are part of its famous tandoori cuisine, named after the *tandoor*, the in-ground oven in which it's made. Brown cardamom is the key spice that gives the distinct taste and texture to the Indian specialties chicken *tikka* and butter chicken. It is sometimes added to rice dishes called *biryanis*, as well as to many other dishes.

The only place you're likely to come across brown cardamom is in an Indian market, a specialty spice retailer, or online. It is only sold in pods, which are similar in texture to green cardamom but tan in color and twice the size. The pods are slightly dull and dusty in appearance.

The first encounter with brown cardamom pods is a culinary adventure. When you open a brown cardamom pod you will find gooey seeds in a sticky membrane. When you remove them they stick together, as well as to your fingers. The way to work with them is to transfer the seeds to a mortar and pestle with other dry spices, which will absorb the stickiness. You can then add them to other spices.

Brown cardamom has not been studied for its medicinal value, but it is in the same family as green cardamom and possesses some of the same volatile oils. It also has a flavor similar to eucalyptus. It doesn't demand nearly the same price as green cardamom—about a third of the cost of green cardamom pods that can sell for upward of $30 a pound. (In Indian markets the cost is much less.)

cream. It gives the distinctive bouquet to India's popular yogurt-based stews called *kormas* and rice dishes called *biryanis*. It is an important ingredient in the Indian hot spiced tea called *chai masala*, which in recent years has gained popularity in the US.

As popular as cardamom is in cooking, 80 percent of the world's cardamom is used by the Arab-speaking nations to make *coffee*. It is a custom in Arab homes to serve cardamom-flavored coffee called *gahira* to guests as a sign of hospitality and generosity. The technique is simple: Push a cardamom pod into the narrow of the coffeepot spout and pour. When the hot liquid passes through the pod, it gives the coffee a refreshing taste. Cardamom is also the flavor that has gained Turkish coffee an international reputation.

The Vikings introduced cardamom to Scandinavia, where it is almost as popular as it is in South Asia and the Middle East. In Sweden, Denmark, and Finland it's mostly used to flavor cakes, sweet breads, pastries (it's what makes a Danish a Danish!), and pickled fruits and vegetables. It is also used to flavor *glögg*, a hot spiced wine popular during the cold winters of Sweden.

In Germany, *kardamom* is a popular spice for making Christmas sweets, especially the popular cookie call *lebkuchen*.

How to Buy Cardamom

The ground cardamom or cardamom seeds you find in the spice aisle of your grocery store appear neither exotic nor out of the ordinary (except, perhaps, for the price). Cardamom *pods*, however, are a different story, and you won't find them in your typical supermarket. You have to go to an Indian market, a specialty spice shop, or an online retailer.

Both the pods and seeds are used in cooking. The best quality pods are small, with a gnarly oval shape and a paper-like husk. They are lime green in color. Look for pods with a vivid, even color; they shouldn't be pale or bleached. Avoid pods that are split open at the corners, which indicates

Cardamom pairs well with these spices:

Allspice	Cumin
Almond	Fennel seed
Cardamom	Ginger
Chile	Mustard
Cinnamon	Star anise
Clove	Turmeric
Coriander	

and complements recipes featuring:

Chicken	Nuts
Citrus fruit	Pudding
Custards	Rice
Ice creams	Tropical fruit,
Lamb	especially mango

Other recipes containing cardamom:

Apple Pie Spice (p. 271)	Los Banos Low-Fat
Baharat (p. 268)	Brownies (p. 97)
Berbere (p. 267)	Ras-el-hanout (p. 266)
Chesapeake Bay	Spicy Vanilla Rice
Seafood Seasoning	Pudding (p. 256)
(p. 273)	
Garam Masala (p. 264)	

that they were harvested late and will have lost some of their volatile oils. "White" cardamom pods are green pods that have been bleached, a custom started and favored by the English. Spice connoisseurs prefer the green pods.

If you can't find pods, buy seeds rather than ground cardamom. The volatile oils in cardamom seeds are sensitive—their pleasant aroma dissipates quickly after exposure to the air (in fact, the aroma starts to fade as soon as the seeds are removed from the pod). When you buy seeds, you can help retain flavor by grinding them only as needed.

Green cardamom seeds are actually brown in color but they're called *green cardamom* (or simply *cardamom*) after the pod in which they come. They should feel slightly oily to the touch and have a scent resembling eucalyptus, with a hint of mint and pepper.

The best cardamom comes from the rainforests of southern India, where the pod is produced by a six-foot shrub with yellow and blue flowers. Cardamom is also cultivated in Thailand and Central America. The majority of the cardamom imported into the US comes from Guatemala, with most of the rest from India and Sri Lanka.

Intact cardamom pods will keep for two years in an airtight container away from sunlight. Seeds will keep up to a year under the same conditions. Ground cardamom has a shelf life of about six months.

In the Kitchen with Cardamom

If you've never smelled a cardamom pod, you haven't experienced the spice's true aroma. It is refreshingly astringent and pleasant to the palate. As a spice, it is quite versatile and can go with almost any sweet or savory dish.

Pods are best used in savory dishes based in liquid. Many ethnic recipes call for using a *bruised* cardamom pod. To bruise a pod, gently thump it with a rolling pin or put it under the flat end of a butcher's knife and give it a gentle push. Bruising releases the oils, allowing their flavors to meld with the other ingredients. For recipes calling for whole seeds, bruising helps release their oils as well. At the end of the cooking, you should discard pods, but not seeds.

Ground cardamom is best for sweet dishes. Use sparingly, however, as it tends to be pungent.

Cardamom is a key ingredient in many traditional spice mixes, so consider using it when making your own mixes.

Here are some ways to get more cardamom in your diet:

- Spice your morning coffee as is the custom in many Arab-speaking countries.

Spiced Milk Tea

Known as chai masala *or simply* chai, *this spiced beverage, which is sold by* chai wallahs *(tea vendors) all over India, is now popular worldwide. Although you can find chai blends in the supermarket, you can create a much better flavor and experience by making your own.*

10 cardamom pods or ½ teaspoon cardamom seeds
1 one-inch cinnamon stick
4 white peppercorns
¼ teaspoon fennel seeds
2 cups low-fat milk
3 tablespoons brown sugar
½ teaspoon ground ginger
2 cups water
4 bags black tea

1. Remove the seeds from the cardamom pods and discard the pods. Dry roast the cardamom seeds, cinnamon stick, peppercorns, and fennel seeds in a hot skillet until they release their fragrance, about five minutes. Transfer to a plate to cool. Put them in a spice grinder or mini food processor and grind to a fine powder.

2. Put the milk in a medium saucepan and bring to a simmer. Add the ground spices, brown sugar, and ginger.

3. Heat the water in another pot and bring to a boil. Turn off the heat and steep the tea bags for three minutes. Pour the tea into the milk mixture and simmer one minute. Let the chai rest for a few minutes. Strain and serve.

Makes 4 servings.

If you don't want to go to the trouble of putting a bruised pod in the neck of a formal coffee pot, drop a crushed pod or two in the brewed pot from your coffeemaker and strain the coffee into your mug or cup. Consider one pod per two cups of coffee.

- Put one or two bruised cardamom pods in the liquid when making rice, or add a pinch of ground cardamom to rice pilaf.
- Sprinkle ground cardamom and a little sugar on grapefruit.
- Add a half teaspoon of ground cardamom to gingerbread or chocolate cake recipes.
- Add crushed cardamom seeds to Bananas Foster and other sweet fruit desserts.
- Add a teaspoon of ground cardamom to your vanilla cupcake recipe and vanilla pie fillings.
- Rub cardamom on a lamb roast before putting it on a spit.

CELERY SEED   *First Aid for Gout*

The celery seed you put in a Bloody Mary for that extra zing has nothing to do with the celery stalk you use to stir it.

Celery seed comes from a sister plant called *smallage* that grows in salt marshes and river estuaries throughout Europe and India. Smallage, also known as *wild celery*, looks similar to the familiar garden-variety celery we eat as a vegetable, but it is so bitter, it's inedible. The seeds, however, are not only edible—they're incredible. The tiniest spice in the world (one pound's worth is 750,000 seeds) may have an oversized talent for healing because it's packed with cell-nourishing phytonutrients—most notably, *phthalides* (the anti-inflammatory substances responsible for giving celery

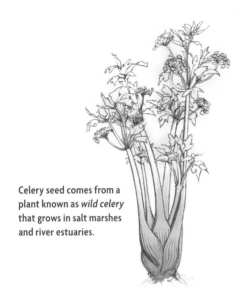

Celery seed comes from a plant known as *wild celery* that grows in salt marshes and river estuaries.

and celery seed their distinctive bite) and the volatile oil *apigenin* (an antioxidant).

Traditionally, healers have used celery seed to treat upper respiratory diseases such as colds, bronchitis, flu, and asthma, as well as indigestion, water retention, and liver disease. Today, celery seed it is best known as a home remedy for the pain and inflammation of arthritis—including its toe-torturing form, gout.

Out with Gout

Gout is caused by a buildup of *uric acid*, a waste product of urine. Over time, the excess acid congeals into sharp-edged *urate crystals* that travel south to the big toe (though they can end up in other joints).

There are many risk factors for gout. They include: too much meat and alcohol (both rich in *purines*, a food component that breaks down into uric acid), overweight, diseases such as type 2 diabetes and high blood pressure that weaken the purine-processing kidneys, and being a guy—three out of four gout sufferers are men. (Blame it on genetics—and beer.)

Gout takes two forms: acute and chronic. Acute gout is an *attack*—pain so severe that brushing your big toe against a sheet can be excruciating.

Chronic gout is a *condition*—the excess uric acid isn't controlled, and crystals form large, painful lumps called *tophi* that gradually deform and destroy joints.

Gout requires medical care: an anti-inflammatory medication to control the pain of a gout attack, and allopurinol (Zyloprim) to stop the body from producing uric acid. But celery seed has long been touted by natural healers (and agonized gout sufferers!) as an effective complement (or even replacement) to medical care, helping calm a gout attack and controlling uric acid long-term. Put the words *celery seed* and *gout* into an Internet search engine, and you'll enter a world of gout-beating claims. Are they true?

James Duke, PhD—a noted expert in botanical healing *and* a long-time gout sufferer—thinks so. "Ever since I started taking celery seed, I've abandoned allopurinol," he said. "For me, celery seed is just as therapeutically effective as its man-made pharmaceutical rival—maybe more so." (Follow his example only with your doctor's approval and supervision.)

And there's some scientific evidence to back up Dr. Duke's anti-gout anecdote.

Noting that celery seeds have been used traditionally for many inflammatory conditions—asthma, bronchitis, osteoarthritis, rheumatoid arthritis, and gout—researchers at Michigan State University decided to chemically dissect the seeds, looking for specific compounds with anti-inflammatory ability. And they found them!

Several compounds in celery seeds "inhibited" *COX-1* and *COX-2*, the cellular enzymes that trigger the inflammation (the hurt, the heat, the redness, the swelling) behind gout and many other pain-causing conditions.

"The biological activities" of compounds in celery seeds "are in agreement with the anecdotal use of celery seeds to alleviate gout and arthritic pain," wrote the researchers in *Phytomedicine*.

Citing this and other research, Michael Whitehouse, MD, PhD, of the University of

Queensland of Australia, touts the anti-inflammatory power of celery seeds in the journal *Inflammopharmacology*. "Extracts from Indian celery seed," he writes, are "powerful nutraceuticals that amplify the potency" of conventional drugs "for treating pre-established chronic inflammation" in diseases such as gout. Celery seed, he concludes, "can be a remarkable resource for supplementing conventional therapy for inflammatory disease." And he hopes the bad news about the class of drugs called COX-2 inhibitors—such as the now-banned rofecoxib (Vioxx) and valdecoxib (Bextra)—will "stimulate serious re-assessment" of celery seed and other "traditional anti-inflammatory therapies."

From Menstrual Disorders to Mosquito Bites

Inflammation Nation. The Inflammation Syndrome. Stop Inflammation Now! The Inflammation Cure. The titles of these and other recent popular health books attest to the fact that inflammation is a big problem. In inflammation, the immune system rushes its warrior-like cells to the site of an injury—from a nasty cut to a nasty accumulation of cholesterol. The resulting collateral damage can cause and complicate many health problems. The diminutive celery seed contains approximately two dozen anti-inflammatory compounds—allowing it to fight not only gout, but many other types of conditions.

Menstrual pain. Researchers studied 180 women with painful menstrual cramps, dividing them into three groups: one took an herbal remedy containing extracts of celery seed, saffron, and anise; one took an anti-inflammatory, pain-reducing drug; one took a placebo. After three months, those taking the herbal remedy and the drug had the same substantial reduction in both the intensity and duration of their menstrual cramps. The findings were published in the *Journal of Midwifery and Women's Health*.

Heart disease and stroke. Several animal studies have found that celery seed extract can significantly decrease total cholesterol, "bad" LDL

Celery seed may help prevent and/or treat:

Arthritis, osteo- and rheumatoid	Liver disease
	Menstrual cramps
Cholesterol problems (high total cholesterol, high "bad" LDL cholesterol)	Mosquito bites
	Stroke
	Ulcer
Gout	Vaginal yeast infection
High blood pressure (hypertension)	

Celery seed pairs well with these spices:

Allspice	Cumin
Black pepper	Fennel seed
Caraway	Ginger
Chile	Sage
Cinnamon	Turmeric
Coriander	

and complements recipes featuring:

Chicken	Fish
Chutneys	Tomatoes
Eggs	

Other recipes containing celery seed:

By-the-Bay Fisherman's Chowder (p. 46)	Spaghettini with Basil-Tomato Sauce (p. 42)
Chesapeake Bay Seafood Seasoning (p. 273)	Spice de Provence (p. 271)

cholesterol, and triglycerides (another heart-hurting blood fat). The extract has also lowered high blood pressure in laboratory animals. And it helped protect the brains of laboratory animals from damage caused by an experimentally induced stroke.

Liver disease. Researchers in India found that celery seed extracts protected experimental animals from liver damage caused by toxic chemicals. The study validates the traditional use of celery seeds in treating and preventing liver diseases, they concluded in the *Journal of Ethnopharmacology*. Another animal study, in *Cancer Letters*, found that celery seed extract protected against liver cancer.

Mosquito bites. Scientists in Thailand put a topical repellent made from celery seed on the skin of volunteers and exposed them to seven different species of mosquitoes—the repellent provided complete protection for three and a half hours. The volunteers successfully continued to use the celery seed repellent for the next nine months.

Drug side effects. A common side effect in men of treatment with the epilepsy drug sodium valproate (Epilim) is damage to the reproductive system from plummeting testosterone levels. In animal research, scientists showed celery seed could block this side effect.

Ulcers. Researchers in England found an extract of celery seed could kill *H. pylori*, the stomach bacteria that cause ulcers.

Yeast infection. Test tube studies show that celery seed can stop the growth of several strains of fungus, including those that cause vaginal yeast infections.

Getting to Know Celery Seed

After their blowout banquets, morning-after ancient Romans often wore wreathes of smallage leaves and celery seed as a hangover "cure." Some moderns also favor celery seed in a hangover "remedy"—the Bloody Mary, a vodka cocktail containing celery seed, horseradish, and ground black pepper.

But although celery seed has been used in traditional medicine for millennia, it wasn't until the Middle Ages that it started to gain favor as a condiment, in France and Italy. Today, celery seed is a popular spice in American and European cooking, sprinkled in tomato juice,

chicken soup, salad dressings, and coleslaw, and as an ingredient in sausage, knockwurst, and corned beef. In the food industry, it's used in bologna, hot dogs, and other processed meats, in non-alcoholic drinks, in soups, in pickles, and in ice cream and baked goods.

Celery seed is also a mainstay of North Indian cuisine, where it's found in curries, pickles, and chutneys.

How to Buy Celery Seed

Celery seed is pungent, with a grassy or hay-like aroma. The miniscule seed is dark brown, with a light hue from tiny ridges you can't see with the naked eye. You'll find them whole in any grocery with a well-stocked spice section.

Because they're so small, grinding isn't necessary, although you can find seeds sold slightly crushed or ground. Best to buy them whole, though, as grinding causes their good-for-you volatile oils to start to dissipate. Whole seeds keep for two years or more. Use ground celery seeds within a few months.

You've probably encountered *celery salt* in the supermarket aisle and recipes. It's a mixture of about 60 percent salt and celery seeds, sometimes with the addition of parsley and dill. If celery seed isn't available, it's an acceptable substitute.

Most celery seeds imported into the US are from India.

In the Kitchen with Celery Seed

Celery seeds are bitter when raw but take on a sweet flavor when cooked. If adding celery seeds to a raw dish, you can mellow the seeds by dry-toasting them slightly. (See the directions on page 11 for dry roasting.) Be careful not to burn them.

Be conservative in using celery seeds—their tiny size belies the impact they can have on a dish. (But do use them. In fact, researchers at the University of Tokyo *proved* that celery seed is indispensable to a flavorful soup—when they asked taste-testers to sample soup broths with

Bloody Mary Soup with Jumbo Lump Crabmeat

In the summer when tomatoes are in season, you can substitute the canned tomatoes with four fresh tomatoes.

1 medium yellow squash, finely diced
1 medium zucchini, finely diced
6 scallions, thinly sliced
1 twenty-eight-ounce can crushed tomatoes
4 cups V-8 juice
3 tablespoons Worcestershire sauce
2 tablespoons toasted celery seeds
1 jalapeño, seeded and diced
1 tablespoon coarsely ground black peppercorns
Coarsely ground kosher salt, to taste

½ pound jumbo lump crabmeat
1 lime cut into four wedges

1. Combine the first 10 ingredients in a glass or ceramic bowl and refrigerate for two hours.
2. Divide the soup into double martini or old-fashioned glasses. Top with the crabmeat. Slice the lime wedges at the center and put one on the rim of each glass.

Serves 4 as a first course or 3 as an entree.

and without celery seed, the testers described the seed-rich broth as thicker, more full-bodied, and more satisfying.)

Here are some ways to put more celery seed into your diet:

- The seeds are a natural with anything containing tomato. Add toasted seeds to

gazpacho, tomato juice cocktails, tomato soups, and tomato sauces.
- They're also a natural with eggs. Add a pinch of celery seeds to scrambled eggs or omelets. Sprinkled toasted seeds on top of deviled eggs.
- Add celery seeds to stocks and chicken soup recipes.

CHILE *Red-Hot Healer*

It's a bit ironic that the hottest spice in the world is called chile. Then there's the ongoing debate as to its spelling. Is it chile, chilli, or chili? (And why not chilly?)

Self-professed keepers of the flame, so to speak, defer to the Spanish *chile*, rather than the English *chili*, or the *chilli* that is synonymous with Mexican cuisine, so chile it shall be. But it really doesn't matter how you spell it as long as you know what it means: *hot*, as in a mouthful of persistent heat that can range from tangy to tongue torching.

Chiles get their trademark fire from *capsaicin*, an alkaloid concentrated mostly in the interior

seeds and membrane. The more capsaicin, the more intense the heat. If there's no heat, there's no capsaicin. If there is no capsaicin, it's not a chile.

Capsaicin is indestructible. Neither cold, nor heat, nor water will douse the fire—a fire so fierce it can incinerate a variety of diseases. And the hotter the chile the more therapeutic it is. But have no fear: you don't need a high pain threshold to benefit. *All* chiles have healing properties.

Chile's healing capsaicin is enhanced by a wealth of antioxidant vitamins. Ounce for ounce, a chile contains nine times more vitamin A than a green pepper, and twice as much vitamin C as an orange. It's also rich in minerals, including potassium and magnesium.

In the last 20 years, thousands of scientific studies have been published describing the medicinal benefits of chiles. Here's the "hottest" research.

A Proven Pain Killer

When you bite into a chile, capsaicin triggers the release of a neurotransmitter called *substance P*, which tells the brain to transmit pain along nerve fibers. Capsaicin, however, builds a tolerance to substance P. As you eat more and more chiles, capsaicin triggers less and less substance P. (At the same time, it also triggers the release of *somatostatin*, a hormone that cools inflammation.) This is why diehard chileheads can down hotter-than-hot habañero hot sauce that leaves neophytes writhing in agony. In effect, your taste buds become desensitized to the burn.

People with a lot of pain have a lot of substance P, and capsaicin affects it in a similar way. When you rub capsaicin cream into the skin at the source of pain, you feel a warm and burning sensation, a sensitivity caused by substance P. However, repeated use, usually over a period of three days, reduces and eventually blocks substance P, numbing the pain, and releases somatostatin, which promotes the healing process.

Studies have found that capsaicin creams, which are approved by the FDA, can have a dramatic and long-lasting anesthetic effect on a variety of painful conditions. Most studies show that capsaicin cream brings relief to nearly 75 percent of people who use it. It even works for extreme pain. Zostrix, for example, is an FDA-approved prescription capsaicin cream for some of life's most painful events, such as nerve pain associated with mastectomy or post-operative amputation.

The one downside to capsaicin cream is the initial heat, which can cause skin redness and irritation in some people. However, a study reported in *Archives of Internal Medicine*

reported that capsaicin cream was the preferred treatment of choice among 100 older patients with severe osteoarthritis in the knees.

These are among the most effective uses for capsaicin creams:

Arthritis. Capsaicin not only offers pain relief to people with osteoarthritis. Studies show that it also increases levels of *synovial fluid*, which lubricates joints and helps prevent the breakdown of cartilage. It all adds up to less pain and increased flexibility.

In a study from researchers at the University of Miami School of Medicine, people with osteoarthritis of the knee applied either a .025% solution of capsaicin or a plain cream to their knees, four times a day. Those who used capsaicin cream had an obvious reduction in pain after two months. By three months, 81 percent reported fewer arthritic symptoms, including morning stiffness. In contrast, only 54 percent of those using the placebo reported feeling better. The study was reported in *Seminars in Arthritis and Rheumatism*.

Nerve pain. A study at the University of California, San Francisco found that high-dose capsaicin cream significantly reduced chronic, debilitating nerve pain (neuropathy) associated with a range of diseases. Seven out of 10 patients improved by at least 50 percent.

A study of 200 patients with nerve damage, reported in the *British Journal of Clinical Pharmacology*, found that capsaicin cream "significantly reduced" shooting pain and numbing pins-and-needle-like sensations.

Postherpetic neuralgia (PHN). Shingles (herpes zoster) is a rash-like outbreak of blisters—typically in middle or old age—sparked by the same virus that causes chickenpox in children. In many people with shingles, the reactivated virus damages the nerves, producing an excruciatingly painful condition that can last for weeks (and sometimes years) called postherpetic neuralgia (PHN). The FDA has approved a prescription patch containing pure, concentrated synthetic capsaicin called Qutenza for relief from PHN.

Diabetic neuropathy. In one study researchers randomly assigned either capsaicin cream or a placebo to treat 250 people with painful diabetic neuropathy, a common complication of diabetes in which nerves are damaged, often in the legs and feet. The patients using the capsaicin cream had nearly a 70 percent reduction in symptoms.

"With the exception of initial transient burning, capsaicin offers several advantages over oral analgesics [painkillers]," wrote the researchers in *Archives of Internal Medicine.* Those advantages included safety, fewer side effects, and fewer drug-drug interactions.

Neck pain. Physicians at Walter Reed Army Medical Center in Washington D.C. treated 23 people with chronic neck pain with a .025% capsaicin cream four times a day. After one month, the doctors asked a number of questions, including: "If your pain returns and you were given a choice, would you choose to use the cream again?" A total of 75 percent said they would. The study was reported in the *American Journal of Physical Medicine & Rehabilitation.*

Headaches. Capsaicin used nasally greatly reduced symptoms among 52 people suffering from one-sided cluster headaches. The researchers, reporting in the journal *Pain,* found 70 percent of the patients benefited when the capsaicin was applied to the nostril on the same side as the headache.

Burning Up Fat

Fiery capsaicin raises your body heat, increases perspiration, and boosts your metabolic rate—an effect that has helped people lose weight and prevented others from gaining it. Eating chiles can benefit weight loss in several ways:

Increases metabolism. Several studies show that eating chiles increases the rate at which you burn calories. The effect can last for 20 minutes to six hours.

Decreases appetite. In a study by Dutch researchers, people who took a capsaicin supplement before meals ate less fat and fewer calories. The findings were in the *International Journal of Obesity.*

In another study, in the *British Journal of Nutrition,* people who ate chiles at breakfast were less hungry and ate less at lunch, and people who ate chiles as part of a dinner appetizer ate fewer calories and fat for the remainder of the meal.

Increases fat burn during exercise. Taking a capsaicin supplement one hour before aerobic exercise increased fat burn, reported a Japanese study in the *Journal of Nutritional Science and Vitaminology.*

Dissolves fat cells. In animal research, eating chiles reduced the number of fat cells and helped prevent new fat cells from forming—even in animals fed a high-fat diet.

Prevent the complications of obesity. Researchers found that capsaicin can reduce insulin resistance and prevent fatty liver disease in animals—two prediabetic conditions common in Americans who eat a high-fat, high-sugar diet.

A Heart-Warming Spice

Population studies conducted around the world show that people living in chile-eating nations have lower rates of cardiovascular disease than people living in nations where the cuisine is bland. Studies show eating more chiles can help:

Prevent blood clots. When scientists looked at medical records in chile-eating countries, they found a much lower incidence of embolisms, or potentially dangerous blood clots, which can lead to a heart attack or stroke. Studies show that capsaicin works like an anticoagulant drug by helping the body dissolve fibrin, a substance that causes the formation of blood clots.

Improve cholesterol. Australian researchers found that healthy adults who added an ounce of chiles to their daily diet increased their resistance to the oxidized blood fats that coat and thicken artery walls, according to a study in the *British Journal of Nutrition.* And a study reported in *Phytotherapy Research* found that

It's the rare person who can down ribs and chicken doused in 10-alarm chile sauce and go back for seconds, or bite into the hottest of the hots—a *naga jolokia*—and keep on grinning.

Chile is said to be an acquired taste, and possessing the tenacity to test the temperature and turn up the heat is like an addiction. There are *thousands* of chile fans who challenge themselves and one another to keep turning it up a notch as if it were a quest to conquer Mount Everest. There is even a scientific method of keeping score called the Scoville heat scale.

The Scoville heat scale measures the levels of capsaicin in a pepper by the amount of sweetened water it takes to dilute it to the heatless state of a bell pepper. One million drops of water moves the index up 1.5 units. This puts bell peppers at 0 units and 100 percent capsaicin at 16 million units. Searing starts at 100,000 units

and goes up to 750,000. A jalapeño, for example, ranges from 2,500 to 8,000 units. The Tabasco chile (with a sauce by the same name) and the cayenne range from 30,000 to 50,000 units. (The cayenne is the chile used in most medical research.)

The Scotch bonnet chile, which is used in Jamaican jerk dishes, ranges from 150,000 to 325,000 units. Tiny bird's eye chiles, used to make Portugal's *piri-piri* sauce and Tunisia's *harissa* comes in at 100,000 to 225,000 units.

The hottest chile is believed to be the *naga jolokia* from India, which hits the scale at over 1 million Scoville units. Of the chiles we're most likely to encounter, the orange habañero is one of the hottest at 150,000 to 325,000 units. However, a few years ago, a hybrid called red savina habañero was designed that tops out at over 500,000 units, one of the highest on record!

---

capsaicin supplements reduced dangerous LDL cholesterol and increased protective HDL cholesterol in test animals.

Reduce heart rate. Healthy men who ate an ounce of chiles a day for a month had a lower resting heart rate (a sign of a stronger, healthier heart) than men who ate a bland diet, according to a study in the *European Journal of Clinical Nutrition*. They also performed better in a stress test that measures heart muscle function.

Prevent arrhythmias. Animal studies found capsaicin reduced ventricular tachycardia and ventricular fibrillation, two serious and life-threatening types of irregular heartbeat. According to the studies, reported in the *European Journal of Pharmacology*, capsaicin worked like calcium blockers, prescription medication used to treat the conditions.

Reduce damage after a heart attack. In an animal experiment, researchers found that capsaicin reduced the damage to heart cells after a heart attack. The researchers, reporting in the journal *Circulation*, believe the capsaicin protected the heart by stimulating nerves in the spinal cord,

which in turn activated survival-oriented nerves in the heart muscle.

Capsaicin and Cancer Prevention

Dozens of studies, including those in my laboratory at M.D. Anderson Cancer Center, have found that capsaicin causes death to tumor cells in test animals and human cell cultures. Earlier studies on cancer and chiles, however, had produced conflicting results, with some suggesting that eating chiles *causes* certain cancers, including colon cancer. However, there is evidence that the commercial capsaicin used in the earlier studies may have been mixed with potentially carcinogenic impurities, whereas recent and current research uses pure capsaicin.

Another conflict arose when researchers at the University of Utah found a correlation between eating chiles and a high incidence of stomach cancer among Mexican-Americans and US Cajun and Creole populations. However, this isn't the case for *all* chile-eating nations, which makes me (as well as many other scientists) believe that something else may be going on in the diet that is raising the cancer risk. Plus, as you're about to read, chiles are actually kind to the stomach.

Truth is, over the last decade, close to 100 test tube and animal studies have found a strong correlation between eating chiles and cancer *prevention*, including cancers of the breast, esophagus, stomach, liver, prostate, and brain, and leukemia. Some of the most promising and extensive research to date has been with prostate cancer.

Prostate cancer. Researchers at Cedars-Sinai Medical Center in Los Angeles found that capsaicin killed 80 percent of cancer cells in test animals medically induced with prostate cancer. Remaining tumors were about one-fifth the size of those in untreated mice. Capsaicin also reduced prostate-specific antigen (PSA), a biomarker that can signal the presence of cancer in men. Dr. H. Phillip Koeffler, director of hematology and oncology at Cedars-Sinai, said it's possible that capsaicin someday may be used to prevent the return of prostate cancer in men treated for the disease.

Breast cancer. Cedars-Sinai is finding similar success with breast cancer. According to the

journal *Oncogene*, capsaicin blocked human breast cancer cells in the test tube and decreased the size of tumors by 50 percent in test animals. Capsaicin has "a potential role in the treatment and prevention of human breast cancer," the researchers reported.

Good for the Stomach

Chiles have a bad—and mistaken—reputation for creating the same fire down below that they do in the mouth. Studies have proven otherwise: they cause neither ulcers nor hemorrhoids. Here's what we know:

Ulcers. Surprise! Not only don't chiles cause ulcers, they actually might *prevent* them.

"Investigations carried out in recent years have revealed that chile and its [active ingredient] capsaicin is not the cause for ulcer formation but a benefactor," Indian researchers reported in *Critical Reviews in Food Science and Nutrition*. "Capsaicin does not stimulate but inhibits acid secretion, stimulates alkali, mucus secretions and particularly gastric mucosal blood flow, which help in prevention and healing of ulcers."

Ulcer-free people eat 2.6 times more chiles than people who come down with ulcers, Malaysian researchers noted in *Digestive Diseases and Sciences*. Researchers in Korea found that capsaicin is even potent enough to kill *H. pylori*, the bacteria that are the leading cause of stomach ulcers.

Animal research in Singapore found that doses similar to typical human chile consumption protected the gastric lining from alcohol-related damage. Another study found the same results on stomach problems related to excess use of aspirin.

Researchers in Singapore found that long-term chile intake protected animals from acute stress ulceration, a serious complication in severely ill patients that often causes stomach hemorrhage, according to a study in the *Journal of Gastroenterology and Hepatology*.

Indigestion. Italian researchers, reporting in the *New England Journal of Medicine*, found that

---

How to Put Out the Fire

Grabbing a glass of water is the worst thing you can do for "chile mouth." This is because chile is not water soluble—in fact, it can make the flame glow even more.

Fat and alcohol are the only substances that can reduce the burn, though they are only mildly effective. Beer, milk, yogurt, peanut butter, and ice cream work the best.

Never rub your eyes or face after handling chiles, as the oil is an irritant and will burn, even hours afterward. If you get chile burn in your eyes, rinse repeatedly with cool water or saline solution until the sting begins to wane.

If your skin burns or is irritated from contact with chile, wash it off with soap and water, or rub it with alcohol, and then dab it with whole-fat milk.

2.5 g of red chili powder a day reduced symptoms in people with functional dyspepsia, a chronic digestive disorder of no known origin with symptoms similar to indigestion. By the third week of treatment, those with dyspepsia reported a 60 percent improvement in their symptoms.

More Hot Discoveries

Psoriasis. Several studies have found that capsaicin cream can help reduce the redness and itching in people with psoriasis, a chronic inflammatory skin condition for which there is no known cure.

In one study, people with moderate to severe psoriasis applied a capsaicin cream containing either .01 or .025% capsaicin to one side of their bodies several times a day and a placebo cream on the other. After six weeks, the capsaicin cream resulted in a 68 percent reduction in scaling, redness, and swelling, compared to 44 percent for the placebo cream. The study was reported in the *Journal of the American Academy of Dermatology*.

Type 2 diabetes. The amount of insulin required to lower blood sugar after a meal was lower in people who ate a meal containing chiles than in people who ate a bland meal, according to an Australian study in the *American Journal of Clinical Nutrition*.

Getting to Know Chile

Chiles are the most widely consumed spice. Worldwide, we eat 20 times more chiles than any other spice!

Millions of people are so passionate about eating fire that there are hundreds of clubs and Web sites for diehards to share their burning desires and recipes, at least two consumer magazines that write about nothing but chiles, a mini-industry of hot sauce products dead set on turning the mouth on fire, and even an international non-profit institute dedicated to preserving the genetic codes of all species while trying to produce even hotter varieties. It's mind-boggling to fathom, but there are more than 3,000 varieties of chiles!

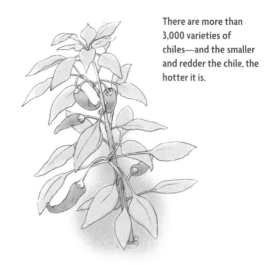

There are more than 3,000 varieties of chiles—and the smaller and redder the chile, the hotter it is.

It is so hard to imagine Indian cuisine without chiles that it is commonly believed that they originated in India. Chiles, however, are from the Americas. Christopher Columbus "discovered" them on his secret route that landed him in the Americas on his quest to find the source of black pepper, which the Arabs had been keeping secret from the Europeans for centuries. He didn't find black pepper (it was 5,000 miles away in India), but he found "red pepper"—the chile. Columbus took chiles back to Spain where they became an immediate sensation as "poor man's pepper." It may be one of the best gifts the New World ever gave to the Old!

By the 17th century, chiles were known around the globe. Today they play a key role in the cuisines of India, Africa, Asia, the Caribbean, Mexico, Central America, and the US South and Southwest. Chiles put heat in South Indian curries, Jamaican jerks, Mexican salsas and moles, Malaysian *sambals*, Korean *kimchi*, Indonesian *rendangs*, Thailand's *nam prik*, North African *harissa*, and Portuguese *piri piri*. They also go in spice blends, relishes, and pastes.

Cajuns, Creoles, and Jamaicans (as well as many others) go to literally painful lengths to see who can create the most searing hell-fire hot sauce. They come in hundreds of different varieties and ranges of heat and are used as condiments all over the Caribbean and America's South, from Louisiana to Arizona.

Mexico is best known for its chile cuisine and rightly so. Mexico is the most advanced chile culture, and Mexicans are said to have the most refined palates in the world for developing chile recipes. Mexicans are masters at using an extraordinary variety of fresh and dried chiles to achieve characteristic flavor, aromas, mouth feel, color, and bite to a whole spectrum of dishes. Mexico alone is home to more than 150 different varieties of chiles. (And thanks to the proliferation of Mexican restaurants in the US, salsa surpassed ketchup in the 1980s as America's favorite condiment.)

India has an infinite variety of chiles, each with its own distinct aroma, flavor, and pungency. Mildly hot green chiles are cooked in butter with tomatoes, molasses, and other spices for a mouth-watering delicacy called *mirchi ki bhaji*. Chiles are stuffed with roasted spices and pickled in mustard oil to make *mirch ka achar*, an all-time favorite eaten with fried bread. The black curries of Sri Lanka contain "bird peppers," possibly the hottest on earth, *and* red-hot cayenne. Indians temper the fire with cooling side dishes called *raitas*, which often include cucumber and yogurt, and with rice dishes.

Chiles put the heat in China's Sichuan and Hunan cuisines. One of the hottest dishes is Kung pao chicken, which contains enough fiery hot chiles in a bean sauce to challenge the taste buds of even the most jaded chile eaters.

Chiles are important in the Caribbean because they add character to otherwise bland starchy staples, such as peas and rice, beans, grains, and yucca. Chiles also produce a sweat, which works like a natural air conditioner in the relentless hot sun.

How to Buy Chile
Chiles are pods with a thick shiny skin covering a hollow that hides a lining of membranes filled with seeds. Chile pods come in an assortment of

Chile may help prevent and/or treat:

Arthritis, osteo-	Heart disease
Blood clots	Indigestion
Cancer	Neck pain
Cholesterol problems (high "bad" LDL cholesterol, low "good" HDL cholesterol)	Nerve pain (neuropathy)
	Overweight
	Postherpetic neuralgia
Diabetes, type 2	Psoriasis
Diabetic neuropathy	Stroke
Headache, tension	Ulcer
Heart attack	

Chile pairs well with these spices:

Allspice	Galangal
Amchur	Garlic
Cardamom	Ginger
Cocoa	Kokum
Coconut	Onion
Cumin	Pumpkin seed
Fenugreek seed	Turmeric

and complements recipes featuring:

Pickles	Salsas
Relishes	Sauces

shapes, colors, and heat levels. They range in size from less than an inch to eight inches or more. But here's the important fact: the smaller and redder the chile, the hotter it is.

Chiles are available fresh, whole dried, crushed (flakes), powdered, canned or jarred, and pickled. You can find many varieties at the market. And what you find—either fresh or dried—depends on your locale, your market, and your area's ethnic population.

Fresh chiles are green until they ripen, after which they turn red, yellow, brown, purple, or

Other recipes containing chile:

black. When buying fresh chiles, look for pods that are firm and have a smooth, glossy outer skin with good color. Chiles should be dry and heavy, not limp, dull, or discolored. Wrinkled skin indicates they have started to dry or may not have ripened on the bush, which is undesirable.

Fresh chiles can be stored loosely in the refrigerator for about two weeks. Wrap them in a paper towel or put them in a plastic bag and leave it partially open. Fresh chiles also freeze well in a sealed freezer bag.

If possible, buy the type of chile called for in the recipe. Though it's always okay to substitute one type of chile for another, remember each has a distinct flavor that can be recognized in the final result.

Most importantly, there is a huge flavor difference between a dried and fresh chile, though the heat is the same. Some have likened it to the difference between a fresh and a sun-dried tomato. Drying caramelizes the sugars and other chemicals in the chile, so a dried chile develops a more complex flavor. If you substitute dry for fresh or vice versa when cooking, expect a very different taste.

Mexico considers this taste difference so important it has given different names to the same chile fresh and dried. For example, a poblano chile is called an *ancho* when dried, and a smoke-dried jalapeño is called a *chipotle*.

You're most likely to come upon more variety by buying dried chiles. Many well-stocked markets carry an infinite variety in cellophane bags. You might even find a garland of dried whole chiles called a *ristra* still hanging from the line on which they were dried. Dried chiles vary in appearance according to the variety. Look for ones that are still vivid in color. If they've lost their color, it's a sign that they have probably lost some of their flavor as well. Dried chiles will keep indefinitely in a dry, dark storage area.

Ground chile is manufactured mainly for using in spice mixes and as a convenience at the stove. In the supermarket it comes in two varieties: chili (not chile) powder or cayenne.

Grilled Pork Chile Adobo

This is one of Mexico's numerous adobos, a vinegar-based all-purpose seasoning designed to give grilled meats a kick. This one is hot, though not fiery, and can be used with any cut of pork. It is traditionally served with guacamole, salsa, and tortilla chips.

¼ cup chili powder
½ cup white vinegar
4 garlic cloves
1 teaspoon dried oregano, preferably Mexican
1 teaspoon salt
1 teaspoon freshly ground black pepper
½ teaspoon ground cloves
½ teaspoon ground cinnamon
4 thick loin pork chops
½ cup chopped cilantro

1. Combine the chili powder, vinegar, garlic, oregano, salt, pepper, cloves, and cinnamon in a blender and process until it becomes a smooth wet paste.
2. Put the pork chops in one layer into a glass or ceramic dish. Spread the marinade on top and refrigerate for at least eight hours, turning every few hours.
3. Remove from the marinade and grill the chops over medium-high heat, three to four minutes on each side. Sprinkle with cilantro and serve.

Makes 4 servings.

Generic chili powder is not pure chile but is made with ground chiles mixed with other spices, such as cumin, oregano, and salt. It's most noted for adding heat to chili con carne. Do not assume it is pure chile unless the label says so.

Cayenne powder is pure chile, ground from the long, red cayenne chile. It is also fiery hot. It can be found in the spice aisle of any supermarket. Many specialty markets carry other pure chile powders in a range of heats. Ground ancho chile powder, for example, is milder than cayenne and is popular in Mexican cooking. The temperature of chile powder ranges in heat according to the ratio of seeds used when the chiles are ground. The hotter varieties are more orange, rather than red. Asian, Indian, and Latin markets sell specialty chile powders by the bag.

You can find virtually any type of dried chile online. Check the "Buyer's Guide" on page 309 for online sources.

Chiles are grown all over the world but the principal growing plantations are found in Mexico, California, Texas, New Mexico, Arizona, Thailand, India, the Caribbean, Africa, and Asia. (India is estimated to be the largest producer of chiles in the world.) In addition to the jalapeño, ancho chiles from Mexico and Anaheim chiles from New Mexico and California are the most commonly used in the US.

In the Kitchen with Chile

Despite all the hullabaloo about heat, chiles add an important *flavor* to food. However, it should never be used alone as a spice. Rather, use it as background to other spices. It goes with virtually any assortment of spices.

You can't take away a chile's heat but you can turn it down by discarding the seeds and cutting away the membrane, the two places where the heat resides. There is more heat in the membrane than the seeds and there's more membrane in the stem, which is why it's the hottest part of the chile. For milder flavor, wash and dry the chile, remove the stem, and slice it lengthwise with a small sharp paring knife under running water.

Dried chiles should be soaked, covered in warm water, for about 20 minutes or until soft and pliable, then chop and use as directed. You can remove the seeds from a dried chile by breaking it and knocking out the seeds by tapping it on its side.

Be forewarned! Capsaicin is volatile and can burn on contact. Always wear plastic or rubber gloves when handing any chile and make sure to keep your hands clear of your skin and eyes. The heat from a habañero, for example, is so intense it has been known to cause blisters in the skin of sensitive individuals. Also, avoid breathing the fumes.

Ideally, you should have a special cutting board and knife to work with chiles. Even after washing, capsaicin residue will remain on the surface of your tools. If disposing of chile seeds and remnants in the garbage disposal, make sure to run the disposal with very cold water. Hot water will give you a backlash as the heat diffuses into the air. (This is why capsaicin is an ingredient in pepper spray.)

If you're tentative about cooking with chiles, always start with a little less. You can always add more heat, but it's hard (though not impossible) to take it out. If a dish tastes too hot, add a little sugar, milk, or cream. An old wife's tale says adding a whole potato to the pot for a half hour will draw out some of the heat.

Dried chiles can be added whole to slow-cooked foods, as the heat will slowly seep out and blend into the dish. You can also soak a chile in hot water to soften it and pierce it with a sharp knife before adding.

To intensify the flavor of dried chiles, dry roast them using the method described on page 11 before soaking. You can get the same effect by running them under a broiler.

To add mild heat to simmering dishes, cut a few slits in a whole fresh chile and add it to the dish while cooking. Remove and discard the chile before serving.

There is no boredom factor when it comes to experimenting with culinary chile creations. With so many different varieties, chiles offer an endless adventure in eating.

CINNAMON *Balancing Blood Sugar*

Maybe it's ironic that cinnamon—the spicy-sweet favorite that cooks use to give sugary confections extra flavor—can help control blood sugar problems. Or maybe—given the fact that 24 million Americans have type 2 diabetes and 57 million have prediabetes—it's Mother Nature's way of cutting us a break.

Defeating Diabetes

The rate of type 2 diabetes in the US has *doubled* in the past two decades, from 5 to 10 percent of American adults, with 1.3 million new cases every year. This disease of chronically high blood sugar (fasting blood sugar levels above 125 milligrams per deciliter, or mg/dL) attacks arteries and veins, increasing the risk of heart disease six-fold. In fact, medical guidelines instruct doctors to treat a patient with type 2 diabetes *as if* he

or she has already had a heart attack! This body-wide circulatory destruction can lead to many other health problems along with heart disease and stroke. They include painful nerve damage, hard-to-heal skin ulcers, vision loss and blindness, kidney failure, and even—as blood flow is choked—the amputation of gangrenous toes, feet, and lower limbs.

Managing type 2 diabetes requires a total approach that typically includes losing weight, eating more whole foods, exercising regularly, and taking (or injecting) glucose-controlling medications such as insulin (the pancreas-manufactured hormone that helps control blood sugar levels). Preventing diabetes or reversing prediabetes (fasting blood sugar levels from 100 to 125) is possible with lifestyle alone—and lifestyle changes are *more* effective than preventive medications, as

Will the Real Cinnamon Please Stand Up?

You know that stuff you sprinkle on your morning toast and oatmeal called cinnamon? It's not *true* cinnamon. It's *cassia*.

Cassia cinnamon (*Cinnamomum cassia*) and true cinnamon (*Cinnamomum verum*) belong to the same botanical family (*Cinnamomum*). They also look alike—it takes a trained eye to tell them apart. But they differ in flavor. Cassia is the sweeter and stronger of the two—and the one preferred throughout most of the world (including the US) as a culinary spice. It's also the version that was used in all the studies discussed in this chapter.

Cassia cinnamon is commonly used in the United States, Europe, China, and Southeast Asia. True cinnamon is found in kitchens in Mexico, Latin America, India, and other nations in South Asia.

In some parts of the world it's actually *illegal* to refer to cassia as *cinnamon*. In Great Britain and Australia, for example, *Cinnamomum cassia* can *only* be sold as cassia, and *Cinnamomum verum* can *only* be sold as cinnamon. In the US, both are legally sold as cinnamon.

France has solved the issue quite nicely—they call the spice *cannelle*, applying the name to both cassia and true cinnamon.

Cassia cinnamon is also called Chinese cinnamon. True cinnamon also goes by the names Ceylon and Sri Lankan cinnamon. You can find cassia cinnamon . . . everywhere. In the US, you can find true cinnamon in Indian marketplaces and specialty spice shops or online.

---

the 10-year Diabetes Prevention Program Study showed. But study after study also shows that cinnamon can play a role in the everyday management of blood sugar (glucose) levels and other cardiovascular disease CVD risk factors.

Long-term blood sugar control. In a recent study from the US, 109 people with type 2 diabetes were divided into two groups, with one receiving one gram of cinnamon a day and one receiving a placebo. After three months, those taking the cinnamon had a 0.83 percent decrease in A1C, or glycosylated hemoglobin—the percentage of red blood cells that have been frosted (glycated) by blood sugar, and the most accurate measurement of long-term blood sugar control. (Seven percent or less means the diabetes is controlled, and a decrease from 0.5 to 1.0 percent is considered a significant improvement.) Those taking the placebo had a 0.37 percent decrease in A1C. "Taking cinnamon could be useful . . . in addition to usual care" of diabetes, concluded the study leader in the *Journal of the American Board of Family Medicine.*

However, cinnamon probably won't work to control blood sugar in type 1 diabetes—an autoimmune disease that attacks the insulin-producing pancreas. In a study by researchers at Dartmouth College in New Hampshire, researchers asked 72 adolescents with type 1 diabetes to take either cinnamon or a placebo. After three months, there was no change in A1C levels in either group, or the amount of insulin they had to take to control the disease.

Heart-protecting power. In another study, 30 people with type 2 diabetes took one to six grams of cinnamon a day (about ¼ to ½ teaspoon). After 40 days, they had decreases up to 29 percent in fasting blood sugar—and decreases up to 27 percent in "bad" artery-clogging LDL cholesterol, up to 26 percent in total cholesterol, and up to 30 percent in triglycerides (another blood fat, with high levels linked to heart disease). "Those who have type 2 diabetes, or those who have elevated glucose, triglycerides or total cholesterol, may benefit from regular inclusion of cinnamon in their daily diet," concluded the researchers in *Diabetes Care.*

The researchers also noted that the study participants had lower levels of blood sugar and blood fats even after 20 days without taking any cinnamon—"indicating that cinnamon would not need to be consumed every day" for health benefits.

They also pointed out that cinnamon worked at every level it was tested, from one to six grams—and that "intake of less than one gram daily is likely to be beneficial in controlling blood sugar and lipid [fat] levels."

Finally, they said that regular inclusion of cinnamon in the diet is probably a good idea not only for those with type 2 diabetes, but for everybody—"cinnamon may be beneficial for the remainder of the population to *prevent* . . . elevated glucose and blood lipid levels." There's a lot of evidence that shows they're right.

Lowering risk factors in prediabetes. Researchers in France studied 22 people who were overweight and had prediabetes, dividing them into two groups. One group took a widely available supplement containing 250 mg of a water extract of cinnamon (Cinnulin PF). The other group took a placebo. After three months, those taking the cinnamon supplement had much lower levels of several biomarkers of *oxidation*—the destructive, cell-destroying process that contributes to the development of both diabetes and cardiovascular disease. And the lower the oxidation levels, the more stable the levels of blood sugar. "The inclusion of water soluble cinnamon compounds in the diet could reduce risk factors associated with diabetes and cardiovascular disease," concluded the researchers in the *Journal of the American College of Nutrition*.

Mastering the metabolic syndrome. This condition—also known as the insulin resistance syndrome and syndrome X—is characterized by blood sugar problems, overweight (especially around the abdomen), high blood pressure, and high triglycerides (but not necessarily high LDL). It's one form of prediabetes, and, needless to say, it's a risk factor for type 2 diabetes and heart disease. Cinnamon can help control it.

In one study, 22 people with metabolic syndrome were divided into two groups: one took 500 mg a day of Cinnulin PF and one took a placebo.

After three months, those taking the cinnamon had significant decreases in average fasting blood sugar (down 8.4 percent, to 106), lower systolic blood pressure (the top reading, down 4 points to 128), and more muscle, or lean body mass. (That's good news, because additional muscle means additional ability to burn up excess blood sugar.) They also had a small drop in body fat. "This naturally-occurring spice can reduce risk factors associated with diabetes and cardiovascular diseases," concluded the researchers.

Stopping spikes in blood sugar after a meal. Swedish researchers studied 14 people, feeding them the same meal twice—rice pudding, with or without a hefty sprinkling of cinnamon. The cinnamon-spiced meal significantly lowered post-meal levels of blood sugar.

Works in healthy people, too. British researchers studied healthy young men, dividing them into two groups. For two weeks, one group received three grams of cinnamon a day and the other a placebo. After two weeks, the men taking the cinnamon supplement had a much improved "glucose tolerance test"—the ability of the body to process and store glucose. They also had better "insulin sensitivity"—the ability of this hormone to usher glucose out of the bloodstream and into cells.

Richard Anderson, PhD, a scientist at the Beltsville Human Nutrition Research Center of the US Department of Agriculture, who has conducted several studies on cinnamon and diabetes, theorizes that the spice mimics the action of insulin, the hormone that regulates blood sugar. It may stimulate insulin receptors on fat and muscle cells the same way insulin does, he said, allowing excess sugar to move out of the blood and into the cells.

And a team of Indian researchers laud *cinnamaldehyde*, cinnamon's active ingredient—which their study on experimental animals with diabetes showed can decrease blood sugar, A1C, total cholesterol, and triglycerides, and increase insulin and "good" HDL cholesterol. The findings were in *Phytomedicine*.

Controlling Polycystic
Ovary Syndrome (PCOS)

There's another disease where insulin and blood sugar levels are haywire and the sufferer is at higher risk for type 2 diabetes, heart disease, and stroke—polycystic ovary syndrome (PCOS). This hormonal disorder, which strikes 5 to 10 percent of women of reproductive age in the US, lines the ovaries with small cysts. Symptoms include menstrual abnormality, extra facial and body hair, acne, and overweight. It's also *the* most common cause of female infertility.

In a study by a team of American researchers from Columbia University, the University of Hawaii, and the US Department of Agriculture, 13 women with PCOS were asked to take either a daily cinnamon supplement (333 mg, three times a day) or a placebo. After eight weeks, those taking cinnamon had a 17 percent decrease in fasting glucose, a significant decrease in insulin resistance, and 21 percent reduction in levels of blood sugar after a glucose tolerance test. The researchers called the findings "interesting" and encouraged other scientists to conduct additional studies to validate their findings, which were reported in *Fertility and Sterility*.

Manhandling Microbes

Cinnamon has the power to fight disease-causing microbes such as bacteria and fungi.

Preserving food. Scientists proved cinnamon's ability to preserve food and help prevent food poisoning in a kitchen experiment with two pots of vegetable broth. They added cinnamon oil to one pot but not the other and let the two sit in the refrigerator—for two months! When they took off the lids, the pot without the cinnamon was teeming with bacteria. The other pot? Good enough to eat. In fact, the scientists said the added cinnamon improved the flavor! (Don't try this at home.)

Fighting fungi. Cinnamon is also effective against *Candida albicans*, the fungus that causes most cases of vaginal yeast infections. In labora-

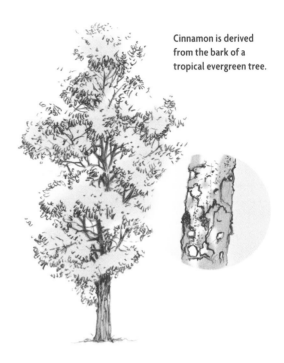

Cinnamon is derived from the bark of a tropical evergreen tree.

tory tests, cinnamon extracts were able to stop the growth of strains of *C. albicans* resistant to fluconazole (Diflucan), the medication commonly used to treat yeast infections.

Beating bacteria. Researchers in Italy found that cinnamon is effective at eradicating *Helicobacter pylori* infection, the bacterial cause of most stomach ulcers and a leading cause of stomach cancer. In fact, their research showed that cinnamon was *more* effective than the antibiotic amoxicillin (Amoxil) at killing *H. pylori*. And the bacteria didn't show any resistance to the spice—important, because *H. pylori* are becoming more and more resistant to standard antibiotic treatment.

Cinnamon, On and On

There are other intriguing areas of research for cinnamon.

Cancer. American researchers found that cinnamon may slow *angiogenesis*, the development of new blood supplies to tumors. They concluded that an extract of the spice "could potentially be useful in cancer prevention and/or treatment." The findings were in *Carcinogenesis.*

Post-stroke protection. Researchers in Korea found that cinnamon protected brain cells in the laboratory from the type of damage caused by a stroke.

Brain injury from liver failure. Similarly, cinnamon protected brain cells from the type of damage seen in *hepatic encephalopathy*—a type of brain damage caused by advanced liver disease.

Wound healing. In a study from Indian researchers, extracts of cinnamon bark improved wound healing in animals.

Getting to Know Cinnamon

Cinnamon's sweet-and-spicy bite is the same as its bark—the spice is derived from the bark of a tropical evergreen tree.

That deliciously aromatic bite has been heralded since the beginning of human history. God commanded Moses to include cinnamon in a recipe for sacred anointing oil. The Song of Solomon praises its scent. The Greeks and Romans offered it to their gods.

The ancient cultures of India and China also used cinnamon—as medicine. The Ayurvedic physicians of India used it (and continue to use it) for respiratory ailments, stomach upset, muscles spasms—and, of course, for diabetes.

Practitioners of traditional Chinese medicine used it (and continue to use it) for its "warming" qualities, particularly for respiratory problems and muscle aches. (It's also a major ingredient in Tiger Balm, the popular Chinese ointment for pain relief.)

Of course, cinnamon is more than medicine—it's a much-beloved ingredient in cuisines around the world. In the United States and Europe, it's most popular in sweet dishes—apple pie, coffee cake, fruit compotes, buns, muffins, doughnuts, cakes, and cookies. It is a key ingredient in apple pie spice and mulling spice. It is sprinkled on toast and whipped cream. Cinnamon sticks are stirred into hot beverages, including mulled cider and wine.

The English are very fond of what they call *cassia.* (For more on the difference between "true cinnamon" and cassia, please see the box on page 80.) Many households keep a large sterling silver canister on the table for sprinkling cassia onto sweets and into beverages. It is an ingredient in English fruitcakes, stewed fruits, and pastries.

In Spain, cinnamon is a popular addition to chocolate dishes and confections. In Germany, it's used in apple strudel, to flavor sweet and sour dishes, and in foods containing raisins. In the Netherlands, cinnamon is the dominant flavor in the Christmas spiced cookie called *speculaas.*

Can Chewing Gum Make You Smarter?

Maybe—if you chew *cinnamon* gum. In fact, you don't even have to chew it. Just smelling cinnamon might boost your thinking ability.

That's the result of a study conducted by Phillip R. Zoladz, PhD, an assistant professor of psychology at Ohio Northern University, who found students scored better on several mental performance tests after smelling or tasting cinnamon.

In the first part of the study, Dr. Zoladz gave a group of students one of the following to chew: cinnamon, peppermint, cherry, or flavorless gum. In the second part, he asked students to sniff cinnamon, peppermint, jasmine, or no odor.

In both parts of the study, the students who chewed the cinnamon gum or smelled cinnamon scored best—with the best memory, the most focused attention, and the fastest reflexes between connecting what they saw and what they had to do.

Dr. Zoladz and his colleagues concluded that cinnamon has potential for decreasing test anxiety—and even preventing age-related memory loss!

Italians put whole cinnamon sticks in *mostarda,* a classic chutney-like condiment.

The French favor *canelle* (their word for cinnamon) in savory foods featuring game, such as duckling à la Montmorency, a classic dish flavored with cinnamon and spiked with cherry sauce. It's one of the four ingredients in the French spice *quatre épices,* which is most often used to enhance game dishes.

In Asia, cinnamon is almost exclusively used in savory dishes. In China, it's used in braises and clay pot cooking, or what is often called "red cooking." In this technique, you simmer cinnamon, star anise, and orange zest in water, rice wine, and soy sauce, then cook a chicken breast side down in the liquid until it is red and cooked through. Cinnamon is also one of the five spices in Chinese five-spice powder.

Cooks in the Middle East use cinnamon as a flavoring in meat stew. It's a popular spice in many Moroccan spice blends, including the famous *ras-el-hanout.* It also gives a tang to Moroccan stews called *tagines.* In Syria, it's one of only two spices found in the kitchen. (The other is allspice.) In Iran it's a key spice in *khoresht,* a thick tart stew made with pomegranate juice.

In India, it's a common spice in curry cooking, and in rich dishes called *biryanis.* Indian cooks fry a whole cinnamon stick in hot oil to release its aroma, then add it to the curry or rice as it is being cooked. It's also used in many Indian spice blends, and is a key flavoring in the ubiquitous *garam masala.*

Vietnamese use it in *pho bos,* long-simmering beef soups, which are served with noodles.

Mexicans are fond of cinnamon tea (*té de canela*), which is made from broken cinnamon quills. It's also an ingredient in Mexican moles.

Cinnamon is also used in a wide array of non-food products. It is put in toothpastes to mask the taste of pyrophosphate, an unpleasant-tasting compound that inhibits the formation of plaque. It is used in making toiletries, pharmaceutical products, and even tobacco.

How to Buy Cinnamon

Virtually all of the cinnamon imported into the United States is *cinnamon cassia.* (For the difference between cassia and so-called "true cin-

Cinnamon may help prevent and/or treat:

Cancer	Insulin resistance (prediabetes)
Cholesterol problems (high total cholesterol, high "bad" LDL cholesterol, low "good" HDL cholesterol)	Metabolic syndrome
	Polycystic ovarian syndrome (PCOS)
Diabetes, type 2	Stroke
Food poisoning	Triglycerides, high
Heart disease	Ulcer
High blood pressure (hypertension)	Vaginal yeast infection
	Wounds

Cinnamon pairs well with these spices:

Allspice	Ginger
Caraway	Mint
Cardamom	Nutmeg
Clove	Star anise
Cocoa	Sun-dried tomato
Coriander	Tamarind
Cumin	Turmeric

and complements recipes featuring:

Apples	Curries
Baked or stewed fruit	Grapes
Bananas	Hot toddies
Cantaloupe	Pastries
Cauliflower	Oranges
Chicken	Pork
Chocolate	Winter squash
Corn	

namon," please see the box on page 80.) If you want to find "true cinnamon," take a trip to an Indian marketplace or shop online. Cassia cinnamon is usually called cinnamon, cassia, or Chinese cinnamon. True cinnamon is usually called true cinnamon, Ceylon cinnamon, or Sri Lankan cinnamon.

Both cinnamon and true cinnamon are harvested from dried bark and rolled, scroll-like, into tight quills—or what we call cinnamon sticks.

Quills of cinnamon are usually cut into four or five-inch pieces that easily fit in a spice jar. The quills are thick and are dark reddish-brown in appearance and deliver a sweet and strong aroma. It is grown in China, Vietnam, and Indonesia.

True cinnamon is cut the same way, but the quills are longer, have a brittle, paper-like appearance, and are light-brown in color. The taste is mild, delicate, and sweet. Though true cinnamon grows wild in South India, the best comes from Sri Lanka, off the coast of South India.

The best quality cinnamon is harvested from the trunk and is graded according to its length, breadth, and thickness.

The best quality quills are tightly rolled, evenly colored, and blemish free. When transported, the quills often break and are then sold as *second-grade quillings*. The next grade is called *featherings*, which are the inner bark of twigs and small shoots that were not large enough to form a full quill. They are still considered cinnamon, but lack the visual appeal of good quality quills. The lowest grade is *cinnamon chips*, made from shavings and trimmings. The lower grade featherings and chips generally come from the Seychelles Islands or Madagascar, which accounts for much of the world's supply of lower-grade cinnamon bark.

Once ground, cinnamon begins to lose the fragrance that comes from its volatile oils, so it's best to buy whole quills and grind them as needed. The quills are somewhat tough, so you'll need a sturdy spice grinder.

If your only option is to buy ground cinnamon, you'll get the most fragrance from the finest quality, which is smooth rather than gritty. Ground cinnamon quills are the best grade, though the spice is also ground from quillings and featherings. Ground cassia, often called "baker's cinnamon," is usually lower-priced than the ground quills of true cinnamon.

Whole quills keep for three years, as long as they aren't in extreme heat. Ground cinnamon begins to fade in flavor after a few months.

In the Kitchen with Cinnamon

All the studies on the health benefits of cinnamon were done on . . . cinnamon (cassia, Chinese cinnamon)—the spice you're familiar with and that is sold in supermarkets. Culinary

Other recipes containing cinnamon:

Apple Pie Spice (p. 271)

Baharat (p. 268)

Berbere (p. 267)

By-the-Bay Fisherman's Chowder (p. 46)

Chesapeake Bay Seafood Seasoning (p. 273)

Chinese Five-Spice Powder (p. 268)

Garam Masala (p. 264)

Grilled Lamb Patty Pockets with Cucumber Mint Sauce (p. 165)

Grilled Pork Chile Adobo (p. 78)

Jamaican Jerk Marinade (p. 269)

La Kama (p. 266)

Malaysian Curry Paste (p. 287)

Mulling Spice (p. 273)

Pears Poached in Port and Star Anise (p. 223)

Pickling Spice (p. 272)

Quatre Épices (p. 271)

Ras-el-hanout (p. 266)

Sambaar Masala (p. 265)

Spiced Milk Tea (p. 66)

Spiced Mixed Nuts (p. 90)

Spicy Vanilla Rice Pudding (p. 256)

Banana Cinnamon French Toast

Cinnamon is a classic on toast—and is even better on a special dish like French toast.

2 large very ripe bananas
1 cup milk
1 teaspoon cinnamon
¼ teaspoon nutmeg
4 eggs, cracked
8 slices thick whole grain bread
3 tablespoons butter
Maple syrup

1. Place the bananas, milk, cinnamon and nutmeg in a blender or food processor. Add the cracked eggs and process until smooth. Transfer to a large baking pan large. Add the bread slices, turning occasionally, under the bread has absorbed most of the mixture, about 30 minutes.
2. Melt the butter in a large skillet over medium head. Add the bread in batches and cook until golden brown, about 3 minutes on each side. Serve with maple syrup.

Makes 4 servings.

experts generally agree (with some dissenters) that cinnamon cassia also has the best flavor—more robust, more perfume. Cassia goes best with other strong flavors, liked dried fruit. The more delicate true cinnamon is a better complement to fresh fruit. But there's no rule that says you can't mix the two and get the best of both worlds!

Ground cinnamon is more commonly used in the US because it is the form that is generally used in baking. Quills are preferred for liquid-based savory dishes; they're used to infuse flavor and are discarded after cooking and before eating.

Whatever form of cinnamon you choose and use, make sure you don't overcook it. Cinnamon turns bitter if it's in the pot too long.

Here are some ideas to help get more cinnamon in your diet:

- Put a cinnamon quill in beef or vegetarian stews, or in lentil soup.
- Make spiced wine: Put a bottle of wine in a large pot and gently simmer it with ½ cup of sugar, a cinnamon stick, and a lemon studded with cloves for 15 minutes.
- Make spiced tea: Put a quart of brewed tea in a pot, add two cups of apple juice, and gently simmer it with a sliced lemon and two cinnamon sticks for 10 minutes.
- Sprinkle some cinnamon into pastry dough for pies and quiches.
- Sprinkle cinnamon on apples, bananas, melons, and oranges.
- Mix cinnamon with mint and parsley in ground beef for burgers or meatloaf.
- Combine equal parts of cinnamon, cardamom, and black pepper and rub it into pork tenderloin or lamb before baking.
- Mix cinnamon into rice pilaf.
- Add cinnamon to hot cocoa to enhance the flavor of the chocolate.

CLOVE *Pain Relief's Loyal Servant*

"Is it not remarkable, simple oil of clove. How amazing the results. Life can be so easy—relief or discomfort."

That could be your dentist talking. But in this case it's Lawrence Olivier, playing a sadistic dentist in the 1976 film *Marathon Man*, as he repeatedly drills into Dustin Hoffman's tooth and then relieves the pain with . . . oil of clove.

Fortunately, oil of clove can relieve dental pain in *real* life. Along with a lot of other health problems.

TLC For Teeth and Gums

The scientific name for oil of clove is *eugenol*. And biting into a clove (the dried flower bud of an Asian tree, and a culinary spice enjoyed around the world) reveals just how powerful eugenol is: there's an instant rush of localized numbness. The eugenol and other aromatic molecules in clove make it one of the most penetrating spices on the planet. And that penetrating power is perhaps nowhere more apparent than in the dentist's chair—or while waiting through a tooth-aching weekend to get into one!

Yes, oil of clove is a mild anesthetic. (In fact, clove oil is just as powerful as benzocaine in numbing oral tissue before needle sticks at the dentist, reported a team of researchers in *Journal of Dentistry*.) *And* it can boost circulation: when it's rubbed around a painful tooth, blood vessels near the gum dilate, bringing blood to the surface with a warm, soothing sensation. *And* it's an analgesic, reducing pain. *And* it's anti-inflammatory, reducing redness and swelling around an injury. *And* it's antibacterial, killing germs.

All those therapeutic powers help explain why eugenol is not only a home remedy for an untreated toothache, but a formidable medicine against many forms of oral disease. It can fight *gingivitis*, the early stage of gum disease, when gums are inflamed. It can fight *periodontitis*, the later stage, when gums recede and bone erodes.

It's also effective against *stomatitis*, a painful inflammation of the mucous lining of the mouth, caused by factors such as medications, poor dental hygiene, or ill-fitting dentures.

"Clove oil has been used to cure dental problems for ages" and is "an integral part of the dentist's kit," said a team of Indian researchers who investigated a long-lasting eugenol-containing treatment to battle periodontal disease, reporting their results in *Drug Development and Industrial Pharmacy*.

Fighting Infections

Eugenol's germ-fighting powers aren't limited to your teeth and gums. It can fight bacteria (and viruses) throughout the body. Such as:

Helicobacter pylori. These bacteria cause stomach ulcers and are also linked to stomach cancer. An international team of researchers from India noted that conventional medical treatment to eradicate *H. pylori* is only 80 to 90 percent effective, and that the bacteria are also developing resistance to various antibiotics. Since eugenol had already proven effective at stopping the growth of so many other types of nasty, disease-causing bacteria—including *E. coli* (food poisoning), *Staphylococcus* (staph infections), *Proteus* (bladder infections), *Klebsiella* (respiratory infections), *Enterobacter* (hospital-acquired infections), and *Pseudomonas* (urinary tract infections)—they decided to test it against *H. pylori* too. And in a laboratory study, they found that eugenol stopped the growth of 30 strains of *H. pylori*—and did so 25 percent faster than amoxicillin (Amoxil), a common antibiotic. And they found that the bacteria didn't develop any resistance to eugenol.

In their discussion of the study, the researchers noted that eugenol is already part of the diet in many countries and is likely to be "non-toxic"; that it was used by modern medicine as early as 1950 to treat ulcers; and that its "benefits could be multiple" because it's also a powerful anti-oxidant. They urge other researchers to duplicate their findings to help establish eugenol as a treatment and overcome the "treatment failures and antibiotic resistance in the area of *H. pylori* management."

Herpes simplex. Japanese researchers found that using the antiviral medication acyclovir (Zovirax) *and* eugenol was more powerful against the virus that causes cold sores (HS-1) than using acyclovir alone, both in the test tube and in animals. Thai researchers found that the virus that causes genital herpes (HS-2) couldn't replicate in the presence of eugenol. And US researchers found that eugenol protected animals against infection with HS-2.

Hepatitis C. Millions of Americans are infected with the hepatitis C virus, which can lead to cirrhosis and liver cancer. Japanese researchers found that eugenol caused near total "inhibition" of the virus. "Natural products" including eugenol "could play a great role as anti-hepatitis C agents," conclude the scientists in *Phytotherapy Research.*

Clove Loves You—All of You

Researchers have found many other ways that eugenol can protect the body.

Mosquito finito. Put away your citronella candles and get out your clove oil—it might be the best way to stop mosquitoes from biting. That's what Thai researchers discovered when they tested 38 different essential oils against mosquito bites, including the popular citronella.

The researchers enlisted volunteers to stick their forearms into an area dense with mosquitoes. Only a few essential oils protected against the bites, including citronella, patchouli, and clove oil, providing two hours of "complete repellency." When those oils were retested, only clove oil gave "100 percent repellency" for four hours.

Stopping blood clots. Blood clots that plug arteries are the cause of most heart attacks and strokes. And blood clots are caused in part by *platelet aggregation*—plate-shaped blood cells become sticky and clump together. Researchers in Denmark tested eugenol against two "blood-thinning" medications that fight platelet aggregation—aspirin and indomethacin (Indocin)—and found eugenol stronger than aspirin and equal to indomethacin.

Anti-cancer. Studies in animals with lung and skin cancer show eugenol can stop cancer cells from multiplying.

Getting to Know Clove

In the ancient days—BT, or Before Toothbrushes —cloves were used to clean teeth and keep breath smelling clean. In the ancient imperial court of China, during the Han Dynasty, no one was

The Coveted Clove

Cloves have a bloody history. They were coveted for their medicinal and culinary use, and brought enormous wealth to the intrepid explorers who went in search of them. Nations fought over them.

At the height of the Spice Wars, in 1605, the Dutch wrested possession of the Moluccas, or "spice islands," from the Portuguese, breaking their 60-year monopoly of the clove trade. Then the Dutch uprooted and burned all the clove trees, and restricted clove plantations to the remote island of Ambon—keeping the source of cloves secret and the price high. Inquisitive explorers in search of the spice were turned away. Anyone caught trying to pirate seedlings from the island was put to death. It took nearly 200 years to break this stranglehold. But in the early 1800s, a Frenchman by the name of Pierre Poivre (Peter Pepper)—the Peter Piper of nursery rhyme fame—managed to smuggle flowering clove buds off the island. Poivre took the buds to the French West Indies in the Caribbean and cultivated the tree there. Eventually, the tree spread to other countries with the right climates for cultivation. Today, cloves grow from South America to North Africa.

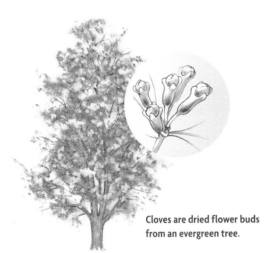

Cloves are dried flower buds from an evergreen tree.

Clove may help prevent and/or treat:

Bad breath	Gum disease (gingivitis and periodontal disease)
Blood clots	
Cancer	
Cold sores	Hepatitis C
Denture problems (stomatitis)	Mosquito bites
	Toothache
Food poisoning	Ulcer
Genital herpes	

Clove pairs well with these spices:

Allspice	Cocoa	Nutmeg
Amchur	Coriander	Star Anise
Cardamom	Cumin	Tamarind
Chile	Ginger	Turmeric
Cinnamon	Kokum	

and complements recipes featuring:

Apple pie	Mincemeat	Red cabbage
Cakes	Orange	Stewed fruit
Chocolate	Pickled eggs	
Ham	Pumpkin	

Other recipes containing clove:

Apple Pie Spice (p. 271)	Garam Masala (p. 264)
Baharat (p. 268)	Grilled Pork Chile Adobo (p. 78)
Berbere (p. 267)	
Caribbean Curry Paste (p. 287)	Mulling Spice (p. 273)
	Pickling Spice (p. 272)
Chesapeake Bay Seafood Seasoning (p. 273)	Quatre Épices (p. 271)
	Ras-el-hanout (p. 266)
Chinese Five-Spice Powder (p. 268)	Spicy Vanilla Rice Pudding (p. 256)
Colombo Powder (p. 270)	

allowed to speak to the emperor without a clove in his or her mouth. And that traditional use has continued to this day in Asia, where cloves are often used as an after-meal breath freshener.

In traditional and folk medicine, clove and clove oil have been used for a variety of ills—indigestion, for nausea, gas, diarrhea, bloating, and colic; against infections of all kinds; for muscle spasms, and to prepare for labor; for skin problems, including acne, ulcers, and sores; as an aid to memory; and even as an aphrodisiac. And, of course, for toothache.

It wasn't until the Middle Ages that clove caught on in the kitchen, and today cloves are a common culinary spice in virtually every cuisine. Spice blends the world over make liberal use of cloves. In China, clove is a key ingredient in Chinese five-spice powder. Clove is found in many of India's spice blends, including the basic blend *garam masala*. Clove is one of the four spices in French *quatre épices*. And it's a key ingredient in the Moroccan spice blend *ras-el-hanout* and the Ethiopian *baharat*.

Cloves are a popular spice in the United States, used in both sweet and savory dishes, with more than 1,000 tons imported every year. Americans stud hams with cloves, include them in apple spice mixes, put them in pickled eggs and soused herring, and add them to homemade

Spiced Mixed Nuts

Nutritionists recommend eating a daily handful of nuts—high in heart-healthy polyphenols and monounsaturated fats—as a wholesome snack. Spicing them with these five healing spices makes them even healthier. These nuts make a nice gift at holiday time.

½ cup sugar
1 teaspoon ground cinnamon
½ teaspoon ground cloves
¼ teaspoon ground allspice
¼ teaspoon ground ginger
¼ teaspoon ground nutmeg
½ teaspoon salt (optional)
1 egg white
2 tablespoons water
2 pounds whole mixed nuts, such as almonds, cashews, pecans, and walnuts

1. Spray two pastry sheets with non-cook spray and preheat the oven to 275°F.
2. Combine the sugar, spices, and salt (if using) in a large bowl. Stir in the egg white and water, and mix. The mixture should resemble a smooth paste. Add the nuts and gently stir so each nut is thoroughly coated with the spice mixture.
3. Spread out the nuts on the pastry sheets, separating them so they don't touch and stick together. Bake for 40 minutes or until the coating is crisp and golden brown. Cool and transfer to an airtight jar.

Makes about 5 cups.

sausages and Christmas fruitcakes. Cloves add to the distinctive flavor of Worcestershire sauce and are reportedly one of the "secret" spices in Heinz ketchup.

The French stud onions with cloves to add aroma to stocks and stews. Germans are fond of adding cloves to pot roast and other long-cooking meat and game dishes. The British put cloves in Christmas pudding and apple tart.

Clove is a key ingredient in mulled wine, and an element of many other alcoholic beverages. Germans use cloves to spike popular fire-tongue punch (*Feuerzangenbowle*), which is made with wine, hot rum, citrus juices, and sugar. The French add cloves to a home-brewed orange liqueur made with coffee beans and vodka. Similar versions are also made in Italy and Spain. Clove is also used in some sweet vermouths.

But for all their culinary popularity, the largest share of the world's cloves goes into producing the popular Indonesian cigarette called *kretek*. The cigarettes contain 40 percent clove, which give the cigarettes a crackling sound as they are smoked.

How to Buy Clove

Clove comes from the Latin word *clavus*, meaning nail—because cloves resemble nails. A clove is the still-closed bud from an evergreen that flowers twice a year. Growing and harvesting cloves is tricky, because they have to be picked by hand at precisely the right time.

Cloves are native to the Malukus ("spice islands") of Indonesia, but the best cloves don't come from there. Among clove aficionados, *penang* cloves from Malaysia are considered the best, followed by cloves from Zanzibar and Madagascar. The majority of the cloves imported into the United States come from Madagascar or Brazil.

The only way to buy cloves by their place of origin is from a specialty spice shop or online. The "Buyer's Guide" on page 309 has a list of recommended dealers.

However, it's not necessary to go out of your way to buy exotic cloves. For culinary flavor, what's most important is keeping cloves as fresh as possible. That means buying them whole and grinding them yourself. Once ground, they start to lose their volatile oil, which weakens their aroma.

When buying, look for cloves that are *large*—meaning you can clearly make out the head and stems. (Penang cloves are the largest.) In fact, you should be able to recognize the four would-be petals of the bud, and the stamen inside them, forming the nail-like head. You don't want to buy cloves that look like little bits of sticks; those are just stems. The color should be reddish-brown.

Whole cloves will keep for a year or more in an airtight container away from light and heat.

In the Kitchen with Clove

Cloves have a distinctive aroma—pungent and somewhat woodsy—and a sweet and musty taste. They will mellow somewhat from cooking, but they can definitely overpower a dish.

The food writer Tom Stobart, author of *Cook's Encyclopedia*, advises, "As a flavoring, cloves are best when kept below the level of recognition." Keep this in mind when using cloves. It takes only a *few* cloves to add aroma to a pot of savory stew, or a *few* ground cloves to flavor a pastry.

When adding whole cloves to a savory dish they should be removed before serving, as unknowingly biting into a whole clove can spoil the taste, not to mention chip a tooth. One way to avoid inadvertent clove-crunching is to stud a small onion with cloves and add it to the broth. When the dish is finished, retrieve the onion and throw it out.

COCOA   *How Sweet It Is!*

When the news first hit more than a decade ago, it seemed too good to be true: chocolate, the confection synonymous with culinary decadence, was actually *good* for you.

One by one, studies started appearing in medical journals—studies so richly provocative they made headlines worldwide. "Chocolate a Health Food?" pondered *The New York Times* in 2000. "Chocolate Is Good for You," announced London's *Sunday Mirror* in 2003. "Chocolate—The Sixth Major Food Group," declared a Washington D.C. weekly in 2008. A year later, a candy industry professional journal wrote a cover story about chocolate bars flying off the shelves all over America. Indeed, the headlines about chocolate as "the new health food" stirred the hearts and minds (and taste buds) of many Americans.

Don't take these headlines too literally, however. It isn't chocolate, per se, that is good for you. It's *cocoa*, the spicy powder that makes chocolate taste like, well, chocolate. *All* the healthful goodness in a chocolate bar is concentrated in the cocoa. Truth is, a piece of chocolate is only as healthy as its cocoa content.

Cocoa—the *spice*—is one of the richest source of *flavanols*, plant compounds that help protect the heart in a variety of ways. Study after study shows that cocoa flavanols can disarm cell-damaging free radicals, preserve cell membranes, protect DNA, prevent the formation of artery-clogging plaque, improve blood flow to the heart, lower high blood pressure, and prevent blood clots that can cause a heart attack or stroke.

The Cocoa-Loving Kuna

We'd still be eating chocolate with a chaser of guilt if it weren't for the Kuna Indians living on the remote San Blas Island off the coast of Panama. Back in 1997, researchers from Brigham and Women's Hospital in Boston (part of Harvard Medical School) were the first to observe that high blood pressure is almost unheard of on San Blas, where cacao trees grow wild and cocoa, which comes from the fruit of the tree, is a staple in the diet. It is common for a

65-year-old (and older) Kuna to have the blood pressure of a 20- or 30-year-old! And it's not due to hypertension-proof genes, because Kunas who move to mainland Panama and adopt the typical Panamanian diet develop the same high blood pressure and heart disease rates that plague the rest of the country.

The reason? Kunas eat a lot of cocoa—so much, in fact, that they have the highest intake of flavanols in the world. The typical Kuna drinks four or five cups of cocoa as a beverage a day! And that doesn't count the cocoa added to food. Researchers believe their cocoa-rich diet also contributes to another phenomenal fact about their health: death rates from heart disease, stroke, diabetes, and cancer on San Blas Island are remarkably lower than in mainland Panama. And most of the world.

That fact surfaced when researchers from Harvard Medical School returned to San Blas Island just a few years ago to compare the causes of death among lifelong residents who had died in the previous few years to those who died in mainland Panama. Compared to the San Blas residents, death rates in Panamanians were six times higher from heart attack, 17 times higher from stroke, and 18 times higher from cancer. In fact, a person living on San Blas Island is more likely to die of malaria, tuberculosis, or the flu than any of the top six leading causes of death in industrialized nations! And much of the credit goes to cocoa.

Why Your Arteries Adore Cocoa

Cocoa's abundance of flavanols protects the *epithelial cells* that line the arteries. These cells produce *nitric oxide*, a compound that is key to the care and feeding of your arteries. Nitric oxide relaxes and widens blood vessels, increasing blood flow and lowering blood pressure. It prevents blood components called *platelets* from becoming sticky, thereby helping prevent the blood clots that cause most heart attacks and strokes.

It stops the smooth muscle cells of the arteries from sprouting plaques. It even helps diminish plaque once it's in place.

And nitric oxide isn't only important for the heart. It also helps regulate the hormone insulin, which ushers blood sugar into cells. Balanced insulin levels are a must for preventing type 2 diabetes. (Prediabetes—blood sugar levels above the normal range but not yet high enough for a diagnosis of diabetes—is also called *insulin resistance*.) Nitric oxide also helps slay cancer cells before they anchor to your body.

High levels of nitric oxide improve your odds for living a long life. High levels of cocoa boost nitric oxide.

Heart-Shaped Healing

Dozens of studies show that people who consume flavanol-rich cocoa—as a powder mixed in water, or eaten in dark chocolate (defined in most studies as 74 percent cocoa)—are in much better cardiovascular shape than those who don't. Here's a representative sampling of the nearly 200 studies on cocoa and cardiovascular disease that have been conducted in the last decade or so:

Lower cholesterol. Japanese researchers gave drinks with either flavanol-rich or flavanol-poor cocoa to 160 people—and those drinking the flavanol-rich cocoa had substantial decreases in "bad" LDL cholesterol and increases in "good" HDL cholesterol.

Reduced LDL oxidation. Artery-choking plaque only happens when LDL cholesterol oxidizes, forming the goo that sticks to artery walls. Researchers at Pennsylvania State University found that adding dark chocolate to the "average American diet" decreased LDL oxidation by 8 percent.

Lower blood pressure. German researchers analyzed 10 studies on flavanol-rich cocoa and high blood pressure, involving nearly 300 people—and found that regular consumption had the power to lower high blood pressure an average of 4.5 mm Hg systolic (the upper reading) and 2.5 mm Hg diastolic (the lower reading).

Better circulation. Researchers in Japan studied 39 healthy men, dividing them into two groups—one ate flavanol-rich dark chocolate and the other ate no-flavanol white chocolate. After two weeks, the men eating dark chocolate had a 22 percent boost in a measurement of blood flow through the arteries. "Dark chocolate intake significantly improved coronary circulation in healthy adults," wrote the researchers in the *International Journal of Cardiology*.

Thinner blood. Doctors at the Center for Thrombosis Research at Johns Hopkins University fed dark chocolate to 28 healthy people for seven days, measuring their level of platelet activity—the tendency of the blood to form artery-blocking clots. Platelet activity fell by 27 percent. (Those eating dark chocolate also had a 6 percent drop in LDL and a 9 percent increase in HDL.)

Increased nitric oxide. German researchers gave small amounts of dark chocolate to 44 men and women, aged 56 to 73. They had a "sustained increase" in a biomarker of nitric oxide levels. And after 18 weeks, the percentage of those in the study with high blood pressure fell from 86 percent to 68 percent.

More flexible arteries. Heart disease used to be called "hardening of the arteries"—stiff arteries are sick arteries. Researchers in Greece studied nearly 200 people and found that higher cocoa intake was linked to "low arterial stiffness." They reported their results in the *American Journal of Cardiology*.

Lower C-reactive protein (CRP). This biomarker of inflammation has been linked to heart disease. When Italian researchers analyzed a year of dietary and health data from nearly 5,000 people, they found that those who regularly ate dark chocolate had lower levels of CRP. "Regular consumption of small doses of dark chocolate may reduce inflammation," they wrote in the *Journal of Nutrition*.

Lower risk of heart disease. All those heart-healthy benefits add up to a very positive result. When researchers in the Netherlands analyzed 15 years of diet and health data in 470 people, age 65 and older, they found that those with diets richest in cocoa were *half* as likely to die from cardiovascular disease, compared to people who consumed little or no cocoa.

And when researchers at the Harvard School of Public Health analyzed 136 studies on flavanols and cardiovascular disease, they found those with the highest intake of flavonols from chocolate had a 19 percent lower risk of coronary heart disease, compared to those with the lowest intake.

Survival after a heart attack. Chocolate is protective even *after* a heart attack. When Swedish researchers looked at eight years of dietary data from participants in the Stockholm Heart Epidemiology Program, they spotted an amazing pattern—of the 1,169 people in the study who had suffered a heart attack, those who had eaten chocolate at least twice a week *before* the attack were 27 percent less likely to die in the eight years afterwards, compared to those who never ate chocolate. "In contrast," they note, "intake of other sweets was not associated with cardiac mortality."

Lower risk of stroke. Canadian researchers analyzed several studies and found that those who ate chocolate once a week were 22 percent less likely to have a stroke than people who didn't eat chocolate, and that regular chocolate-eating also lowered the risk of death after a stroke by 46 percent.

Chocolate Goes to Your Head

Blood flow isn't only crucial for the heart. It's also a must for a healthy *brain*.

Nourishing your gray matter. Sixteen healthy people downed a flavanol-rich cocoa drink and then performed a mental task—while researchers watched the activity inside their brains, using functional magnetic resonance imaging (fMRI). And those researchers saw a big boost in blood flow. "Flavanol-rich cocoa can increase the cerebral flood flow to gray matter, suggesting the potential of cocoa flavanols for treatment of . . . dementia and strokes," concluded the researchers in the *Journal of Cardiovascular Pharmacology*.

"The prospect of increasing cerebral perfusion [blood flow to the brain] with cocoa flavanols is extremely promising," said researchers from Harvard Medical School, in another scientific paper in the same issue of the journal.

More mental energy. When 30 people drank cocoa flavanols before taking six 10-minute mental tests over an hour, they performed better on some of the tests and had less mental fatigue.

Smarter seniors. Researchers in Norway gave several standardized tests for mental ability and memory to more than 2,000 people, aged 70 to 74, who were participants in a long-running health study tracking their diets. Those who had the highest dietary intake of chocolate performed best on the tests.

More Cocoa Cures

Is cocoa good for what ails you—no matter what ails you? Plenty of people would say yes—without any scientific evidence whatsoever! They might not be far from the truth.

Diabetes. When healthy people ate an ounce of flavanol-rich dark chocolate every day for a week they had improved "insulin sensitivity"— the ability of cells to respond to the hormone that controls blood sugar. As mentioned earlier, *insulin resistance* is one of the first signs that type 2 diabetes is developing.

Wrinkles. *Photoaging* is the scientific name for wrinkles, age spots, and other skin damage from a lifetime of exposure to the sun's ultraviolet (UV) rays. In a study of 30 people, eating high-flavanol chocolate for three months more than *doubled* their skin's resistance to UV-caused damage. "Our study demonstrates that regular consumption of a chocolate rich in flavanols confers significant photoprotection and can thus be effective at protecting human skin from harmful UV effects," concluded the researchers in the *Journal of Cosmetic Dermatology*. "Conventional chocolate has no such effect."

Softer skin. In another study on cocoa and skin, women who consumed a high-flavanol cocoa powder drink for three months had less skin roughness and scaling, compared to women who consumed a low-flavanol cocoa powder drink.

Preeclampsia. This condition of high blood pressure during pregnancy strikes 5 percent of pregnant women and can threaten the life of both mother and baby. Researchers from Yale University studied nearly 3,000 pregnant women and found that those who routinely ate chocolate had a lower risk of developing preeclampsia than those who never ate chocolate—19 percent lower in the first trimester of pregnancy, and 40 percent lower in the third trimester.

Endurance. Nine top cyclists were asked to cycle to exhaustion on a stationary bike—but those who drank chocolate milk before starting were able to cycle up to 51 percent longer than those who drank other types of sports drinks.

With Chocolate, You Want to Be in the Dark

Want to protect your heart, nourish your brain, balance your blood sugar, and brighten your skin? Then *don't* eat chocolate. Milk chocolate or white chocolate, that is. Remember, health benefits from chocolate are from the flavanols in cocoa— and flavanol-rich cocoa powder or dark chocolate (the type that contains at *least* 60 percent cocoa, and ideally no less than 74 percent) is the only way to get those flavanols into your body.

Researchers from Pennsylvania State University proved this when they measured the amount of flavanols in the blood of two groups of chocolate lovers: one eating 3½ ounces of dark chocolate a day and one eating the same amount of milk chocolate. After two weeks of chocolate-eating, the blood levels of flavanols in people eating dark chocolate shot up by 20 percent, but stayed the same in those eating milk chocolate.

The milk in milk chocolate might even foil flavanols. That's the finding of researchers in Italy and Scotland, who discovered that when milk is added to make smoother, creamier chocolate, it binds with flavanols, interfering with their absorption. When the researchers had people wash down dark chocolate with a glass of milk, blood levels of flavanols *didn't* go up.

Cocoa, on the other hand, gives you concentrated flavanols—without the fat and calories found in a chocolate bar. One ounce (one serving) of Dove dark chocolate, for example, contains 155 calories, 9 grams of fat, and 185 mg of flavanols. One tablespoon of Mars Cocoapro cocoa powder—used in many of the research studies—has about 20 calories, less than 1 gram of fat, and approximately 1.8 grams of flavanols. Just like other spices, cocoa itself has virtually no impact on your daily calorie count, but can make your levels of health-protecting nutrients soar.

In other words, you *can* consume cocoa without gaining weight! In a study conducted by researchers at the Yale University School of Medicine, 44 overweight people drank a cocoa beverage, with or without sugar, for six weeks—and didn't gain weight. "Our study suggests that healthy overweight adults can make cocoa ingestion part of their daily diet routine without adverse effects on body weight," concluded the researchers in the *International Journal of Cardiology*.

Getting to Know Cocoa

Throughout this book, you'll find condensed histories of spices that feature the ancient civilizations of Egypt, Greece, Rome, India, and China. But the Mayans, Aztecs, and other ancient peoples of Mexico and Central and South America also had thriving civilizations—and the spice they revered was *cacao*.

The Aztecs called it "the food of the gods," honoring their deities with a ceremonial drink called *tchacahoua*. Concocting the drink was an elaborate ritual—seeds were extracted from cacao pods, roasted, and reduced to powder with giant stones; the powder was added to boiling water, along with honey, ground maize, annatto, and red chiles; the mixture was slowly stirred over a fire until it became a frothy blend. The Aztec leader Montezuma is said to have drank

50 cups of *tchacahoua* out of a golden goblet on one occasion.

Chocolate was imported to Europe by the Spanish in the 15th century (where it was reserved for royalty and aristocrats). By the 17th century, cocoa houses were opening in England—where chocolate was available to anybody who could pay for it.

The British Royal Navy brewed a cocoa drink called *kye* to keep sailors awake on night watch. Making the brew was considered an art that required an apprenticeship to perfect. Kye was considered potent enough to drink when it was thick enough to hold a spoon standing straight up.

Some of the first European imbibers of cocoa praised its healthful properties, with one text claiming it "comforted the liver, aided in digestion, and made one happy and strong," according to the book *The True History of Chocolate*. (The same text also presciently said cocoa healed "heart pain.")

Europeans also adopted the spice into their cuisines. An old Sicilian lasagna recipe, for example, includes crumbled unsweetened chocolate in the meat sauce. Spanish cooks braise rabbit and squab in wine and chocolate. The Spanish also combine powdered chocolate, milk, and butter and pour it over steamed lobster.

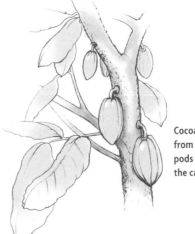

Cocoa is derived from beans in fruit pods produced by the cacao tree.

Needless to say, cocoa is still immensely popular in the Americas. Cocoa with cinnamon is one of the most popular beverages in Mexico, where many drink it daily. Cocoa is added to fish soups, corn chowders, spicy sauce bases called *sofritos*, and spice blends called *recados*. It is also a key ingredient in *mole*, a popular hot sauce. (One of the most complex of those sauces is *mole negro*, from Oaxaca, Mexico, which includes more than 20 ingredients and takes hours to make.)

In America, cocoa is best known for its presence in innumerable sweet treats. (But the secret to many of the chili recipes that win awards in the contests conducted each year in towns throughout the US is a dash—or more—of cocoa powder.)

How to Buy Cocoa

The cacao tree—small trees that sprout large fruit pods containing cocoa beans—are indigenous to Mexico and Central and South America, but are now cultivated in West Africa, Sri Lanka, Java, and Malaysia.

Unprocessed, cocoa beans are extremely bitter and virtually inedible. To turn them into chocolate, the beans are fermented, dried, and roasted. Then the shells are removed, revealing the *nibs*, which are again ground and liquefied, resulting in chocolate liquor. That liquor is further refined into either cocoa solids or cocoa butter; the latter is the ingredient found in most chocolate confections.

Chocolate gets its strong astringent flavor from the flavanols in the cocoa. The higher the percentage of cocoa in a chocolate product, the higher the level of flavanols and the stronger the flavor.

But those healthy flavanols in chocolate get diluted as sugar and milk are added. *Dark* chocolate is chocolate in its purest and healthiest form. The most healthful dark chocolates contain 74 percent or more cocoa solids. If you're interested in a healthier heart, don't buy anything under 60 percent cocoa.

Many European (and some US) brands of

Cocoa may help prevent and/or treat:

Alzheimer's disease	High blood pressure (hypertension)
Cholesterol problems (high "bad" LDL cholesterol, low "good" HDL cholesterol)	Insulin resistance (prediabetes)
	Memory loss (age-related, mild cognitive decline)
Dementia (non-Alzeheimer's)	
Diabetes, type 2	Preeclampsia
Fatigue, mental and physical	Stroke
	Wrinkles and aging skin
Heart disease	

Cocoa pairs well with these spices:

Allspice	Curry leaf	Mint
Almond	Fennel seed	Nutmeg
Aniseed	Garlic	Onion
Cinnamon	Ginger	Vanilla
Clove	Lemongrass	

and complements recipes featuring:

Carrots	Oranges
Cheese	Sauces for desserts
Fish	Savory sauces
Ground beef	Sweet potatoes
Nuts	

Other recipes containing cocoa:

All-American Chili con Carne (p. 110)	Cocoa Rub (p. 270)

cocoa undergo a process called *dutching* to give the cocoa a milder flavor. However, the process also reduces flavanols. Dutched cocoa runs in shades from light brown to dark brown to almost black. The darker the color, the milder

Los Banos Low-Fat Brownies

This traditional brownie recipe cuts saturated fat by substituting monounsaturated canola oil for butter and cocoa for chocolate squares. The spices help enrich their delicate flavor.

1 cup white flour
1 teaspoon baking powder
Pinch sea salt
1 cup sugar
2 large eggs, room temperature
⅔ cup canola oil
½ cup unsweetened cocoa powder
¼ cup crystallized ginger, diced
1 teaspoon amchur (optional)
½ teaspoon ground cardamom
1 teaspoon vanilla extract
¼ cup toasted almonds, chopped

1. Preheat the oven to 350°F. Spray an 8"×8" baking pan with non-stick spray.
2. Mix the flour, baking powder, and salt in a small bowl. Beat sugar into the eggs in a large bowl. Stir the oil, cocoa powder, ginger, amchur, cardamom, and vanilla into the egg mixture. Add the dry ingredients all at once and mix well. Add the almonds and blend.
3. Scrape mixture into the pan and bake 20 minutes or until a toothpick comes out nearly clean. Let cool to warm or room temperature before serving.

Makes about 16 brownies.

the flavor—and the less flavanol in the product.

The rule of thumb for buying and using cocoa: the higher the percent of cocoa, the richer the chocolate flavor.

In the Kitchen with Cocoa

Raw cocoa is astringent and strong, but it takes on a subtly sweet flavor during cooking, and melds nicely with other spices in savory dishes. In Italy and Spain, cooks add a little unsweetened cocoa to the garlic-and-onion base for fish and meat dishes.

You can get more flavanols and save on calories and fat by substituting unsweetened cocoa for chocolate in most any recipe. For every 1-ounce chocolate square, substitute 4 tablespoons unsweetened cocoa powder.

Food scientists used to think that most of the flavanols were lost during the baking process. However, recent testing found that using baking powder in recipes retains all the flavanols, though using baking soda results in some losses. Because baking soda is needed for cakes to rise, substituting baking powder for half the soda will result in a high cake and also retain almost

all the flavanols, according to the study in the *Journal of Food Science*.

Here are easy ways to get more cocoa into your diet:

- Cocoa goes well with naturally sweet vegetables, such as carrots and sweet potatoes. Add a teaspoon of unsweetened cocoa powder when making glazes for these vegetables.
- Add a tablespoon of unsweetened cocoa powder to chili con carne.
- Make a healthy Mexican hot chocolate by adding 1½ tablespoons of unsweetened cocoa powder, 1 tablespoon sugar, ½ teaspoon vanilla extract, ¼ teaspoon ground cinnamon, and a pinch of cloves to 8 ounces of hot water.
- Make a low-fat chocolate glaze for cupcakes by combining ½ cup of unsweetened cocoa powder with 1 cup of granulated sugar and ½ cup of water in a saucepan, and stirring until it spins. Remove from the heat, stir in 1 tablespoon of butter until smooth and thick.

COCONUT   *The Fat that Burns Calories*

Several things go by the name "coconut"—the tree, the fruit, the candy. And the spice.

Coconut *spice* is the dried shredded meat from the fruit of the majestic palm tree that grows in subtropical and tropical regions around the world. Though people in these regions use coconut to spice savory foods, we mostly identify coconut with yummy sweets (and all the calories they deliver)—a dietary habit that may have led to the common perception that coconut is bad for you.

True, coconut contains a *lot* of fat. Coconut is 82 percent fat, 76 percent of which is saturated, the type we're told to minimize because it clogs arteries. But here's the surprise: the saturated fat is what makes coconut a super-spice! Because the saturated fat in coconut *isn't* the same as the saturated fat in meat and milk.

The saturated fat in coconut is what's called a *medium-chain triglyceride* (MCT). To understand why that's important, let's take a closer look at fat.

Put a tiny drop of fat under a powerful microscope that displays atoms and molecules, and you'll see *triglycerides*—three (tri) fatty acids hooked up to a molecule of glycerol. Those fatty acids form chains, linked together by carbon atoms. Some chains are short, with four to six carbon atoms. Some chains are long, with 24. And some chains are medium-sized, with 8 to 12.

Ninety percent of fats—like those in meat and milk—are long-chain fatty acids (LCT). To process them, the body hooks them up with transport molecules in the bloodstream called *chylomicrons* and sends them off to fat cells.

But MCT isn't digested that way. The body shunts MCT directly from the stomach to the liver, where it's metabolized in a flash. And that super-rapid metabolic action actually *burns more calories* than the fat contains. Studies show that people who get lots of dietary MCT burn an average of *100 extra calories a day*, compared to folks who don't eat an MCT-rich diet. And coconut contains more MCT than any other food.

Yes, you heard right: the fat in coconut can *help* you burn calories, so that you maintain or lose weight. Sound too good to be true? Scientists don't think so.

The Belly-Friendly Fat

Canadian researchers asked 12 healthy women to eat one of two strange diets for two weeks. Both diets contained 15 percent protein, 45 percent carbohydrates, and 40 percent fat—normal enough. But half the women ate 80 percent of their daily fat from beef tallow, while the other half ate their fat from a combination of butter and coconut oil. In other words, both groups ate plenty of LCT-containing saturated fat, but only one group also ate saturated fats with MCT.

After two weeks, those eating MCT were burning up about 45 percent more LCT!

No one lost (or gained) weight—the study wasn't designed as a weight-loss experiment. It was designed to prove the hypothesis that MCT are potent fat-burners—and it proved just that.

"The capacity of MCT" to increase fat-burning of long-chain saturated fatty acids "suggests a role for MCT in body weight control over the long term," concluded the researchers in the *International Journal of Obesity and Related Metabolic Disorders*.

And in a study in the journal *Lipids*, Brazilian researchers studied 40 women, dividing them into two groups—one group took supplements of soy oil, while the other group took coconut oil. After three months, both groups lost a little weight. But only those taking the coconut oil had much trimmer tummies. (Abdominal fat isn't only unsightly. The fat around your gut has the bad habit of pumping out inflammatory compounds that increase the risk for heart disease and stroke.) Coconut, concluded the researchers, may "promote a reduction in abdominal obesity."

Importantly, the researchers found the coconut oil *didn't* increase heart-hurting LDL cholesterol, and *did* increase heart-helping HDL cholesterol.

Coconut & Co.—
In the Business of Better Health

Helping you stay slim isn't the only health-promoting power of coconut.

Antibacterial. Coconut milk contains the MCT lauric acid, which the body breaks down into *monolaurin*. In a study by Philippine researchers, monolaurin killed off several types of disease-causing bacteria, including *Staphylococcus aureus*, *Streptococcus*, *Enterobacter*, and *Enterococcus*.

Monolaurin "might prove useful in the prevention and treatment of severe bacterial infections, especially those that are difficult to treat and/or are antibacterial resistant," said a team of researchers from Georgetown University Medical Center, who also studied the compound.

Acne. Researchers at the University of California, San Diego found that a compound containing lauric acid was uniquely effective in killing the bacteria that cause acne. The compound has "great potential of becoming a safe and effective therapeutic medication for acne," they concluded.

Antifungal. Researchers in Iceland found that lauric acid and capric acid (another MCT in coconut) killed *Candida albicans*, the fungus that causes yeast infection.

Colon cancer. Coconut is rich in *catechins*, cancer-fighting antioxidants. In an Indian study, the addition of coconut to the diet of laboratory animals "markedly reduced" the development of chemically induced colon cancer.

Alzheimer's. An international team of researchers induced menopause in laboratory animals and then divided them into four groups, feeding one group coconut water. After five weeks, they found the coconut-fed animals had

higher blood levels of estrogen *and* less destruction of brain cells—showing that coconut water has "estrogen-like characteristics" and may play a role in preventing Alzheimer's and other types of dementia after menopause.

Crohn's disease (inflammatory bowel disease). Researchers in Spain used coconut oil to reduce the rate of chemically induced Crohn's disease in experimental animals. The oil worked by reducing inflammation. There may be a "primary therapeutic effect of MCT in human Crohn's disease," they wrote in the *Journal of Nutrition*.

Pain relief. A tea popular in northeast Brazil made from coconut husk fibers is popularly used to "treat several inflammatory disorders," said Brazilian researchers. When they tested the tea in the laboratory on experimental animals, they found it not only reduced inflammation—it also relieved pain in the same way as morphine. The study "confirms" the use of the tea for reducing inflammation, said the researchers in the *Journal of Ethnopharmacology*.

Getting to Know Coconut

It's not surprising that the coconut palm is called the "tree of life." A typical tree produces anywhere

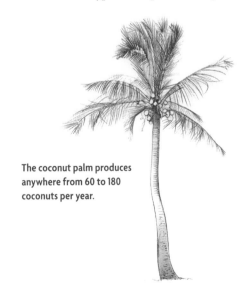

The coconut palm produces anywhere from 60 to 180 coconuts per year.

from 60 to 180 coconuts a year—the dietary mainstay for millions of people in South and Southeast Asia, the South Pacific, and the Caribbean, where the equivalent of a coconut a day is eaten as coconut water, milk, oil, and spice.

Coconut water is the juice found inside young (but not mature) coconuts. It's a popular drink throughout the tropics—in Brazil, for example, it's second only to orange juice.

Coconut milk is made by pouring hot water or coconut water over shredded coconut and squeezing it to extract the milk. It's sweet and milky-white, with an almond-like flavor. It's widely used as a spicy flavoring in cooking throughout Southeast Asia, South India, Indonesia, South America, the Pacific Islands, and the Caribbean.

Coconut milk gives distinctive flavor to *saté lalot*, grilled meatballs popular on the Indonesian island of Madure, near Java. It's widely used in *Bahian* cooking, a Cajun-like cuisine of Brazil, and is in the base of the much-beloved Bahian peanut sauce, which also features garlic, tomato, and cilantro.

In Sri Lanka, coconut milk is used with toasted spices to mellow and give body to hot curries. Coconut milk is also used in *hoppers*, steamed fermented breads made with rice flour and served for breakfast.

Coconut cream—a thicker, more paste-like version of coconut milk—is used in many dishes in Kerala, an area of South India known for its wonderful fish curries.

Coconut spice (dry, grated) is an essential ingredient in curries and vegetables in Indonesia and Malaysia, along with coconut milk. The spice is also used in the beef dish called *rendang*. And it's used to make rice pudding and *dadar*, pancakes with a sweet coconut filling.

Fish and seafood cooked with rice and shredded dried coconut form the daily diet of people living along India's tropical Malabar Coast. Dried coconut is used extensively in South Indian cooking, especially curries. (South India is famous for its coconut chutney.)

Coconut may help prevent and/or treat:

Acne	Infection, bacterial
Alzheimer's disease	Overweight
Cancer	Pain
Crohn's disease (inflammatory bowel disease)	Vaginal yeast infection

Coconut pairs well with these spices:

Allspice	Galangal
Asafoetida	Garlic
Basil	Ginger
Black pepper	Lemongrass
Cocoa	Sun-dried tomato
Cumin	Turmeric
Curry leaf	Vanilla

and complements recipes featuring:

Beef	Curries	Potatoes
Chicken	Fish and seafood	Vegetables
Chocolate		
Chutney	Lentils	

Other recipes containing coconut:

Black Mango Chutney (p. 51)	Mussels with Thai Red Curry Sauce (p. 156)
Madras Beef Curry (p. 106)	Thai Coconut Chicken Soup (p. 126)

Vegetarian dishes generally feature toasted desiccated coconut.

Coconut oil is the most popular frying medium in South Indian cuisine.

How to Buy Coconut

Aside from Floridians and Hawaiians, most of us only encounter fresh coconuts and taste

Coconut Meatballs with Peanut Sauce

These meatballs are based on sate lalat, *a dish that is popular on the Indonesian island of Java. (However, the dish originated on the island of Madura, off the coast of Java.) It makes a nice hors d'oeuvre. The peanut sauce gives the meatballs a tropical flavor, but they are moist enough to serve without it.*

Peanut sauce:
1 cup unsweetened coconut milk
½ cup creamy peanut butter
1½ tablespoons brown sugar
1 tablespoon Asian fish sauce
1 tablespoon soy sauce
1 tablespoon Thai curry paste (optional)
½ teaspoon *Madras Curry Powder* (p. 284) or
**   commercial curry powder**
½ cup warm water
Meatballs:
1 pound 90 percent lean ground beef
1 cup dried or fresh (sweetened or unsweetened)
**   shredded coconut**
2 tablespoons minced fresh ginger
2 tablespoons black vinegar or 1 tablespoon
**   balsamic vinegar**
1 teaspoon turmeric
1 teaspoon ground allspice
1 teaspoon ground cumin
2 tablespoons extra-virgin coconut oil or olive oil
2 teaspoons fresh lime juice
½ teaspoon freshly ground black pepper
Salt to taste

1. *To make the peanut sauce:* Combine the coconut milk, peanut butter, brown sugar, fish sauce, soy sauce, curry paste (if using), and curry powder in a medium saucepan over low heat. Stir with a wooden spoon until smooth.

2. Gradually whisk in the warm water and simmer, stirring occasionally, for 15 minutes. Set aside to cool. Serve room temperature.

3. *To make the meatballs:* Combine the beef, coconut, ginger, vinegar, turmeric, allspice, cumin, one tablespoon of the oil, the lime juice, pepper, and salt in a large bowl. Form into one-inch meatballs. Keep your hands moistened with water to roll the balls.

4. Heat the remaining oil in a large skillet over medium-high heat and fry the meatballs, turning frequently, until lightly browned and cooked through, about 10 minutes.

Makes about 30 meatballs and 2 cups of sauce.

coconut water on a trip to the tropics. But fresh and dried shredded coconut is readily available in most supermarkets, and is sold desiccated, toasted, sweetened, and unsweetened. It's available in three grades: fine, medium, and coarse. (The grading reflects texture, not quality.) Look for it in the baking section.

You'll find the largest selection of shredded coconut in Asian and Indian markets. You can also purchase it online.

Coconut milk can be found sweetened or unsweetened in a can, or as a concentrated paste that must be reconstituted. Look for it in the Asian section of most well-stocked supermarkets, or in Asian and Indian markets. Once the can is open, you can freeze any unused portion. Coconut milk freezes well and will keep for several months.

In the US, coconut oil is rarely used in cooking—because it's unfamiliar, and out of concern for its high level of saturated fat. As news of the fat-burning powers of MCT spread, coconut oil may become a "functional food" like olive oil—widely understood to taste good *and* do your health good. For cooking, virgin coconut oil is considered superior to regular oil.

In the Kitchen with Coconut

A lot of Americans know coconut best as *Coco Lopez*, the thick, canned mix of sugar cane and coconut cream that is the basis of the tropical rum drink piña colada. Cooks are familiar with coconut as an ingredient in cakes, candy, and other confections.

Throughout the coconut-growing nations of the world, coconut is used more in savory dishes. (Americans are perhaps most familiar with the savory use of coconut in the popular appetizer coconut shrimp, which is deep fried in hot oil.) Don't hesitate to give coconut a try—it complements almost any kind of food, especially red meat, poultry, and fish.

Other than making cookies and cake, here are some ideas to extend your use of coconut in the kitchen:

- Sprinkle toasted coconut on curries at the end of cooking or add shredded coconut to meat, fish stews, and curries.
- Sprinkle coconut over hot chocolate. Better yet, make hot cocoa with coconut milk instead of cow's milk. Add a cinnamon stick for stirring.

CORIANDER *Taming Tummy Troubles*

First, let's define terms.

The strongly-scented leaves of the coriander plant are *cilantro*. They're not a spice, they're an herb. And they're not uniquely healthful.

The sweet, nutty seeds of the coriander plant are the spice coriander. And they're really good for you.

Coriander is one of the world's oldest spices—seeds were found in a Neolithic archeological dig dated around 7000 BCE. They were also in Tutankhamen's tomb. Coriander is mentioned in Exodus (the Bible, not the movie) and was used as a spice in ancient Greece.

In ancient Asia, practitioners of Chinese medicine used the seeds to treat all varieties of digestive ills. (It's still an ingredient in over-the-counter preparations for relieving gas and constipation.) The Ayurvedic physicians of India used it for many purposes, including as a diuretic. A quick tour through the annals of planetary folk medicine shows it's been used for a variety of other health problems, including bladder and urinary tract infections, allergies, diabetes, anxiety, high blood pressure, insomnia, and vertigo. Today, scientists are discovering *why* it's an effective healer.

Coriander is 85 percent volatile oils, containing at least 26 of these energetic compounds. Two of those oils—*linalool* and *geranyl acetate*—are powerful, cell-protecting antioxidants, and are probably behind many of coriander's curative powers. Such as its ability to soothe digestive ailments.

Ending Digestive Woes

Coriander is a classic remedy for tummy troubles.

Soothing irritable bowel syndrome. Gastroenterologists studied 32 people with irritable bowel syndrome (IBS), a chronic digestive complaint that afflicts 10 to 20 percent of Americans, two-thirds of them women. The symptoms of IBS include abdominal pain, cramping, and bloating, along with diarrhea and constipation (usually one or the other, but sometimes both, alternating). They divided them into two groups: one received Carmint, a preparation that contains coriander; the other received a placebo. After eight weeks, those taking Carmint had three times more improvement in abdominal pain and discomfort than the placebo group. The findings were published in *Digestive Diseases and Sciences*.

Easing chronic constipation. In another study on digestive ills, 86 residents at a nursing home in Pennsylvania were given either a coriander-containing laxative tea (Smooth Move) or a placebo tea. Over the next month, those drinking Smooth Move had more bowel movements.

Stopping intestinal spasms. "Coriander is traditionally used for various digestive disorders," observed a team of scientists from Pakistan and Morocco in the *Journal of Ethnopharmacology*. In an experiment with laboratory animals, they found the spice works like an antispasmodic drug, relaxing the contracted digestive muscles that cause the discomfort of IBS and other "overactive gut disorders." (That same relaxing effect—working on arteries—may be one reason why the spice can help lower blood pressure, they noted.) They also found the spice delayed the movement of food from the stomach—a possible explanation for why it's effective in easing indigestion and gas.

More proof. Researchers in Saudi Arabia also found that coriander protected animals against laboratory-induced stomach ulcers, confirming "the traditional use" of coriander for stomach problems. It's probably the powerful antioxidants in coriander that protect the stomach lining, they theorized.

Commission E agrees. It's no surprise that the German Commission E—which helps guide physicians and other health professionals in Germany in the medical use of natural remedies—declared that coriander is safe and effective for the treatment of digestive complaints, loss of appetite, bloating, flatulence, and cramplike stomach upsets.

Coriander's Curative Cornucopia

Coriander passes the gut check. But its soothing powers don't stop there.

Reducing the redness in inflammatory skin diseases (eczema, psoriasis, rosacea). Dutch researchers asked 40 volunteers to expose small patches on their backs to intense UV radiation— the same type of radiation from the sun that causes sunburns, wrinkling, and skin cancer. After the exposure, the researchers applied coriander oil—and it significantly reduced redness. Coriander "could be useful in the . . . treatment of inflammatory skin diseases" such as

eczema, psoriasis, and rosacea, concluded the researchers.

Diabetes. Coriander is a traditional remedy for "indigestion, diabetes, rheumatism, and pain in the joints," noted a team of researchers in *Phytotherapy Research*. Testing an extract of the spice on animals with laboratory-induced type 2 diabetes, they found it decreased blood sugar levels and increased insulin (the hormone that controls blood sugar).

Decreasing "bad" LDL, increasing "good" HDL. "Coriander has been documented as a traditional treatment for cholesterol," said a team of researchers in India in the *Journal of Environmental Biology*. In their study, animals given coriander had a decrease in "bad" LDL cholesterol and an increase in "good" LDL cholesterol—that type of change would dramatically lower the risk of heart disease in people.

In another study on blood fats, coriander's cholesterol-lowering powers led researchers to conclude, "Coriander has the potential to be popularized as a household remedy with preventive and curative effect against" high cholesterol.

Coriander may help prevent and/or treat:

Bloating	High blood pressure (hypertension)
Cholesterol problems (high "bad" LDL cholesterol, low "good" HDL cholesterol)	Indigestion
	Insomnia
Colic	Irritable bowel syndrome
Colon cancer	Lead poisoning
Constipation	Liver disease
Diabetes, type 2	Psoriasis
Diarrhea	Rosacea
Eczema (atopic dermatitis)	Stomachache
	Ulcer
Flatulence	Vaginal yeast infection

Insomnia. "Coriander has been recommended for relief of anxiety and insomnia in . . . folk medicine," noted a team of Middle Eastern researchers in the *Journal of the American Medical Directors*. In a study on laboratory animals, the researchers found the spice was a potent sedative and muscle relaxant.

Colon cancer. In an animal study, Indian researchers blocked the development of tumors in chemically-induced colon cancer. Their conclusion in the *Journal of Ethnopharmacology*: "The inclusion of this spice in the daily diet plays a significant role in the protection of the colon against . . . carcinogenesis."

Liver disease. Researchers in India found that coriander extracts protected the liver from damage. They noted that the powerful antioxidants in coriander not only protected the "integrity" of cells in the liver, "but at the same time increased the regenerative and reparative capacity of the liver"—good news if you're one of the tens of millions of Americans with nonalcoholic fatty liver disease (NAFLD), hepatitis C infection, or cirrhosis.

Yeast infection. Brazilian researchers tested coriander essential oil against *Candida albicans*, the fungus that causes yeast infections, and found coriander could limit its growth. Coriander essential oil "could be used . . . to treat or prevent Candida yeast infections," concluded the researchers in *Food Chemistry*.

Lead poisoning. Researchers in India found that coriander extracts could "significantly protect" laboratory animals from the damage caused by lead exposure. In a second group of animals, the extracts also *reversed* damage from lead exposure. The mechanism: coriander's power as an antioxidant, said the researchers in *Biological Trace Element Research*.

Getting to Know Coriander

Coriander is the seed from the pink and mauve flowers of a delicate plant that resembles parsley (and is from the same botanical family). When ripe, coriander seeds are deliciously sweet, with

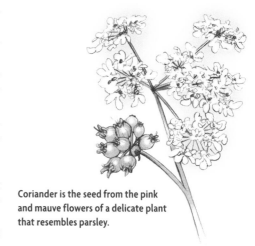

Coriander is the seed from the pink and mauve flowers of a delicate plant that resembles parsley.

a nutty taste of sage and orange. (When unripe, they have an unpleasant bug-like smell—perhaps the reason the Greeks called it *koris*, meaning bedbug.)

Even in the unlikely event that coriander isn't in your spice cabinet, it is in your diet. Americans eat a *lot* of coriander—more than 900,000 pounds a year, much of it used to flavor some of America's favorite foods, including hot dogs, sausages, lunch meats, pastries, and cookies. It's also a flavoring in gin and other types of alcohol.

Coriander seeds are used extensively in sweet and savory dishes in cuisines around the world—in Europe, India, Latin America, Mexico, North Africa, and the Middle East.

In Europe, the French flavor cheese with coriander. It's also the flavoring in the French liqueur Chartreuse. It is a key ingredient in the Spanish hot sausage chorizo.

Coriander is one of the most popular spices in Indian cuisine and is a key ingredient in all forms of curry spice mixes. Indians use the entire plant—seed, root, stem, and leaf—to make chutneys and sauces.

In Java, an island of Indonesia, both coriander and cilantro are rubbed into *satay*, a meat dish.

Moroccans rub the ground seeds into meat

and put them in couscous, stews, and salads. Coriander is a key ingredient in North African spice blends, including *baharat*, *tabil*, and *ras-el-hanout*. In Yemen, cooks mix coriander with dried fruits, green chiles, and other spices to make a condiment called *jhoug*, which is also popular as a dip. It is also used to flavor Turkish coffee.

Mexicans make liberal use of cilantro—in salsa, to make a hard sugar candy called *cola-ciones*, and in bread pudding.

Coriander pairs well with *all* spices, but particularly well with:

Allspice	Cumin	Sun-dried
Cardamom	Fennel seed	tomato
Clove	Garlic	Turmeric
Coconut	Ginger	

and complements recipes featuring:

Beans	Lentils	Poultry
Cakes	Mushrooms	Potatoes
Fish	Pastries	Spice mixes
Fruit, especially apples	Pork	Vegetables

Other recipes containing coriander:

Apple Pie Spice (p. 271)	Madras Curry Paste (p. 286)
Baharat (p. 268)	
Berbere (p. 267)	Madras Curry Powder (p. 284)
Caribbean Curry Paste (p. 287)	
	Malaysian Curry Paste (p. 287)
Chaat Masala (p. 256)	
Cocoa Rub (p. 270)	Ras-el-hanout (p. 266)
Colombo Powder (p. 270)	Sambaar Masala (p. 265)
Dukkah (p. 268)	Tabil (p. 267)
Garam Masala (p. 264)	Thai Red Curry Paste (p. 286)
Ginger Carrot and Squash Soup (p. 140)	Vindaloo Curry Paste (p. 286)
Hot Curry Powder (p. 284)	

How to Buy Coriander

Coriander seeds come in two main varieties: European and Indian. European is more flavorful because of its higher concentration of volatile oils, including a large proportion of linalool. Indian coriander, however, contains oils not found in European coriander, giving it a more lemony scent. Both are used the same way in cooking.

Most of the coriander found in American markets is European. You can tell the difference between the two by their size and color. European coriander is a spherically-shaped, ribbed seed, about a quarter-inch in diameter, and tan in color. Indian coriander is slightly smaller, more egg-shaped, and pale yellow with a greenish tinge.

Other varieties of coriander come from Morocco and Romania. Moroccan seeds are larger than European seeds, and Romanian coriander is the smallest.

Whole coriander seeds are a husk with two dry seeds inside. The seeds should appear uniform in color and clean, with no signs of grit. (A tiny tail on the end of the seeds is natural and *not* a sign of grit.)

Coriander is sold powdered, but it's best to buy whole seeds, as the oils dissipate fairly quickly once ground. (If you purchase coriander ground, buy it in small quantities.) The seeds stay fresh for a year a more, but ground seeds are only good for a few months.

You can buy dried parsley but you can't buy dried cilantro—the leaves don't hold up in the drying process. When buying fresh cilantro, try to buy leaves with their roots intact, which keeps leaves freshest the longest. Store the leaves upright in water in the refrigerator and cover them with a plastic bag. They'll stay fresh for several days.

Madras Beef Curry

This classic Indian curry is quick-and-easy to prepare. It's even faster if you already have the curry mix pre-made. This dish will develop a more intense flavor if made a day or two ahead of time.

2 tablespoons canola or vegetable oil
2 tablespoons Madras Curry Paste (p. 286)
2 cups chopped onions
3 garlic cloves, crushed and chopped
2 pounds beef cubes
2 large tomatoes, chopped
1 cup coconut milk
1 cup beef stock
1 teaspoon lemon juice
½ cup cilantro

1. Heat the oil in a large heavy Dutch oven. When it is hot, add the curry paste and stir until the spices release their oils and flavor, about three minutes. Add the chopped onions and fry, stirring frequently, until the onions are golden, about seven minutes. Add the garlic and fry one minute more.

2. Add the beef cubes and stir to coat in the spices and onions. Add the tomatoes, coconut milk, and stock and bring to a boil. Reduce the heat and simmer, covered, for two hours, stirring occasionally. Add the lemon juice and cook 10 minutes more. Serve over rice sprinkled with the cilantro.

Makes 6 servings.

In the Kitchen with Coriander

Coriander is a versatile and useful spice that mixes well with everything—and is at its *least* flavorful by itself. Always combine it with other spices—especially with its favorite companion, cumin.

It's almost impossible to use too much coriander. (In North African cuisine, some recipes call for it by the cupful!) In fact, coriander can fix a lot of errors in cooking. If you've gone too heavy on a particular spice in a dish, add the same amount of ground coriander, which should correct the flavor. This works particularly well when you've overdone a strong spice such as clove or cinnamon.

For a more intense aroma, always roast coriander seeds before they are ground. You can dry roast them (directions on page 11) or toast them in oil. The seeds are easy to grind with a mortar and pestle.

The seeds create a complex aroma when added to long-cooking braises, casseroles, or stews. When making sweet dishes, however, you should only used ground coriander.

The papery husks and coarse grain-like consistency of the ground seeds absorb moisture; use them to thicken sauces and gravies.

Cilantro is too delicate to withstand heat. Sprinkle it on a finished dish or add it during the last few minutes of cooking.

Here are some ways to add more coriander to your diet:

- Add whole or ground seeds to stews, casseroles, marinades, vinaigrettes, and pickled dishes.
- Coarsely grind coriander and rub it into meats or fish before cooking.
- Mix coriander seeds with peppercorns in the peppermill you use at the stove.
- Make a classic Moroccan rub: mix coriander with garlic, butter, and paprika and rub it on lamb before roasting.
- Sprinkle coriander on sautéed mushrooms.
- Add cilantro (fresh coriander leaves) to salad dressings or stir into mayonnaise.
- Add ground coriander toward the end of steaming rice or couscous.
- Add whole seeds to chicken casseroles.

CUMIN *Keeping Diabetes Under Control*

Cumin is a commoner. Sitting in the jar, it isn't much to look at—just kind of brown and drab. It isn't pleasant to touch—a little too oily. Its flavor won't send your taste buds into orbit—it's bitter and stale. And the aroma is akin to musty old pine.

But once it's out of the jar and into the cooking pot, its transformation is akin to Cinderella's, as the pungent and bitter smell mellows to a rich, nutty aroma that brings to mind the scent of a Mexican cantina. That's because while chile gives Mexican food the fire, cumin gives the zest—it is *the* most popular spice in Mexican cuisine.

Cumin has a flavor unlike any other because it's loaded with *cuminaldehyde*, a compound with medicinal qualities that are active as, well, Mexican jumping beans.

Fighting Diabetes

Diabetes is a disease of chronically high levels of blood sugar (glucose). And that flood of extra sugar damages blood vessels throughout the body, increasing the risk for heart disease and stroke (the cause of death in 75 percent of people with diabetes), blindness, and kidney disease. Cumin to the rescue . . .

In a study from India, scientists treated laboratory animals with type 2 diabetes with either cumin or glibenclamide (Diabeta), an antidiabetes drug. They found that both worked equally well to reduce levels of cholesterol and triglycerides, heart-damaging blood fats common in people with diabetes. The animals also had a "significant reduction" in blood sugar, lowered levels of A1C (the amount of glucose attached to red blood cells, a measure of long-term blood sugar levels), and lower levels of damaging fat and inflammation in the cells of the pancreas, the organ that manufacturs insulin, the hormone that controls blood sugar levels.

Cumin "supplementation was found to be more effective than glibenclamide in the treatment of diabetes mellitus," concluded the researchers in *Pharmacological Research*.

People with diabetes have a 60 percent higher risk of developing cataracts, a vision-clouding covering on the lens of the eye. In another animal study from India, researchers tested cumin against the eye disease. They found that feeding cumin powder to diabetic rats delayed the progression of cataracts—by preventing changes in the lens caused by high blood sugar. Dietary cumin "was able to delay the diabetes-caused cataract progression and maturation," said the researchers.

Researchers at India's National Institute of Nutrition found that cumin (along with cinnamon, black pepper, and green tea) can cut the formation of AGE, or advanced glycation endproducts, by 40 to 90 percent. AGE are toxic cellular time bombs that form when an overdose of glucose warps proteins. "The inhibition of the formation of AGE is believed to play a role in the prevention of diabetic complications," wrote the researchers in the *British Journal of Nutrition*.

Will the Real Cumin Please Stand Up?

Cumin suffers from a bit of an identity crisis . . .

It's not caraway. In Europe, its popularity has lost out to caraway seed—but caraway can't stand in for cumin in dishes such as chili and curry.

It's not black cumin. Cumin isn't the same as (nor is it a substitute for) black cumin. Black cumin is English for the Indian spice *kolonji*. Black cumin seeds are jet black, and are sometimes called imperial cumin (because black cumin is somewhat pricey compared to cumin).

It's not curcumin. Cumin has no relationship to curcumin, the principal ingredient in the spice turmeric.

Protecting Bones

Eating more soy protein or taking soy supplements is commonly suggested as a way to prevent, delay, or even reverse osteoporosis, the bone-thinning disease that afflicts tens of millions of Americans. That's because soy is a *phytoestrogen*, a plant compound that helps keep calcium in bones. Well, now researchers are looking at cumin as a possible bone-protector, because it's also rich in phytoestrogens.

In a study from India, researchers tested the ability of cumin to stop bone loss in laboratory animals with induced osteoporosis. They found those given the spice had greater bone density than those who didn't receive cumin. In fact, the spice's "osteoprotective effect" was comparable to that of the hormone estradiol (Estrace), which was popular for the prevention of osteoporosis before researchers discovered it also increased the risk of heart disease and breast cancer.

The researchers' remarkable conclusion: "Cumin can help postmenopausal women from losing their bone and seems to be a potential candidate for the development of new herbal approaches for osteoporosis treatment without any serious side effects."

Combating Cancer

Cumin's volatile oil and rich content of vitamins C and A make it a potent antioxidant—and a potential cancer-stopper. Animal studies have found that cumin:

- Prevented the formation of colon tumors in rats fed cancer-causing substances.
- Reduced the risk of cervical cancer by 82 percent compared to animals not receiving the spice.
- Significantly decreased the incidence of stomach and liver cancer.

Cumin to the Max

Other conditions that cumin may help control include:

Epilepsy. Researchers in the Middle East found

Cumin may help prevent and/or treat:

Cancer	Food poisoning
Diabetes, type 2	Osteoporosis
Epilepsy	Tuberculosis

Cumin pairs well with these spices:

Ajowan	Fenugreek seed
Allspice	Garlic
Basil	Ginger
Black pepper	Mustard
Caraway	Onion
Chile	Oregano
Cinnamon	Pumpkin seed
Cocoa	Saffron
Coriander	Tamarind
Fennel seed	Turmeric

and complements recipes featuring:

Black beans	Potatoes
Chile con carne	Tomatoes
Curries	Tex-Mex dishes
Mexican food	

---

that cumin suppressed convulsions in animals with chemically induced seizures.

Food poisoning. In India, researchers found that cumin was the most effective spice in blocking the action of the bacteria that cause food poisoning.

Tuberculosis. Cumin boosts the infection-fighting power of *rifampicin*, a antibiotic used to treat tuberculosis.

Getting to Know Cumin

Like most popular spices, cumin has a world-historical pedigree. Ancient Greeks kept cumin on the dining table in its own box, just as they

Other recipes containing cumin:

Adobo (p. 270)

Alamelu's Salt Substitute (p. 289)

Baharat (p. 268)

Black Pepper Rice with Almonds (p. 57)

By-the-Bay Fisherman's Chowder (p. 46)

Caribbean Curry Paste (p. 287)

Chaat Masala (p. 256)

Cocoa Rub (p. 270)

Coconut Meatballs with Peanut Sauce (p. 101)

Colombo Powder (p. 270)

Dukkah (p. 268)

Garam Masala (p. 264)

Garbanzo Beans with Mushrooms and Toasted Almonds (p. 29)

Green Pumpkin Seed Sauce (p. 200)

Grilled Lamb Patty Pockets with Cucumber Mint Sauce (p. 165)

Hot Curry Powder (p. 284)

Madras Curry Paste (p. 286)

Madras Curry Powder (p. 284)

Onion and Tomato Chutney (p. 113)

Panch Phoron (p. 266)

Potato Cauliflower Curry (p. 252)

Ras-el-hanout (p. 266)

Sambaar Masala (p. 265)

Spicy Hash Brown Potatoes (p. 151)

Vindaloo Curry Paste (p. 286)

Yucatan Pickled Red Onions (p. 21)

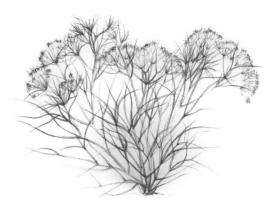

Cumin comes from a flowering plant that thrives in hot, arid lands.

did with pepper. It was currency for the early Romans, who used it to pay taxes. (If only we could send a jar of cumin seeds to the IRS!)

Today cumin is a staple in the kitchens of North Africa, western Asia, India, Greece, Turkey, and, of course, Mexico and Latin America. However, those countries south of the border didn't use cumin until it was brought to the Americas by merchants from India.

India has appreciated cumin for millennia, for both its aroma and medicinal qualities. Cumin is one of the essential ingredients in curry powder and most curry spice mixes. It is also a key ingredient in *garam masala*, the Indian basic spice mix. The whole seeds are used in the spice mixes *chaat masala* and *panch phoron*.

In Mexico, cumin is used in tacos, enchiladas, and burritos, as well as other popular dishes. It is as essential as chili powder in making Mexican chili (and Texan chili con carne).

In the Caribbean, the seeds are a main ingredient in Colombo powder, a super-hot spice blend.

The Dutch make a cumin-flavored cheese. Cumin bread is a regional French specialty. In Spain, cumin is cleverly combined with cinnamon and saffron to flavor casseroles.

In Morocco it is used in couscous (cracked wheat steamed in spices) and is a main ingredient in *ras-el-hanout*, the famous Moroccan spice blend. Iranians use it to make pickles.

How to Buy Cumin

Americans know cumin best as a dark powder that feels somewhat oily to the touch. However, cumin starts out as seeds, which is the way it is sold in Indian markets, where it is referred to as *jeera*. Indian as well as many Asian cuisines use the seeds whole.

Buying whole seeds is better than buying ground cumin, and both are available in most

All-American Chili con Carne

We call this all-American because it combines the best of this country's chilies, from Texas, Arizona, and (believe it or not) Cincinnati, Ohio, which claims to have more chili parlors than anywhere else in the country. The secret ingredient in Cincinnati chili is the allspice. Make chili at least a few hours ahead and let the aromas meld. Reheat before serving.

2 tablespoons olive oil

2 large onions, chopped

5 cloves garlic, minced

2½ pounds extra-lean ground beef or ground turkey

3 tablespoons chili powder

1 tablespoon ground cumin

1 tablespoon dried Mexican oregano or other oregano

2 teaspoons dried basil

1 teaspoon ground allspice

1 teaspoon unsweetened cocoa powder

1 teaspoon turmeric

½ teaspoon salt

½ teaspoon freshly ground black pepper

1 twenty-eight-ounce can crushed tomatoes, chopped

½ cup red wine vinegar

3 cans red kidney beans

2 or more jalapeños, seeded and diced

½ cup Monterey Jack cheese (optional)

½ cup sour cream (optional)

½ cup diced onions or sliced scallions (optional)

1. In a large heavy-bottom casserole, heat the olive oil. Add the onions and cook until soft but not brown. Stir in the garlic and cook one minute more.

2. Add the ground beef or turkey, breaking up the pieces with a wooden spoon, until just brown. Combine the chili powder, cumin, oregano, basil, allspice, cocoa, turmeric, salt, and pepper and add to the meat. Blend well and cook one minute.

3. Add the canned tomatoes, red wine vinegar, kidney beans, and jalapeños and stir. Bring to a simmer, lower the heat, cover, and cook for 30 minutes. Serve with the optional ingredients on the side.

Makes 8 servings.

supermarkets. If you are cooking ethnic dishes, chances are you'll need a jar of whole seeds. Once the seeds are ground the flavor starts to deteriorate. (If you've had a bottle of cumin for a year or more, throw it out. Ground cumin doesn't retain its quality for more than a few months.)

Cumin seeds should be dry roasted before they're ground, which will intensify the flavor. For instructions on how to dry roast see page 11.

Cumin seeds are yellowish-brown and oval shaped and somewhat resemble caraway seeds. If you can't find the seeds in the supermarket, you can buy them in an Indian market or via the Internet. The "Buyer's Guide" on page 309 can help you find a retailer.

In the Kitchen with Cumin

Cumin is one of the most frequently used spices and is found in virtually every cuisine in the world. The reason: its versatility. Though the ground spice is quite pungent, keep in mind that it mellows when cooked.

Use cumin in stews and casseroles and any long-cooking food that requires liquid. It pairs well with other strong spices, especially chili powder. In fact, cumin can come in handy if you find a dish you are making is too strong or "off" the intended aroma. Adding a pinch of cumin will help even out the flavor. Here are some other ways to enjoy cumin:

- Make a glaze for roasted vegetables by combining ½ cup canola oil with ½ cup orange juice and 1 tablespoon of ground cumin. Season with salt and freshly ground black pepper.

- Use it as a flavoring in cheese sauces.
- Sprinkle it in a cheese omelet.

- Add roasted seeds to marinades.
- Make a spice blend with ½ cumin and ½ chili powder.
- Use cumin to help spice up creamy dips.
- Add toasted seeds to lentils and rice pilaf.

CURRY LEAF *From Mother Nature's Branch of Medicine*

As with a few other spices in this book, the first step in talking about curry leaf is clearing up a bit of confusion.

Curry *leaf* isn't curry *powder*. It doesn't look like curry powder or taste like it. But curry leaf has a lot to do with curry *dishes*. The wonderfully fragrant, tangerine-like flavor of the curry leaf is as common in South Indian curries as bay leaf is in American stews.

Curry leaf is also a standard remedy in Ayurveda, the traditional medicine of India, where it's used to control diabetes, heart disease, infections, and inflammation. In the 1950s, scientists began discovering the biochemical details underlying its therapeutic powers, and in the subsequent decades dozens of studies have demonstrated that it's loaded with healing compounds.

Just like many green leafy vegetables, curry leaf is rich in the antioxidants beta-carotene and vitamin C. But when Indian researchers measured the antioxidant *power* of curry leaf— its ability to gobble up the malicious molecules called *free radicals* that injure cells and their precious genetic cargo—they found it outperformed three other leafy greens popular in Indian cuisine. The reason: an elite team of antioxidants called *carbazole alkaloids* that are abundant only in curry leaf.

Relief from a Leaf

It's no surprise that curry leaf might help hinder a range of diseases linked to the oxidative damage from free radicals—type 2 diabetes, heart disease, and cancer.

Diabetes. Type 2 diabetes—the disease of chronically high blood sugar—afflicts more than 24 million Americans, damaging blood vessels and causing heart attacks, strokes, kidney failure, blindness, hard-to-heal foot ulcers, and other circulatory disasters. More curry leaf in the diet might help.

In a study on mice bred to develop diabetes, high cholesterol, and obesity, researchers at the Tang Center for Herbal Medicine Research at the University of Chicago used curry leaf to reduce levels of high blood sugar (glucose) by 45 percent. And cholesterol dropped by 35 percent—another important finding, since high cholesterol is a major risk for the heart attacks and strokes that kill three out of four people with type 2 diabetes.

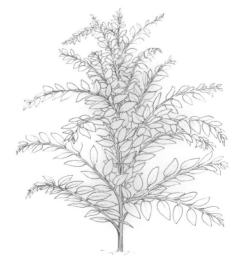

Curry leaf—with a flavor half lemon and half tangerine—is from a tree that is a member of the citrus family.

Curry leaf may offer help in "improving the management" of type 2 diabetes and high cholesterol, the researchers concluded.

Indian researchers, at the Alternative Therapeutics Center of the University of Allahabad, used curry leaf extracts to lower glucose 48 percent in experimental animals. The spice also lowered total cholesterol by 31 percent, triglycerides (another heart-damaging blood fat) by 23 percent, and raised "good" HDL cholesterol by 30 percent. Curry leaf has a "favorable effect in bringing down the severity of diabetes," they concluded in the *Journal of Ethnopharmacology*.

Memory loss. When Indian researchers added curry leaf to the diets of laboratory animals, they found the spice improved their memories—and the more spice the animals ate, the better they could remember. The researchers also found the spice boosted *cholinergic activity* in the brains of the animals, the same activity that progressively decreases with the step-by-step onset of age-related memory loss, mild cognitive impairment, and Alzheimer's disease. Curry leaf might have "therapeutic potential . . . in the management of Alzheimer patients," concluded the researchers in *Phytotherapy Research*.

Colon cancer. Indian researchers found that curry leaf extract significantly reduced the number of tumors in experimental animals with chemically induced colon cancer. Including curry leaf in the "daily diet plays a significant role in the protection of the colon" against cancer, concluded the researchers.

Getting to Know Curry Leaf

The curry tree—a member of the citrus family that grows in the backyards and the back country throughout India—produces a leaf with a flavor that's half lemon and half tangerine.

That flavor adds zest not only to the cuisines of India and Sri Lanka, but also to the cuisines of Burma, Malaysia, and Singapore. And it's an essential spice not only in curries, but also in *dals* (lentil stews), *samosas* (deep-fried appetizers, usually vegetarian), *sambars* (chowder-like broths), chutneys, and breads. It's also an ingredient in South Indian curry powder.

How to Buy Curry Leaf

Curry leaf is incomparable fresh, but the only place you're likely to find it fresh is in an Indian

Curry leaf may help prevent and/or treat:

Alzheimer's disease	Diabetes, type 2
Cholesterol problems (high total cholesterol, low "good" HDL cholesterol)	Memory loss (age-related, mild cognitive decline)
	Triglycerides, high
Colon cancer	

Curry leaf pairs well with these spices:

Allspice	Fennel seed	Onion
Chile	Fenugreek seed	Sun-dried tomato
Cinnamon		
Clove	Garlic	Tamarind
Coriander	Ginger	Turmeric
Cumin	Mustard seed	

and complements recipes featuring:

Beans	Lentils
Cabbage	Okra
Chutneys	Rice
Curries	Seafood
Eggplant	Soups

Other recipes containing curry leaf:

Black Pepper Rice with Almonds (p. 57)	Hot Curry Powder (p. 284)
Brussels Sprouts Kulambu (p. 123)	Sol Kadhi (p. 152)

market. If you're lucky enough to live near one, you'll find curry leaves in the produce section, packaged on the stem, in clear wrap. The leaves look like small, thin bay leaves. Don't pass up an opportunity to buy fresh curry leaves—they're not expensive, and they won't go to waste because you can freeze them. (If you don't see them, ask for them. They're almost always available.)

To keep curry leaves fresh and fragrant, keep them on the stem until you're ready to use them. Then pull them off one by one, as needed. They keep in the refrigerator for about a week. As mentioned, they freeze well, too—just pop the bag in your freezer and pull off the leaves as needed. They will keep in the freezer for about two months. Once frozen, they form dark spots and can turn almost black, but this change in appearance doesn't decrease flavor. It's best to chop up darkened, thawed curry leaves.

Curry leaf is also available dried or as a powder. You can purchase both in Indian markets or online, through Web sites that sell Indian spices. (See the list of retailers in the "Buyer's Guide" on page 309.) Both dried and powdered curry leaf keeps for about a year, in an airtight container away from heat and light.

In the Kitchen with Curry Leaf

Use curry leaves as they're used in Indian cooking—sautéed in sizzling oil, at the beginning of cooking. They'll splatter, so cover the pan. Sautéed leaves add crunchiness and aroma to your dishes. In South Indian cooking, fresh curry leaves are most often paired with mustard seed.

Fresh curry leaf adds a deeply fragrant and distinctive flavor to food—which is mostly lost when the spice is dried. If you're using dried curry leaves, add a handful to get the same flavor you'd get from one fresh leaf.

Here are ways to add more curry leaf to your diet:

Onion and Tomato Chutney

This deliciously spicy Indian chutney was developed by my friend Alamelu Vairavan, a native of South India, for her book Healthy South Indian Cooking. *Serve it as a snack with bread or crackers or as an accompaniment to grilled beef, chicken, or fish. Add more or less red chile depending on your personal preference for the heat.*

2 tablespoons canola oil
¼ teaspoon asafoetida powder
5 fresh curry leaves
2–4 whole dried red chiles
1 teaspoon black mustard seeds
1 teaspoon *urad dal* (split white lentils) or
   1 teaspoon cumin seed
1 cup coarsely chopped onions
1 cup chopped fresh tomatoes
3 garlic cloves, peeled
¼ teaspoon tamarind paste
½ teaspoon salt

1. Heat the canola oil in a small skillet or wok over medium heat. When the oil is hot but not smoking, add the asafoetida powder, curry leaves, red chiles, mustard seeds, and urad dal. Cover and heat until the mustard seeds pop and the urad dal turns golden brown, about 30 seconds.

2. Add the onions, tomatoes, and garlic cloves and stir-fry until tender.

3. Add the tamarind paste and salt. Stir and cook for a few minutes until the mixture is well blended. Remove from heat.

4. Transfer the ingredients to a blender or food processor. Add 1 cup of warm water and grind until the ingredients are ground thoroughly and reach a thick consistency.

Makes 2½ cups.

- Add fresh curry leaves to salads and salad dressing.
- Add them to seafood or meat stews.
- Try them in chili.
- Add a few fresh leaves to chicken soup, or ladle the soup and add a fresh leaf to each bowl of soup.

- Use it instead of bay leaf, for a change of pace and taste.
- The citrus-like flavor of curry leaf makes it a natural for marinades.
- Add a curry leaf or two to pickling recipes.

FENNEL SEED *Calming Cramps and Colic*

Fennel is one of the few plants that has it all—it's a vegetable, herb, *and* spice.

Every fall, the ground-level bulb (vegetable) sprouts celery-like stalks with willowy fronds (herbs) that flower and produce aromatic seeds (spice). And vegetable, herb, and spice all carry the sweet scent of licorice.

Fennel isn't the most popular bulb in the batch—not everyone likes a licorice-tasting vegetable or herb. But the seeds are definitely in demand—they're the spice that makes Italian sausages and pepperoni pizza world-famous.

The familiar tang of licorice when you bite into a fennel seed comes from the volatile oil *anethole*, the same compound that gives anise its licorice-like flavor. Fennel seeds are teeming with anet-

Fennel is a bulb that sprouts stalks with willowy fronds that flower and produce aromatic fennel seeds.

hole and dozens of other potent phytochemicals. That includes *phytoestrogens*, estrogen-like compounds found in plants. Once a month, those phytoestrogens might be a woman's best friend.

Relieving Menstrual Pain

Menstrual cramps—or *dysmenorrhea*, in medical terminology—affect more than 50 percent of menstruating women, with 10 percent having pain so severe they're incapacitated for a few days each month.

In a study in the *International Journal of Gynecology and Obstetrics*, doctors treated 30 high school students with moderate to severe menstrual cramps, using either an extract of fennel or a non-steroidal anti-inflammatory drug (NSAID) similar to ibuprofen. Both the drug *and* fennel effectively relieved menstrual pain. "The essence of fennel can be used as a safe and effective" treatment for menstrual cramps, the researchers concluded.

In a similar study, involving 110 high school girls, fennel outperformed the NSAID, providing "complete pain relief or pain decrease" to 80 percent of the girls, compared to 73 percent taking the drug.

And in a study in the journal *Phytomedicine*, doctors found that a topical version of the fennel extract reduced the diameter of hairs in women with *hirsutism* (unwanted, excess hair, such as facial hair), a problem caused by imbalanced hormones.

Calming Colic

Your baby cries inconsolably for hours at a time, arching his back or pulling his legs up. And it's been going on and on—a couple of days a week, week after week. It might be colic. The good news: your baby *isn't* in pain, says Laura Riley, MD, medical director of labor and delivery at Massachusetts General Hospital in Boston, and assistant professor of obstetrics, gynecology, and reproductive biology at Harvard Medical School. But that doesn't mean you don't want to stop the crying.

In a study published in *Alternative Therapies in Health and Medicine*, doctors treated 125 infants (2 to 12 weeks of age) with colic, dividing them into two groups: one received a product containing fennel seed oil (PediaCalm) and the other received a placebo. The fennel seed product *eliminated* colic in 65 percent of the babies given it, compared to 24 percent of those given the placebo. In another study, Italian researchers gave either a placebo or a formula containing fennel, and the herbs chamomile and melissa, to 88 colicky infants. One week later, the daily crying time of the infants taking fennel had decreased from a daily average of 3½ hours to 1¼ hours. Meanwhile, the crying time of the placebo group went from 3½ hours a day to just under 3 hours.

A Powerful Anti-inflammatory

Fennel seed is a powerful antioxidant—in fact, one study shows it's *more* powerful than vitamin E (famous as an antioxidant) in defeating free radicals, those oxidizing molecules that damage cells and DNA. Fennel seed is also a powerful anti-inflammatory. Oxidation and inflammation are the evil twins that cause many chronic diseases, including heart disease, type 2 diabetes, Alzheimer's, cancer, and arthritis. That's why fennel may help tame them all.

Alzheimer's disease and non-Alzheimer's dementia. Approximately one-third of 75-year-olds have dementia—the near-total loss of memory—and Alzheimer's disease is the most common form of dementia, comprising 80 percent of all cases.

Fennel seed may help prevent and/or treat:

Alzheimer's disease	Glaucoma
Arthritis, osteo- and rheumatoid	Heart disease
	High blood pressure (hypertension)
Cancer	
Colic	Hirsutism (unwanted hair growth in women)
Colitis (inflammatory bowel disease)	
	Menstrual cramps
Dementia, non-Alzheimer's	Stroke

In a study by Indian researchers, an extract of fennel seed "profoundly" improved long-term memory in laboratory animals. It also boosted the activity of the brain chemical *acetylcholine*, the same mode of action as donepezil (Aricept), a drug used to treat Alzheimer's. Fennel extract "can be employed in the treatment of cognitive disorders such as dementia and Alzheimer's disease," concluded the researchers in the *Journal of Medicinal Food*.

Cancer. A daily diet containing fennel seeds inhibited the formation of tumors in experimental animals exposed to cancer-causing chemicals. "The inclusion of fennel seeds in the diet is likely to reduce the risk of cancer in the human population," concluded the researchers in *Food and Chemical Toxicology*.

Arthritis. Korean researchers found fennel extract significantly decreased swelling and pain in animals with experimentally induced arthritis. Fennel's anti-inflammatory activity "may reduce the risk of inflammatory-related diseases" such as osteoarthritis, rheumatoid arthritis, and lower back pain, concluded the researchers.

Heart disease and stroke. Moroccan researchers found that fennel lowered systolic blood pressure (the upper number in the reading) in animals with laboratory-induced high blood pressure. High blood pressure is a leading risk

Fennel seed pairs well with these spices:

Allspice	Cumin	Onion
Bay leaf	Fenugreek	Rosemary
Black cumin	seed	Sun-dried
seed	Galangal	tomato
Cardamom	Garlic	Tamarind
Cinnamon	Ginger	Turmeric
Clove	Marjoram	
Coriander	Mustard seed	

and complements recipes featuring:

Cheese	Poultry	Shad
Curries	Salmon	Tomatoes
Mushrooms	Sausage	
Pasta	Satay	

Other recipes containing fennel seed:

By-the-Bay Fisherman's Chowder (p. 46)	Pickling Spice (p. 272)
	Ras-el-hanout (p. 266)
Chinese Five-Spice Powder (p. 268)	Roast Chicken with 40 Cloves of Garlic (p. 134)
Dukkah (p. 268)	Roasted Tomato Soup with Fennel and Mint (p. 231)
Hot Curry Powder (p. 284)	
Malaysian Curry Paste (p. 287)	Spiced Milk Tea (p. 66)
Panch Phoron (p. 266)	

factor for heart disease and stroke. Their results were published in *Clinical and Experimental Hypertension*.

In another animal experiment, researchers in Italy found that both anethole and a fennel extract inhibited *platelet aggregation*—the clumping of blood compounds that can trigger an artery-clogging blood clot. And unlike aspirin (often used to decrease platelet aggrega-

tion and "thin" the blood), neither anethole or fennel extract caused any stomach damage—in fact, they *protected* the lining of the stomach against damage!

Inflammatory bowel disease. In folk medicine, fennel has been used to soothe digestive upsets of all kinds, including abdominal bloating and gas. It works because it relaxes the lining of the intestines and douses inflammation. Perhaps the worst digestive problem of them all is *inflammatory bowel disease* (IBD), with urgent bowel movements and diarrhea as the main symptoms. IBD is called *colitis* when it mainly afflicts the colon (large intestine), and *Crohn's disease* when patches of inflammation afflict the small and large intestine.

Researchers in Bulgaria gave a formula including fennel to 24 people with colitis. "Palpable pains along the large intestine disappeared in 96 percent of the patients by the 15th day" of the treatment, the researchers wrote. "Defecation was normalized in patients with diarrhea syndrome."

Glaucoma. In glaucoma, the canals that drain fluid from inside the eyeball clog up, producing pressure inside the eye that damages the optic nerve. Indian researchers gave drops of a fennel extract to animals with experimentally induced glaucoma. The extract decreased intraocular pressure by 31 percent—the same level of relief provided by an antiglaucoma drug. Fennel may find a place "in the arsenal of antiglaucoma drugs prescribed by physicians," the researchers concluded.

Getting to Know Fennel Seed

Fennel is widely used in Mediterranean cuisines, particularly in Italy—where *finnochio* is regarded as *delizioso*. In Florence, a highly regarded variety of fennel has been cultivated since the Middle Ages. The national liqueur, sambuca, is flavored with fennel. And the seeds are the hallmark spice used to make Italian sausages, meatballs, salami, and pepperoni.

The French in Provence grow *fenouil* to use

fresh in pastas and salads or as a vegetable. A Provencal specialty is *poisson au fenouil*: a whole fish is laid on a bed of fennel stalks on an open grill, giving off a smoky, sweet, licorice-like aroma as the stalks burn under the fish. The seeds are mostly used in sauces and pasta dishes.

The English use the seeds in soups. Germans put them in breads, fish dishes, and sauerkraut. The Spanish use fennel seed to flavor cakes and other baked goods. Scandinavians use fennel as the seed on rye bread.

In India, fennel seed is a key ingredient in many spice blends, including Indian curry powders and the seed blend *panch phoron*. Indians add fennel seeds to pickles, curries, soups, and lentil and rice dishes. It is also used in a specialty dessert called *malpoora*, which is a deep-fried pancake flavored with fennel and pistachio. Many Indian restau-

rants offer sugar-coated fennel seeds at the end of dinner with coffee and the check. Recently, India has cultivated its own fennel seed, Lucknow, named after its town of origin. Lucknow fennel has a sweeter flavor, closer to anise, and is favored as an after-dinner digestif.

In China and throughout Asia, fennel seeds are used in sweet-and-sour dishes and rich fish sauces. Asians toast the seeds before using, imparting a more vibrant flavor.

Fennel seed is found in the Moroccan spice blend *ras-el-hanout* and in Middle Eastern *dukkah*. Arabs sprinkle it over salads and bake it into bread.

How to Buy Fennel Seed

Fennel seeds are about a quarter-inch long, oval-shaped with vertical hairlines, and yellow, tinged

---

Penne and Sausage with Fennel Tomato Sauce

This recipe bridges the Mediterranean influences of both French and Italian cuisines. If tomatoes are out of season, use canned.

1 pound sweet Italian sausage
2 teaspoons fennel seeds
2 cloves garlic, diced
3 tablespoons tomato paste
1 cup chopped tomatoes, fresh or canned, with
    their juices
½ cup chopped Kalamata olives
1 cup Chianti or other dry red wine
1 bay leaf
½ teaspoon dried marjoram
½ teaspoon dried rosemary
1 pound penne pasta
2 eggs
¼ cup freshly grated Parmesan or Romano cheese
Freshly ground black pepper

1. Remove the sausage from its casing and coarsely chop. Brown the meat in a large non-stick skillet over low heat. Continue to break up the pieces until browned, about three or four minutes. Add the fennel seeds and cook until they release their oils, about 30 seconds. Add the garlic, stir and cook one minute. Add the tomato paste and coat to blend. Increase the heat to medium and cook two minutes.

2. Add the tomatoes, olives, Chianti, bay leaf, marjoram, and rosemary. Bring to a simmer, cover, and cook for 15 minutes.

3. Meanwhile, bring water to a boil for the pasta and cook to firm, according to package directions. Drain.

4. While the pasta is cooking, beat the eggs in a small bowl with a whisk. Whisk in the cheese and freshly ground pepper.

5. Remove the bay leaf from the sausage mixture. Add the pasta and toss to mix. Remove the skillet from the heat and add the egg and cheese mixture, tossing with two large forks to incorporate.

Makes 6 servings.

with green. Look for that tinge when buying, as it indicates top quality. Check to make sure the package of seeds is free of grit. (The small seeds are difficult to separate from dirt and other extraneous matter.) Look for seeds that are whole, rather than broken.

You can find fennel seeds whole or ground in most supermarkets. The volatile oils start to dissipate as soon as the seeds are ground, so buying them whole and grinding them just before using guarantees the most flavor.

If you shop for fennel seeds in an Indian market, you may come across Lucknow fennel, which may be labeled *Lakhnawi saunf*. These seeds are almost half the size of regular fennel seeds and mostly all green, like the brilliant lime green of cardamom pods.

Fennel seeds will keep for up to three years in an airtight container, in a cool place, away from sunlight. Ground seeds start to lose their intensity after six months or even sooner.

The fennel plant is cultivated in moderate climates around the world, including Italy, France, India, Morocco, Egypt, and Taiwan. Most of the fennel seed used in the US is imported from Egypt.

In the Kitchen with Fennel Seed

Fennel seed is strong-flavored, and works equally well in savory and sweet recipes. It can perk up the taste of a wide range of dishes, from meats to cakes to beverages. The seeds help add balance to almost any spice blend. Use them in the same way you use anise, cumin, and caraway seeds.

Fennel seeds don't have to be toasted as most other seeds do, but doing so intensifies and sweetens their flavor. Toasted seeds have an aftertaste similar to brown sugar. Dry-fry them, according to the directions on page 11, but make sure not to burn them, even slightly—they'll have an unpleasant, bitter taste.

Fennel seed works well with many foods from the Mediterranean diet, such as tomatoes, ripe olives, olive oil, basil, grilled meat, and seafood. They also combine well with fatty fish, such as salmon and tuna.

Here are some ways to add more fennel seed to your diet:

- Fennel can turn ordinary bread into something special. Try mixing a tablespoon of seeds into your favorite dough.
- Brush commercial French or Italian bread with lightly beaten egg, sprinkle with fennel seeds, and bake at 400°F until the seeds set.
- Dry and crush toasted fennel seeds and steep them in tea.
- Sprinkle fennel seeds on top of cakes and muffins before baking.
- Add fennel to fruit salads and compotes.
- Add ground fennel to scrambled eggs.
- Make spiced olives by marinating 2 cups of olives in ½ cup of extra-virgin olive oil and 1 teaspoon each of fennel seeds, dried oregano, and dried thyme.

FENUGREEK SEED *Defeating Diabetes*

New Yorkers like to say that they've seen it all, but apparently they haven't *smelled* it all. One night a few years ago, the city's hotline was flooded with phone calls about a mysterious odor reminiscent of maple syrup wafting across the western end of lower Manhattan. It wasn't the first time such an "incident" was reported, and the mayor promised city officials would get to the bottom of it.

A few days later, the mayor called a press conference. With pointer in hand he spent the next 20 minutes aiming at dots on a map where the smell was reported and at arrows showing wind patterns coming across the Hudson River from northern New Jersey. The odor, said the mayor, occurred on days when the wind speed was moderate and the air somewhat humid. His investigators had traced the odor to a plant in north Jersey that manufactures flavors for the food, beverage, and fragrance industries. The maple syrup-like scent, he revealed, was the smell of *fenugreek seeds* being processed.

"I can think of a lot of things worse than maple syrup," the mayor told a reporter. "It just happens to be one of the aromas that we're going to have to live with in a city like New York."

From Folk Medicine to the Medicine of the Future

What's fenugreek?!?, you say? Fenugreek, for sure, is Greek to most of the Western world (even New Yorkers), but it is a common culinary spice in South Asia, East Asia, and the Middle East. It also has a storied history as a medicinal spice: since ancient times (and right up to the present), fenugreek has been used as a folk remedy for an astonishingly long list of ills.

Fenugreek is a legendary aphrodisiac. Men have used it to grow hair and women to increase bust size. (Its rich content of the hormone-like compound *diosgenin* is probably responsible for any effects fenugreek might have on increasing libidos or bustlines.) It's been used to help regulate menstrual cycles, ease labor pains, and encourage milk flow for breastfeeding. Soaked in water, the seeds soften and swell, and are used to normalize digestion, countering both constipation and diarrhea. It has battled asthma, allergies, and other respiratory ills. And in Ayurveda, the traditional medicine of India, it's a classic "drug" for blood sugar (glucose) control—a use that modern science has strongly seconded.

Good News for Glucose Control

The body works best on a steady supply of blood sugar: not too much, not too little, but just right. The hormone insulin, manufactured by the pancreas, keeps levels normal, ushering glucose into liver cells for processing, muscle cells for instant energy, and fat cells for storage. But the standard American diet—loaded with sugars and refined carbohydrates that turn into a flashflood of glucose—overwhelms the insulin-generating capacity of the pancreas. And all the fat in the American diet clogs insulin receptors on cells. The end result is chronically high levels of blood sugar: 57 million Americans have *prediabetes* (fasting blood sugar levels 100 to 125 mg/dL), and another 24 million have type 2 diabetes (fasting blood sugar levels above 125 mg/dL). The long-term consequences of diabetes are disastrous: year after year, extra blood sugar batters blood vessels, leading to heart disease, stroke, blindness (from damage to the vessels of the retina), kidney disease (from damage to these vessel-rich organs), nerve pain (from damage to the tiny vessels called capillaries that nourish nerves), and amputations (from poor circulation to the feet and legs).

Fenugreek to the rescue. More than 100 scientific studies—mostly in animals with experimentally induced diabetes—show that fenugreek has the power to regulate blood sugar. Fenugreek can: balance daily blood sugar levels, lower A1C (the percentage of red blood cells that have been frosted by hemoglobin, the best measurement of long-term blood sugar control), increase enzymes that help regulate blood sugar, and activate insulin signaling in cells. Fenugreek can also help control the circulatory aftershocks of high blood sugar: high total cholesterol, high "bad" LDL cholesterol, high triglycerides, and low "good" HDL cholesterol.

In the most recent study on people, researchers in the Food Science Department at Louisiana State University (LSU) made flour from fenugreek seeds, baked up a batch of fenugreek bread, and fed two slices a day to eight people with type 2 diabetes. The bread lowered *insulin resistance*—the inability of cells to use the hormone insulin. Another demonstration, said the researchers in the *Journal of Medicinal Food*, that fenugreek "will reduce insulin resistance and treat type 2 diabetes."

In another recent study, this one in the

Fenugreek seed may help prevent and/or treat:

Cancer	Infection, bacterial and viral
Cataracts	
Cholesterol problems (high total cholesterol, high "bad" LDL cholesterol, low "good" HDL cholesterol)	Insulin resistance (prediabetes)
	Kidney stones
	Liver disease
	Overweight
Diabetes, type 2	Triglycerides, high
Gallstones	

International Journal of Vitamin and Nutrition Research, scientists studied 18 people with type 2 diabetes, feeding them powdered fenugreek seeds in either yogurt or hot water. After two months, there was a 25 percent decrease in fasting blood sugar, a 30 percent decrease in triglycerides, and a 30 percent decrease in "bad" LDL cholesterol. "Fenugreek seeds can be used . . . in the control of type 2 diabetes," the researchers concluded.

In China, researchers studied 69 people with type 2 diabetes that wasn't well-controlled with a standard diabetes drug. They divided them into two groups—one group continued taking the drug; one group took the drug *and* fenugreek seeds. After three months, those taking the drug and fenugreek had "remarkable" results, said the researchers: much lower fasting blood sugar, lower blood sugar levels after meals, lower A1C, and fewer symptoms of diabetes (such as fatigue). The combined therapy of an anti-diabetes drug and fenugreek "could lower blood glucose and ameliorate clinical symptoms in the treatment of type 2 diabetes," said the researchers in the *Chinese Journal of Integrative Medicine*.

Indian researchers gave 60 people with type 2 diabetes a mixture that included fenugreek seeds. After three months, many in the study had either lowered their dose of glucose-controlling medication or gotten off the medication completely.

In another study from India, doctors at the Jaipur Diabetes and Research Centre studied 25 people newly diagnosed with diabetes, dividing them into two groups. Half received an extract of fenugreek seeds and half were treated with diet and exercise. After two months, those on the fenugreek had more normal levels of glucose and insulin, a bigger drop in triglycerides, and a bigger increase in HDL. "Use of fenugreek seeds improves glycemic control and decreases insulin resistance in mild type-2 diabetic patients," the researchers concluded.

Why is fenugreek so effective in controlling type 2 diabetes? "Fenugreek stimulates the insulin signaling pathway," said the researchers from LSU. In other words, it helps cells respond to the hormone that moves glucose out of the blood, said the researchers. Fenugreek also stimulates insulin secretion from the pancreas, slows the absorption of glucose from the intestines, and helps generate enzymes that regulate the use of glucose for energy in muscle cells. And, they note, "fenugreek is very safe."

Fenugreek: Multi-Tasking Natural Medicine

The LSU scientists point out that "fenugreek has other beneficial effects in addition to its effect on diabetes"—including stopping kidney stones, helping with weight loss, and controlling fatty liver disease. Let's look at these and other benefits of the spice.

Weight loss. Researchers from the University of Minnesota studied 18 obese people (body mass index over 30), dividing them into three groups: at breakfast, one group took four grams of fenugreek fiber powder with orange juice, one took eight grams, and one didn't take any. Between breakfast and lunch, the group taking eight grams of powder had a greater feeling of fullness, felt more satisfied (satiety), and felt less hungry—*and* they ate 10 percent fewer calories for lunch! "Fenugreek fiber may have a role in the control of food intake in obese individuals," said the researchers in *Phytotherapy Research*.

Fenugreek fiber powder—also called *galacto-mannan*—is widely available as a supplement.

In another experiment on fenugreek and food consumption, French researchers found that people taking fenugreek seed extract (about 600 mg a day) ate 17 percent less fat and 12 percent fewer calories. Fenugreek seed extract might help with "weight reduction in the long term, particularly in some . . . overweight or obese patients for whom a low-fat diet is recommended," the researchers concluded in the *European Journal of Clinical Pharmacology*.

Cancer. In a paper called "Fenugreek: A Naturally Occurring Edible Spice as an Anti-cancer Agent," scientists at the Sidney Kimmel Comprehensive Cancer Center at Johns Hopkins University discuss how their studies have shown fenugreek seed extract can slow or stop the growth of breast, pancreatic, and prostate cancer cells. "These studies add another biologically active agent to our armamentarium of naturally occurring agents with therapeutic potential," said the scientists in *Cancer Biology and Therapy*.

High cholesterol. Fenugreek doesn't just lower cholesterol in people with type 2 diabetes. Indian doctors studied 20 healthy people, dividing them into two groups—one took fenugreek seed powder and one didn't. After one month, there was a "significant reduction in total cholesterol and LDL levels," wrote the researchers in *Plant Foods in Human Nutrition*.

Fatty liver disease. An estimated one-third of Americans have *non-alcoholic fatty liver disease* (NAFLD): at least 20 percent of liver cells are filled with fat globules. The causes: overweight, insulin resistance, and diabetes. Another 10 million Americans have *alcoholic fatty liver disease*, caused by heavy drinking (more than two drinks a day for a woman and more than three drinks a day for a man). Fatty liver can progress to cirrhosis and liver cancer. In an animal study, Canadian researchers found that fenugreek seeds prevented or reversed fatty liver. "These findings . . . provide a strong impetus to explore the therapeutic benefit of fenugreek and its active com-ponents in [fatty liver disease] associated with obesity and insulin resistance," the researchers said in the *International Journal of Obesity*.

Cataracts. Researchers in India used a chemical to induce cataracts in the eyes of two groups of experimental animals—one that was fed fenugreek seeds and one that wasn't. Fenugreek seed *completely prevented* the development of cataracts; 72 percent of the animals not eating fenugreek developed the disease. The researchers found a high level of antioxidant activity in the eyes of the fenugreek-fed animals.

Kidney stones. Eighty percent of kidney stones are made of calcium oxalate. Noting that fenugreek seeds are "widely used in Morocco" to prevent the development of kidney stones in those prone to form them, Moroccan researchers tested the seeds on experimental animals. Fenugreek decreased the deposition of calcium oxalate in the kidney by 27 percent.

Gallstones. Researchers in India induced gallstones in experimental animals and then divided them into three groups: one group received a high dose of fenugreek seed powder, one group received a low dose, and one didn't receive any powder. Fenugreek reversed gallstones by 64 percent in the high dose group and 61 percent in the low dose; there was no reversal in the other group. Fenugreek could help prevent gallstones, shrink ones that already exist, and prevent recurrence, the researchers concluded.

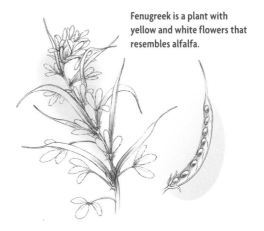

Fenugreek is a plant with yellow and white flowers that resembles alfalfa.

Fenugreek seed pairs well with these spices:

Asafoetida	Clove	Mustard seed
Black cumin seed	Coriander	Onion
	Curry leaf	Star anise
Black pepper	Garlic	Tamarind
Chile	Ginger	Turmeric

and complements recipes featuring:

Bread	Pickles	Tomatoes
Chutney	Potatoes	Vegetables

Caution: Pregnant women should not eat fenugreek seeds, because they contain *saponins*, an active compound that is found in oral contraceptives. Research indicates that fenugreek could induce a miscarriage.

Other recipes containing fenugreek seed:

Berbere (p. 267)	Toasted Almonds (p. 29)
Caribbean Curry Paste (p. 287)	Hot Curry Powder (p. 284)
Colombo Powder (p. 270)	Panch Phoron (p. 266)
Garbanzo Beans with Mushrooms and	Sambaar Masala (p. 265)

Infections. Researchers in India fed experimental animals a fenugreek extract and tested their immune systems. They found the spice increased the activity of *macrophages*, white blood cells that gobble up bacteria and viruses. "Overall, fenugreek showed a stimulatory effect on immune functions," they wrote, a result that "strengthens the rationale of its use in several Ayurvedic drugs."

Getting to Know Fenugreek Seed

Fenugreek—known to botanists as *Trigonella foenum-graecum*—is a plant with yellow and white flowers that resembles alfalfa. In fact, its Latin name means "Greek hay," and it was grown by the ancient Egyptians as fodder for animals. Today, fenugreek is grown around the world—in South Asia, the Middle East, South America, Europe, and China.

As a spice, fenugreek is popular in India, Egypt, Saudi Arabia, Armenia, Iran, and Turkey, where it is used to make curries, chutneys, pickles, relishes, and an array of vegetarian dishes.

In India, the seeds are dry roasted or fried in hot oil and used whole to flavor curries (especially fish curry), broth-based stews called *sambars*, and fermented flat breads, such as *dosas* and *idlis*. It is also an ingredient in many Indian spice mixes, including curry powder. A few fenugreek seeds are always added to starchy vegetables and hard-to-digest legumes, especially if asafoetida is not available.

In the Middle East, seeds are soaked overnight in cold water and mixed into a paste with other spices to make a condiment called *hilbeh* and a sweetmeat called *halva*. Cooks also grind fenugreek into a paste and rub it into salted meat, which is then dried.

In Yemen, fenugreek is mixed with other spices to make *zhug*, which is put on top of stews. Armenians mix it with garlic and red chile to make a peppery spice mix called *chemen*, which is used to spice beef. The Greeks boil the seeds and eat them with honey.

How to Buy Fenugreek Seed

Fenugreek seeds are hard, yellowish-brown ovals that resemble tiny pebbles. You can recognize them by the deep furrow across one side. They are sold whole or ground in Indian markets. Fenugreek is also available in specialty spice shops and online, usually ground. (To find whole seeds, see the "Buyer's Guide" on page 309.)

In terms of quality, one batch of fenugreek seeds is pretty much like another. But double-check for cleanliness. Because the seeds *look* like stones, it's not uncommon to find them contaminated with little stones and grit. Examine them

Brussels Sprouts Kulambu

Kulambu is a sweet-and-sour stew popular in India. This authentic Indian recipe, courtesy of Alamelu Vairavan's Healthy South Indian Cooking, is a vegetarian entree to be served over rice. You can also serve it as a side dish to a roast. Check the "Buyer's Guide" section to find some of the more unusual ingredients.

2 tablespoons canola oil
¼ teaspoon asafoetida powder
4 to 6 curry leaves (optional)
½ teaspoon fenugreek seeds
1 teaspoon black mustard seeds
1 teaspoon *urad dal* (split white lentils)
½ cup chopped onion
½ cup chopped tomato
¼ teaspoon turmeric
2 teaspoons *sambaar masala* (p. 265) or
  commercial curry powder
1 cup tomato sauce
1 teaspoon salt
¼ teaspoon tamarind paste
1½ cups brussels sprouts, cut in half (if large, cut
  into quarters)

1. Place oil in a saucepan over medium heat. When the oil is hot, but not smoking, add the asafoetida powder, curry leaves, fenugreek seeds, mustard seeds, and urad dal. Cover and fry over medium heat until the mustard seeds pop and urad dal is golden brown, about 30 seconds.
2. Add the onions, tomato, and turmeric, stirring constantly.
3. Add the sambaar masala, tomato sauce, and salt. Stir well. Add 2 cups of warm water to the saucepan. Stir and cook for a few minutes.
4. Add tamarind paste and mix thoroughly.
5. When the mixture in the saucepan begins to boil, add the brussels sprouts. Cover and cook over low heat until the brussels sprouts are just tender, about 10 minutes. Be careful not to overcook.

Makes 4 servings.

---

carefully before putting them in your grinder so you don't damage it.

Whole seeds stay fresh for three years, as long as they're kept in an airtight container and out of sunlight. Fenugreek's flavor dissipates once the seeds are ground, and ground seeds keep for only a few months.

In the Kitchen with Fenugreek Seed

Don't eat fenugreek seeds raw—hard as a rock, they're impossible to chew. Cooking turns their pungent, slightly bitter taste into a nutty, maple syrup-like flavor. It also softens the seed, so it's easier to grind. A light roasting of a minute or two is all that's needed. (For directions on how to roast spices, see page 11.) Be careful, however, not to burn the seeds, which makes the flavor so bitter it's unpalatable. You can also soak the seeds overnight to make them soft and jelly-like.

Add fenugreek to a dish *cautiously*—the strong flavor can overtake other flavorings.

Here are some ways to get more fenugreek into your diet:

- Add a sprinkling of ground seeds to the breading for fried foods.
- Sprinkle a few seeds in vegetable casseroles.
- Add a pinch of ground fenugreek to cookie recipes.
- Add a pinch or two to mayonnaise to give it a mustard-like bite.
- Mix roasted ground seeds with dried, ground chiles and other spices, and use as a dipping sauce for bread.
- Add roasted and coarsely chopped seeds to salads, which adds an interesting crunchiness.

GALANGAL *Better Health, Courtesy of Thailand*

If you enjoy Thai food, then you know galangal, even if you've never heard of it. This knobby root, a relative of ginger, is to Thai cooking what the chile is to Mexican cooking. Thai food wouldn't taste "Thai" without it.

While the Chinese favor ginger, Thais prefer the taste of galangal, which is ginger-like—but with a sinus-penetrating, spicy-hot sensation. Its unique "mouth feel" has been likened to the quick heat of a chile without the lingering aftermath.

Though galangal is virtually unheard of in the Western world, people in Thailand, Indonesia, and other parts of Southeast Asia have been relying on it for centuries—and not only as a culinary spice. In Asia, galangal is actually *better* known as a medicine. Traditional healers have used it to treat arthritis, skin problems, digestive ills, diabetes, and even cancer.

Easing Arthritis
Galangal's therapeutic powers come from a unique set of anti-inflammatory compounds known as *galangal acetate*. So it's no surprise that it might be effective against a common inflammatory disease—arthritis.

Researchers at the University of Miami studied 261 people with "moderate to severe" pain from knee osteoarthritis, giving them either a ginger/galangal formula or a placebo. After six weeks, those taking ginger/galangal had less knee pain on standing, less knee pain after walking, were taking less medicine for acute pain from arthritis, had less stiffness, and could function better during the day. The findings were in the journal *Arthritis and Rheumatism*.

In another study, researchers from Johns Hopkins University tested the power of a ginger/galangal formula on *synoviocytes*, the cells of the lubricating synovial fluid inside the joint. They found the formula decreased the production of *chemokines*, one of the components of the immune system that powers inflammation. "This formulation may be useful for suppressing inflammation due to arthritis," concluded the researchers in the *Journal of Alternative and Complementary Medicine*.

Researchers in Thailand tested an extract of galangal on *chondrocytes*—the cells in cartilage, the part of the joint that erodes in arthritis, causing bone-on-bone pain. The extract boosted the release of three compounds linked to stronger, healthier cartilage (hyaluronan, glycosaminoglycans, and metalloproteinases). An extract of galangal is "a potential therapeutic agent for treatment of osteoarthritis," the researchers concluded in *Phytochemistry*.

Rooting Out Cancer
Scientists from around the world—including myself and my colleagues at M.D. Anderson Cancer Center—are investigating galangal as a cancer-fighter.

In my laboratory, we found that a compound in galangal—*acetoxychavicol acetate* (ACA)—turned off cancer genes, limiting the cellular growth of breast, skin, lung, and blood cancer.

Japanese researchers found that a galangal extract prevented skin cancer in laboratory ani-

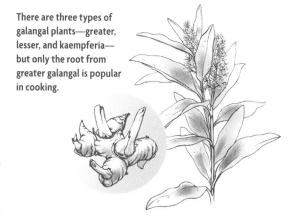

There are three types of galangal plants—greater, lesser, and kaempferia—but only the root from greater galangal is popular in cooking.

mals. "Galangal may have potential importance for cancer chemoprevention [prevention by a natural compound]," the researchers concluded in the *Journal of Natural Medicine.*

Neuroblastoma is a childhood cancer. In the laboratory, Taiwanese researchers found that a galangal extract killed neuroblastoma cells. Galangal "may be useful for the treatment of patients with neuroblastoma," the researchers concluded in *Anticancer Research.*

Researchers in Thailand wondered why the inhabitants of that country had a *high* rate of infection with *Helicobacter pylori* (HP)—a bacteria that lives in the stomach and that can cause stomach ulcers and stomach cancer—but a *low* rate of stomach cancer, compared to other developing countries where HP infection is also common. They found that several plants and spices used in Thai cuisine and medicine—including galangal—are powerful inhibitors of HP.

In England, researchers found that an extract of galangal triggered enzymes that help cells rid themselves of carcinogens, and that it also killed breast and lung cancer cells. "This dual action is quite rare among traditional anti-cancer medicines," said Peter Houghton, PhD, the study leader. "Normally, extracts are able to boost healthy cells' natural defenses against cancer *or* kill cancer cells—but galangal seems to do both."

More Protection from Galangal
Other diseases that galangal might help prevent and/or treat include:

Diabetes. Researchers in Pakistan found that galangal powder lowered blood sugar (glucose) levels in laboratory animals as effectively as the diabetes drug gliclazide (Diamicron). They theorize that antioxidants in the spice stimulate the pancreas to release more insulin, the glucose-lowering hormone.

Ulcers. Japanese researchers found that galangal "completely inhibited" stomach ulcers in experimental animals, and did it better than three anti-ulcer drugs: omeprazole (Prilosec),

Galangal may help prevent and/or treat:

Allergies	Osteoarthritis
Cancer	Ulcer
Diabetes, type 2	

Galangal pairs well with these spices:

Allspice	Fenugreek seed
Black cumin seed	Garlic
Cardamom	Lemongrass
Chile	Mustard seed
Cinnamon	Onion
Clove	Tamarind
Coconut	Turmeric
Coriander	

and complements recipes featuring:

Asian stir-fries	Sambals
Chicken	Soups
Curry blends	Stews

Other recipes containing galangal:

Ras-el-hanout (p. 266)	Thai Red Curry Paste (p. 286)

cimetidine (Tagamet), and cetraxate hydrochloride (Zydis).

Allergies. Researchers in Japan found that a galangal extract hampered the cellular process that causes allergic symptoms such as nasal congestion.

Getting to Know Galangal
There are three types of galangal plants—greater, lesser, and kaempferia—but only the root from greater galangal is popular in cooking. That's because greater galangal is the mildest of the three. Lesser and kaempferia have an abrasive

Thai Coconut Chicken Soup

This soup is called tom kha kai *in Thailand (kha meaning galangal) and it is one of the country's national dishes. It is found on the menu of most Thai restaurants. The Thai ingredients can be found in Asian markets.*

2 cups coconut milk
1 two-inch piece galangal, cut into thin slices, or 1 tablespoon galangal (Laos) powder
2 stalks lemongrass, cut into 1" pieces
5 fresh kaffir (lime) leaves, chopped
1 pound boned chicken breast, thinly sliced
1 cup chicken stock
2 teaspoons diced fresh red chiles
¼ cup Asian fish sauce
2 tablespoons sugar
½ cup lime juice
1 teaspoon black chili paste
½ cup cilantro, chopped

1. Combine 1 cup of coconut milk, the galangal, lemongrass, and kaffir leaves in a large saucepan and bring to a simmer.
2. Add the chicken, stock, chiles, fish sauce, and sugar. Simmer for 10 minutes or until the chicken is cooked through.
3. Add the remaining coconut milk and heat just to a boil but don't let it boil. Stir in the lime juice and chili paste and simmer a few minutes. Serve sprinkled with the cilantro.

Makes 4 servings.

flavor, and are used more for medicinal purposes than for cooking.

Greater galangal is used abundantly in the cuisines of Thailand, Malaysia, Vietnam, Singapore, Cambodia, and Indonesia, in curries, soups, stir-fries, and rice dishes. It is used fresh or powdered in most Thai recipes, where it's the key ingredient in red and green curry pastes, and in the renowned coconut chicken soup called *tom kha gai*. (*Kha* means galangal in Thai.) It is also a key ingredient in Indonesian fiery-hot *rendangs*, meat-and-coconut slow-cooked stews served on festive occasions.

Galangal's warming effect make it the perfect ingredient for imparting the mouth feel of alcohol to low-alcohol and alcohol-free beverages. In a taste test, when galangal was added to a 40-proof alcoholic beverage, the alcohol level was perceived to be greater than 60-proof. In another taste test, it made an alcohol-free beverage taste just like an alcohol-containing drink.

Native to Java, the galangal plant—about six feet tall, with pretty greenish-white, orchid-shaped flowers—is grown in many Southeast Asian countries, including Thailand, Indonesia, and the Philippines, and in China and India. It also goes by the names of galingale, galanga, callangall, and Thai ginger.

How to Buy Galangal

Galangal looks like a giant version of its well-known cousin ginger, but it's much more fibrous and dense. You can purchase it fresh, frozen, canned, pickled, or dried; whole, in slices, or pulverized into a powder—though it's next to impossible to find it in *any* of these forms except in an Asian market, or online through a Web site specializing in Thai foodstuffs.

When buying fresh galangal, buy it *young*. The young root provides optimum flavor and texture, and is the easiest to slice and work with. Young galangal has yellowish-brown skin with reddish-brown hues and a creamy beige interior. Look for a root that is firm, with smooth skin. Wrinkled skin is a sign of age.

Fresh galangal isn't very perishable, so you can purchase it online. Put it in the refrigerator, wrapped in plastic, where it will keep for about two weeks. (Frozen, it keeps for about two months.)

Dried galangal usually comes in a package of chunks that look like old pieces of wood. It's *very* hard: soak it in boiling water for 20 to 30 minutes before using. Dried galangal will keep for years, as long as it's protected from moisture and heat.

If you're unaccustomed to working with galangal, your best bet is to buy a powder. It's often sold by the name *Laos powder*. But be careful when you cook with it! Powdered galangal is stronger than fresh, and it can really punish your sinuses if you get too close and take a sniff. Use half the amount of powder as you would fresh galangal. The powder keeps for about a year.

In the Kitchen with Galangal

By itself, galangal isn't much to look at and offers little taste. But once it's added to other spices and ingredients in a dish, it produces a flavor that is hard to match.

Thai cooks use it unpeeled and thinly sliced in dishes. If you find this unattractive, you can scrape or cut off the skin. You can also finely grate it.

Use galangal much the same way you'd use ginger in curries, stews, and soups. It offers a unique spicy taste to mayonnaise, sour cream, and ketchup. Just be careful not to overdo it, as it can take on a medicinal flavor.

Experts differ on whether or not ginger is a good substitute for galangal in a recipe. It doesn't offer the same flavor, but because both flavors are distinct, I prefer substituting ginger rather than omitting galangal totally from the recipe.

GARLIC   *Strong Enough to Battle Heart Disease*

When scientists in England entered the words "diet" and "anti-aging" into the search engine of a medical database, up popped studies on garlic—study after study after study.

"The accumulated knowledge over the last few years suggests that intake of garlic by humans may either prevent or decrease the incidence of major chronic diseases associated with old age, such as atherosclerosis, stroke, cancer, immune disorders, cerebral [brain] aging, arthritis, and cataract formation," concluded the researchers.

That's a powerful statement for a spice popularly called "the stinking rose." But garlic works *because* it "stinks"—its explosive aroma is based on its most active ingredient, *allicin*, which transforms into *organosulfurs*, and those are the very compounds that minimize the oxidation, inflammation, and other cell-destroying processes underlying every one of the "major chronic diseases" on the researchers' list. In addition, garlic is brimming with vitamins, minerals, and other powerful antioxidants that guard against heart disease and cancer.

In short, garlic is one of the world's most potent natural medicines. The medical database of the National Institutes of Health contains more than 3,200 studies on the therapeutic power of garlic. Many of those studies are about preventing, slowing, and reversing *cardiovascular disease*— the heart attacks and strokes that kill more Americans than any other health problem.

Help for Your Heart

Back in 3000 BCE, Charak, the father of India's Ayurvedic medicine, claimed that garlic "strengthens the heart and keeps blood fluid."

Here in 2010, a team of medical researchers reviewed what they called the "vast scientific literature" about garlic and heart disease, and declared, "Garlic consumption has a significant protective effect against atherosclerosis."

And when a team of researchers analyzed the garlic-rich Mediterranean diet—often equated

Masking Garlic Breath

Garlic's reputation for being a strong spice is well deserved. Even though it mellows when it is cooked, your garlic dinner can "hang around" for days. This is especially true if you eat it raw.

If you or others in your company are offended by the lingering smell of garlic, here are a few tried-and-true home remedies to diminish the odor:

• Drink red wine with your garlic meal.
• Add parsley to garlicky dishes.
• Chew on fresh parsley sprigs at the end of the meal.
• Chew a few roasted fennel, anise, or cardamom seeds.

To get the smell of garlic out of your hands after working with it:

• Wash your hands with water and lemon juice.
• Rub your hands with a stainless steel spoon, then wash both your hands and the spoon.
• Moisten your hands and rub baking soda between your palms.

with heart health—they figured out that if everybody ate one or two garlic cloves a day, the worldwide risk of heart disease would drop by 25 percent. (But you don't have to eat fresh cloves to get an effect. Many studies show that dried or powdered garlic is *more* therapeutic than fresh.) Let's look at all the ways garlic can help your heart.

Lower blood pressure. High blood pressure is a major risk factor for heart attacks and strokes. In a recent "meta-analysis" of 11 studies on garlic supplements and high blood pressure, garlic lowered systolic blood pressure (the upper number in the reading) by an average of 8.4 mm Hg and diastolic blood pressure (the lower number) by an average of 7.3 mm Hg—*very* significant decreases. "Garlic preparations are superior to placebo in reducing blood pressure in indi-

viduals with hypertension," the researchers concluded in *BMC Cardiovascular Disorders*.

In a study from Poland, researchers found that garlic supplements not only lowered blood pressure, but also prevented DNA damage from oxidation. "These findings point out the beneficial effects of garlic supplementation in reducing blood pressure and counteracting oxidative stress, and thereby offering cardioprotection in hypertensives," concluded the researchers in *Molecular and Cellular Biochemistry*.

Thinner blood. People take baby aspirin to help prevent heart attacks because it "thins" the blood, reducing the risk of artery-plugging blood clots. Specifically, aspirin reduces the stickiness of *platelets*, blood compounds that can clump together to form a clot, a process called *platelet aggregation*. Garlic can thin blood, too.

Researchers in England gave people daily supplements of aged garlic extract for 13 weeks, measuring their levels of platelet aggregation at the beginning and end of the study. The garlic supplements "significantly inhibited" the percentage of platelets that were aggregating and the speed at which they were aggregating. Aged garlic extract "may be beneficial in protecting against cardiovascular disease as a result of inhibiting platelet aggregation," the researchers concluded in the *Journal of Nutrition*.

Lower total cholesterol. Okay, garlic *doesn't* lower "bad" LDL cholesterol. At least that was the result of a recent and much-publicized six-month study conducted by researchers at Stanford Prevention Research Center, who gave nearly 200 people with high LDL a daily dose of either raw garlic, powdered garlic supplement, aged garlic extract, or a placebo. "None of the forms of garlic used in the study had clinically significant effects on LDL," concluded the researchers in the *Archives of Internal Medicine*.

But when researchers at the University of Connecticut analyzed this *and* 28 other studies on garlic and cholesterol in a meta-analysis, they reached a more positive conclusion. Garlic, they found, significantly reduced total cholesterol and triglycerides (another heart-hurting blood fat), even though it had no effect on "bad" LDL or "good" HDL.

Less artery-clogging plaque. Year by year, *plaque* can build up inside arteries, narrowing the passageway—and a chunk of that plaque can break off, clog the artery, and trigger a heart attack or stroke. That plaque-accumulating process is called *atherosclerosis*—and garlic can stop, slow, or reverse it.

Research in the Division of Cardiology at UCLA gave 23 people with heart disease a daily supplement containing aged garlic extract. After one year, those taking the placebo had *triple* the rate of plaque progression as those taking garlic. In another year-long study by the same researchers, involving a supplement

DURING THE MIDDLE AGES,
GARLIC WAS HUNG ON
DOORS AT NIGHT TO REPEL
EVIL SPIRITS.

containing aged garlic extract, B-vitamins and an artery-nourishing amino acid, the progression of plaque was "significantly lower" in those taking garlic. Aged garlic extract therapy, with additional nutrients, "reduced progression of atherosclerosis," the researchers concluded in *Preventive Medicine*.

And in a German study, 142 people took garlic powder tablets daily. After four years, they had 5 to 18 percent *less* plaque in their arteries. "Not only a preventive but possibly also a curative

Elephant Garlic: A Big Mistake

If you come across elephant garlic at the market, there's no reason to think you've stumbled upon something special. You haven't, if *garlic* is what you're looking for. Elephant garlic only *looks* like garlic—huge garlic, weighing up to a pound. But it doesn't have anything like the flavor of garlic, and cooks consider it inferior. In fact, elephant garlic is botanically related to a leek and should be used like a leek: braised or baked like a vegetable or sliced into a salad.

role in atherosclerosis therapy may be ascribed to garlic," wrote the researchers in the medical journal *Atherosclerosis*.

More flexible arteries. The lining of the artery is called the *endothelium*, and it generates a compound (nitric oxide) that relaxes and widens the blood vessel. Researchers in New Zealand gave 15 men with heart disease either a garlic supplement or a placebo. After two weeks, the "endothelium-dependent dilation" of the arteries of those taking garlic had increased by 44 percent. And those men were *already* taking aspirin and a statin.

Lower risk of heart attack. Russian researchers gave either a garlic supplement or a placebo to 51 people with heart disease. A year later, they calculated the supplement had reduced the risk of a heart attack by an average of 40 percent.

Colon Cancer Is No Match for Garlic

There are more than 600 scientific studies—in cells, on animals, and in people—on the power of garlic to prevent and treat cancer. Some highlights:

Preventing colon cancer. In a meta-analysis of 18 studies by researchers at the Washington University School of Medicine in St. Louis, people with the highest consumption of garlic had a 41 percent lower risk of colon cancer, compared to those with the lowest intake.

Stopping the advance of early colon cancer. Japanese researchers studied 51 people with colorectal adenomas—pre-cancerous lesions of the colon. They divided them into two groups, giving one group aged garlic extract and one group placebos. After one year, those on the placebo had *more* adenomas, and garlic had "significantly suppressed both the size and number of colon adenomas," wrote the researchers in the *Journal of Nutrition.*

Preventing stomach cancer. Researchers in China studied more than 5,000 people, giving half a high-dose garlic supplement and half a placebo. After five years, those taking garlic had a 47 percent lower rate of stomach cancer.

Preventing endometrial cancer. Researchers in Italy analyzed diet and health data from 454 women with endometrial cancer and 908 free of the disease—and found that those who ate the most garlic were 38 percent less likely to develop endometrial cancer than those who ate the least.

Preventing other cancers. Other studies show a link between increased intake of garlic and decreased risk for lung cancer (22 percent less), prostate cancer (36 percent less), and brain cancer (34 percent less).

How does garlic work to block cancer? Doctors from the International Agency for Research on Cancer say garlic can help:

- stop carcinogens from damaging DNA.
- boost the activity of enzymes that detoxify carcinogens.
- clean up free radicals—cell-damaging, cancer-causing molecules.

Fighting Infection

Garlic has a storied history as an infection-fighter. Louis Pasteur discovered its antibacterial activity. It was on the frontlines in World War I, helping prevent gangrene and blood poisoning. The Russians relied on it so heavily during World War II that it was dubbed "Russian penicillin." And several recent studies confirm its power to fight bacteria and viruses.

Preventing airborne infection. Finnish researchers studied 52 airplane travelers, giving half a garlic-containing nasal spray (Nasaleze Travel) and half a placebo. Those taking the placebo had nearly three times more infections after traveling.

Preventing colds. Researchers in England studied 146 people from November to February, giving half a garlic supplement and half a placebo. In total, those taking the placebo had 65 colds, compared to 24 for those taking garlic.

And Russian researchers studied 600 children, aged 7 to 16, giving some a garlic supplement and some a placebo. Those taking the placebo had four times as many colds.

I recommend a clove of garlic a day to help reduce your risk of cold or flu—and for general good health.

Garlic Galore

There are many other possible benefits to a garlic-rich life:

Diabetes. Researchers in Russia studied 60 people with type 2 diabetes, dividing them into two groups—one received garlic supplements with timed-release garlic powder and the other a placebo. After one month, those taking garlic

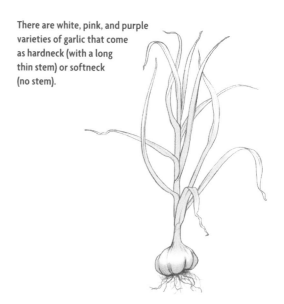

There are white, pink, and purple varieties of garlic that come as hardneck (with a long thin stem) or softneck (no stem).

had a healthy drop in fasting blood sugar, from 138 mg/dL to 113 mg/dL.

Prostate problems. Researchers in Italy studied more than 1,800 men and found that those who ate the most garlic were 28 percent less likely to develop *benign prostatic hypertrophy*—the enlarged prostate that causes urinary difficulties in older men.

Aging skin. German researchers found that taking garlic powder boosted blood flow to the skin—a must for a youthful, glowing complexion.

Oral candidiasis. Researchers in India found that garlic paste was just as effective as a conventional drug in clearing up oral candidiasis (thrush), a yeast infection of the mucous membranes of the mouth.

Sickle cell anemia. Researchers at the UCLA School of Medicine found that four weeks of supplementation with garlic extract decreased by 30 percent the number of damaged red blood cells that are characteristic of this disease.

Alopecia areata. In this disease of patchy hair loss, adding garlic gel to the standard treatment regimen improved results.

Getting to Know Garlic

As medicine and food, garlic goes way back. It was featured in ancient medical textbooks from Egypt, India, China, Greece, and Rome. The ancient Egyptians fed it to the slaves who built the pyramids, and it was part of the diet of Olympic athletes in ancient Greece. During the Middle Ages, people put it on their door at night to repel evil spirits.

Today, garlic flavors virtually every cuisine in the world—and it's the signature spice in the cuisines of Mexico, India, Asia, Greece, and Italy.

Garlic is synonymous with Italian cuisine and goes in just about every savory dish. Well-known Italian-based garlic sauces include *pesto*, which also features basil and olive oil, and *gremolata*, which also contains parsley, and is traditionally served with the famous slow-cooked veal shank called *osso bucco*.

Garlic may help prevent and/or treat:

Aging	Flu
Alopecia areata (generalized hair loss)	Heart disease
	High blood pressure (hypertension)
Benign prostatic hypertrophy	Sickle cell disease
Blood clots	Stroke
Cancer	Thrush (oral candida infection)
Cholesterol problems (high total cholesterol)	Triglycerides, high
Colds	Wrinkles and aging skin
Diabetes, type 2	

Garlic pairs well with virtually *all* spices, but particularly well with:

Ajowan	Marjoram
Basil	Mint
Caraway	Mustard seed
Chile	Oregano
Coriander	Parsley
Cumin	Rosemary
Curry leaf	Sun-dried tomato
Kokam	Thyme

and complements virtually *all* savory dishes, especially:

Marinades	Spice blends
Lamb	Stir-fries
Soups	

The French aren't known for garlicky food, but they have three famous garlic sauces: *Aioli* is a garlic mayonnaise used in enrich fish soups and flavor vegetables; *pistou* is the French version of *pesto* and goes in a vegetable soup by the same name; and *rouille* is a garlic, red pepper, and saffron-based mayonnaise that is stirred into bouillabaisse, bourrides, and other fish stews and soups. *Persillade* is a French-inspired garlic sauce used in Louisiana cooking.

The Greeks enjoy *skordalia*, a garlic sauce made from almonds, olive oil, and soaked bread that is served with salt cod or as a dip. In Serbia, people consume garlic as a snack with *slivovitz*, a strong plum brandy.

Garlic is also a key ingredient in the popular Middle Eastern side dish *hummus*, which also includes chickpeas, olive oil, and pine nuts. It is also an ingredient in Tunisia's infamous fiery condiment *harissa*, and in the Moroccan meat marinade *chermoula*. *Cacik* is a Turkish garlic sauce based on yogurt and olive oil, and served as a side dish.

Thai cuisine is loaded with garlic—virtually no savory dish is made without it.

How to Buy Garlic

The taste of fresh garlic ranges from mild and sweet to strong and pungent, depending on the type of garlic and where it was cultivated. There are white, pink, and purple varieties that come as hardneck (with a long thin stem) or softneck (no stem). Hardneck is the most pungent.

Ninety percent of the garlic sold in the United States is softneck white, and comes from California. Its taste is strong and pungent. All garlic, however, mellows when cooked, turning mild to slightly sweet.

According to top chefs, the best garlic comes from France, with a taste and aroma very different from California garlic. If you come across French garlic, it's well worth trying. You can recognize it by its pink-tinged skin. Other varieties of note include Prussian white and Spanish red (*roja*).

For the best flavor, buy fresh bulbs. They vary in size, containing anywhere from a few cloves to two dozen. When it comes to taste, however, size doesn't matter—taste is determined by the *freshness* of the bulb. For maximum freshness, look for bulbs that are plump, dry, and don't have broken skin. Buying bulbs with large cloves makes working with them in the kitchen easier.

You can also purchase fresh garlic in a jar

Other recipes containing garlic:

Adobo (p. 270)

All-American Chili con Carne (p. 110)

Basic Barbecue Rub (p. 272)

Berbere (p. 267)

Boeuf Bourguignon (p. 240)

By-the-Bay Fisherman's Chowder (p. 46)

Caribbean Curry Paste (p. 287)

Chicken Oreganata (p. 186)

Chimichurri Sauce (p. 190)

French Onion Soup (p. 181)

Garbanzo Beans with Mushrooms and Toasted Almonds (p. 29)

Green Pumpkin Seed Sauce (p. 200)

Grilled Lamb Patty Pockets with Cucumber Mint Sauce (p. 165)

Grilled Pork Chile Adobo (p. 78)

Hungarian Goulash (p. 61)

Jamaican Jerk Marinade (p. 269)

Madras Beef Curry (p. 106)

Madras Curry Paste (p. 286)

Malaysian Curry Paste (p. 287)

Mediterranean Vinaigrette (p. 160)

Mussels with Thai Red Curry Sauce (p. 156)

Onion and Tomato Chutney (p. 113)

Penne and Sausage with Fennel Tomato Sauce (p. 117)

Pizza Spice Blend (p. 272)

Pomegranate Guacamole (p. 197)

Potato Cauliflower Curry (p. 252)

Prawns with Almond Hot Pepper Sauce (p. 26)

Shellfish in Saffron Broth (p. 211)

Sol Kadhi (p. 152)

Spaghettini with Basil-Tomato Sauce (p. 42)

Spicy Hash Brown Potatoes (p. 151)

Tabil (p. 267)

Tamarind Sauce (p. 236)

Thai Red Curry Paste (p. 286)

Yucatan Pickled Red Onions (p. 21)

preserved in liquid, crushed, sliced, minced, chopped, or in a tube.

Dried garlic comes powdered, granulated, flaked, ground, minced, or chopped. You can also find garlic salt and garlic juice.

You can find just about any type of garlic in most supermarkets.

Store fresh garlic uncovered, in a cool place away from heat and direct sunlight. It shouldn't be refrigerated; it will sprout. You can also freeze fresh garlic, although that alters the taste and texture somewhat.

Untouched, fresh bulbs keep for about two weeks. Once you break open a bulb, you reduce its shelf life to about a week. Once it starts to sprout, throw it out, because sprouted garlic turns bitter when cooked.

Before they sprout, garlic cloves start to turn green. Always cut away any green (or any discoloration) on the cloves. For the best flavor, use only white flesh.

Store dried garlic, garlic powder, and garlic salt in an airtight container in a dark, cool place. Dried garlic should keep for about a year, and garlic salt will keep for several years. But when powder or salt start to clump, they've absorbed moisture; throw them away.

If you don't get garlic regularly in your diet, consider taking garlic supplements, especially if you have one or more risk factors for heart disease, such as high blood pressure, high cholesterol, overweight, diabetes, or you're over 65. The most-studied form is aged garlic extract. Follow the dosage recommendations on the label, or your doctor's recommendation.

In the Kitchen with Garlic

Garlic is extremely versatile and goes with just about anything savory. It can be used raw, where you'll experience its strong, lingering flavor. Garlic has little smell when whole, but it releases its notoriously strong aroma when crushed. When cooked, the aroma and flavor mellows, becoming slightly sweet.

To work with garlic, pull the cloves from the

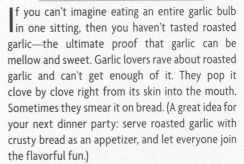

Roasted Garlic: Spice Heaven

If you can't imagine eating an entire garlic bulb in one sitting, then you haven't tasted roasted garlic—the ultimate proof that garlic can be mellow and sweet. Garlic lovers rave about roasted garlic and can't get enough of it. They pop it clove by clove right from its skin into the mouth. Sometimes they smear it on bread. (A great idea for your next dinner party: serve roasted garlic with crusty bread as an appetizer, and let everyone join the flavorful fun.)

Making roasted garlic is simple. Keep the bulb intact, but remove the loose paper skins. Line one or more bulbs up on tinfoil large enough to completely enfold them. Sprinkle them with olive oil, fold tightly, and roast them on a cookie sheet in a 424°F oven for 30 minutes.

head. Unless you are preparing a dish in which the cloves are intended to be eaten whole, you need to remove the papery skin. This is an arduous task *only* if you try to peel it with a paring knife, as you would an apple or onion. Instead, do it as chefs do: set a clove flat on a cutting board and set the flat side of a chef's knife on top, with the blade point away from you. Grip the handle securely with one hand and give the knife a good thump with the base of the palm of your other hand. The paper-like sheaths will come undone. Just pull them off and throw them away. Snip off any parts of the clove that are discolored or green, as they make garlic bitter. (Don't use a wooden cutting board when working with garlic, as the oil will get in the wood and leave a lingering aroma.)

To dice, cut the cloves into thin slices, then into thin slivers.

Be careful when browning garlic—burning makes it bitter. When a recipe calls for browning onions or other vegetables and garlic, it's best to start the onions first, then add the garlic when the other ingredients are already softened. Cook for just one minute.

Roast Chicken with 40 Cloves of Garlic

This is a classic French dish that is special enough to serve at a dinner party. Encourage your guests to eat the garlic; it's the most interesting part of the meal. Serve with a big green salad and crusty French bread. You can substitute chicken pieces for the whole chicken, but brown the chicken pieces before putting in the oven.

1 whole chicken, about 3 pounds
1 teaspoon dried rosemary
1 teaspoon dried sage
1 teaspoon dried thyme
1 teaspoon dried parsley
1 teaspoon ground roasted fennel seed
½ teaspoon salt
½ teaspoon freshly ground black pepper
1 tablespoon olive oil
1 lemon, quartered
2–3 heads of garlic with large plump cloves
   (about 40)
1½ cups chicken stock
1 cup white wine

1. Rinse and dry the chicken. Combine the rosemary, sage, thyme, parsley, fennel, salt, and ground pepper in a small bowl and add the oil. Rub the spice mix- ture into the flesh of the chicken. Place the lemon quarters in the cavity. Truss the chicken, if desired, and place in a casserole dish. Cover and refrigerate for four hours.

2. Remove the chicken from the refrigerator and bring to room temperature. Remove and separate the cloves of garlic but do not remove the skins. Scatter the cloves around the chicken. Combine the stock and wine and pour around the chicken. Place in a 425°F oven, covered, for 15 minutes. Reduce the heat to 375°F, uncover, and cook, basting occasionally, for 40 minutes or until an instant-read thermometer registers 175°F. Let the chicken sit for 30 minutes to let the juices settle before slicing. Serve with several bulbs of garlic on each plate.

Makes 4 servings.

Here are a few of the innumerable ways to add more garlic to your diet:

- To make garlic bread, blanch unpeeled garlic cloves in water for five minutes to soften them. Cool and remove the paper skins. Slice a loaf of crusty Italian bread lengthwise, brush the bread with olive oil, spread the cloves over top, sprinkle with dried rosemary and thyme, and bake on a cookie sheet in a 400°F oven for 10 minutes.
- Make tiny little pockets in red meat roasts with the tip of a chef's knife. Slice a few garlic cloves and stuff a sliver in each "pocket."

- Slice or press fresh garlic into extra-virgin olive oil to use in a marinade, salad dressing, or as a dipping sauce.
- Blanch garlic cloves as above for garlic bread and mash them into potatoes to make garlic mashed potatoes.
- Try this specialty from Trinidad: slice an eggplant into thick slices, stud the slices with garlic cloves, sprinkle with ground coriander and ground ginger, and grill until tender.
- Add a little extra spice to your salads by rubbing the bottom and sides of the salad bowl with garlic before adding the greens and dressing.

GINGER   *Quieting That Queasy Feeling*

Nausea is a possible symptom of dozens of conditions and diseases, from Addison's disease to traumatic brain injury. But it's a prominent symptom of several.

There's motion sickness, when a disconnect between what you see and the way your body is moving confuses the balance center in your inner ear, producing nausea.

There's morning sickness, the nausea of early pregnancy that bedevils so many mothers-to-be.

There's medication-induced nausea, from anesthesia or chemotherapy.

And there's nausea from digestive upset, such as food poisoning.

For thousands of years—in China, India, the Middle East, and the Roman Empire—traditional healers have turned to ginger to help quiet that queasy feeling. For the past few decades, scientists around the world have been *proving* that ginger works.

Saying No to Nausea

No matter the type of nausea, ginger just says no.

Motion sickness. "Nausea associated with motion sickness is unpleasant." That's the scientific understatement of a team of gastroenterologists from the University of Michigan and National Ying-Ming University in Taiwan. But standard over-the-counter and prescription medications for motion sickness aren't particularly pleasant either, they add—not only do they "produce incomplete symptom control," but they also have "significant side effects, such as dry mouth, lethargy, and drowsiness."

Ginger, however, is a traditional Chinese remedy for motion sickness, said the researchers. And they set out to see not only *if* it worked, but *how* it worked.

To do so, they asked 13 volunteers with a history of motion sickness (from car, boat, or plane travel) to sit in a spinning chair. Needless to say, they all became nauseated. But when the volunteers took either 1,000 or 2,000 milligrams (mg) of ginger *before* they sat in the chair, it took them 35 percent longer to develop nausea, the nausea was less intense by 30 percent, and the nausea was far less severe 15, 30, and 45 minutes after the chair stopped spinning. (Both doses of ginger worked equally well.)

In their study, the researchers also measured blood levels of *vasopressin*, a key hormone that helps regulates levels of water, salt, and blood sugar, and that the researchers theorized might

---

GINGER IS A PROVEN REMEDY

TO EASE MOTION SICKNESS

FROM BEING ON A BOAT.

---

play a role in nausea from motion sickness. They found ginger limited the release of vasopressin during "circular vection." (Yes, there is a scientific term for sitting in a spinning chair.)

The researchers also measured electrical activity in the stomach (tachygastria) during circular vection—and found ginger kept the activity "relatively stable" as compared to "chaotic" activity without the spice.

"Ginger is effective in preventing motion sickness, possibly by suppressing vasopressin release from the central nervous system," said the researchers. "Ginger may act as a novel agent in the prevention and treatment of motion sickness."

(And maybe in the prevention and treatment of other problems, too. The researchers noted that Chinese healers have used ginger for thousands of years as a remedy for nausea *and* stomach upset *and* diarrhea *and* arthritis *and* toothache.)

Those researchers weren't the first to test ginger for motion sickness. In an earlier study, navel cadets who took ginger on their maiden voyage had less motion sickness—less nausea, vomiting, dizziness, and cold sweats.

Morning sickness. Morning is the worst time of day for an estimated 50 to 80 percent of pregnant women during the first trimester. They're suffering with morning sickness—the nausea and vomiting that experts say is triggered by pregnancy's sudden flood of hormones. Are experts saying anything about *solving* the problem? Some of them are saying: Take ginger.

"Ginger has been shown to improve the symptoms of nausea and vomiting compared with placebo in pregnant women," wrote a team of researchers in the *Annals of Pharmacotherapy*, after analyzing nearly 40 years of studies on the spice.

"Ginger may be an effective treatment for nausea and vomiting in pregnancy," wrote Italian scientists in *Obstetrics and Gynecology*, after evaluating data from six studies on ginger and morning sickness, involving 675 women. They also noted that there was an "absence of significant side effects or adverse effects on pregnancy outcomes" from taking supplements of the spice.

"Ginger offers the clinician and pregnant woman a safe alternative to prescription medications for nausea," said Eva Bryer, CNM, a midwife in California, in a review of ginger and morning sickness in the *Journal of Midwifery and Women's Health*.

Ginger may help even the most severe form of morning sickness, *hyperemesis gravidarum*. In a Danish study of women with the problem, ginger provided "greater relief of symptoms" than a placebo.

Homegrown Ginger

Here's a unique way to keep fresh ginger root at home:

Take fresh ginger root you purchased at the store and break off a piece at least two inches long. Place it in a pot filled with sandy soil, such as cactus soil. Water occasionally to keep it slightly moistened. The root will start to grow in four to five weeks. Whenever you need ginger, just dig up the root and break off a small portion. The root will continue to grow.

In the most recent study on ginger and morning sickness, researchers divided 67 pregnant women into two groups: one took 250 mg of ginger four times a day, and the other took a placebo. After four days, those taking ginger had 41 percent less vomiting. "Ginger is an effective remedy for decreasing nausea and vomiting during pregnancy," concluded the researchers in the *Journal of Alternative and Complementary Medicine*.

Nausea after surgery. Researchers analyzed data from five studies on ginger and post-operative nausea, involving 363 people, and found that a daily dose of 1,000 mg of the spice reduced the likelihood of postoperative nausea and vomiting by 31 percent. "Use of ginger is an effective means for reducing postoperative nausea and vomiting," they wrote in the *American Journal of Obstetrics and Gynecology*.

Chemotherapy-induced nausea. "Nausea that develops during the period that begins 24 hours after the administration of chemotherapy is called delayed nausea, and occurs in many patients with cancer," wrote a team of researchers in the *Journal of Alternative and Complementary Medicine*. When they gave a high-protein drink spiced with ginger to people with chemotherapy, they found they had less nausea and used less anti-nausea medication than people not getting the drink. "Protein with ginger holds the potential of representing a novel, nutritionally-based treatment for the delayed nausea of chemotherapy," they concluded.

Ginger may help prevent and/or treat:

Arthritis, osteo- and rheumatoid

Asthma

Cancer

Cholesterol problems (high total cholesterol, high "bad" LDL cholesterol, low "good" HDL cholesterol)

Heart attack

Heartburn (gastroesophageal reflux disease, or GERD)

Indigestion

Migraine

Morning sickness

Motion sickness

Nausea (chemotherapy-induced and postoperative)

Stroke

Triglycerides, high

Ginger pairs well with these spices:

Allspice	Cumin	Sesame seed
Cardamom	Curry leaf	Star anise
Chile	Fennel seed	Tamarind
Cinnamon	Garlic	Turmeric
Clove	Mustard seed	Vanilla
Coconut	Onion	
Coriander	Parsley	

and complements recipes featuring:

Ale or beer	Pumpkin
Chicken	Shellfish
Chutney	Sushi
Duck	Sweet potatoes
Oranges	Winter squash
Pork	

And while a study by doctors at the University of Michigan found that ginger didn't help with nausea and vomiting after chemotherapy, those who took the spice had "significantly less fatigue" (a big problem for cancer patients) and also fewer overall "adverse effects" from chemotherapy.

Ginger Aid

Ginger is rich in phytonutrients called *gingerols*, which are antioxidant, anti-inflammatory, antibacterial, antiviral—and anti-disease.

Arthritis. Researchers at the University of Miami studied 247 people with osteoarthritis of the knee, dividing them into two groups. One took a ginger extract, while the other took a placebo. After six weeks, those taking ginger had 31 percent less knee pain on standing, 42 percent less knee pain after walking 50 feet, and they took less pain medication. "Ginger extract had a statistically significant effect on reducing symptoms of osteoarthritis of the knee," wrote the researchers in *Arthritis and Rheumatism*.

Cancer. Dozens of cellular and animal studies show that ginger may be anti-cancer—for lung, breast, prostate, skin, bladder, kidney, pancreatic, and ovarian cancers. In our lab in the Department of Experimental Therapeutics at the University of Texas M.D. Anderson Cancer Center, we have conducted several cellular and animal experiments on cancer and *zerumbone*, a ginger extract.

In a study in *Cancer Research*, we showed that zerumbone activated genes that lead to the death of human colon cancer cells—and could also activate the same cell-killing genes in kidney, breast, and pancreatic cancer cells. Zerumbone also activated a "tumor suppressor" gene.

In an animal study in *Cancer Research*, we found zerumbone could help prevent bone loss in breast cancer—a common problem. (We theorized that zerumbone might also battle osteoporosis.)

In another study in *Cancer Research*, we found zerumbone could "down-regulate" a gene that plays a role in *metastasis*, the spread of cancer beyond the organ it first targets.

And in a study in the journal *Oncogene*, we showed that zerumbone helped stop the activation of NF-kB, a protein complex that activates cancer-causing, cancer-spreading genes.

Migraine. "Treatment of migraine is often delayed due to . . . unwanted consequences from prescription medication," wrote researchers from the Headache Care Center in Springfield, Missouri. To find out if ginger could provide an alternative to those medications, they gave 29 people with migraines either a placebo or a supplement with feverfew and ginger (Gelstat Migraine therapy). "Two hours after treatment, 48 percent were pain-free, with 34 percent reporting a headache of only mild severity," said the researchers. They noted that nearly 60 percent of those who took the remedy said they were satisfied with it, and 41 percent felt it was equal to their medication. Not bad for an herb-and-spice combo.

Asthma. Researchers in the UK noted that drugs used to treat asthma often produce "suboptimal" results, and that "many patients harbor misgivings about conventional" drugs such as inhaled corticosteroids, which have many short- and long-term side effects. To find out if a non-drug approach might help control asthma, they gave 30 adults with mild to moderate asthma either a placebo or a natural formula that included 130 mg of a ginger extract standardized to contain gingerols. After three months, those taking the formula had "clinical improvements" in asthma symptoms, their overall health was better, and they were coughing less.

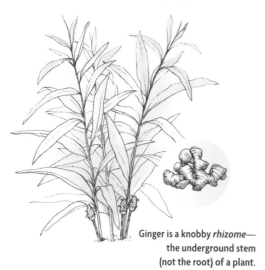

Ginger is a knobby *rhizome*—the underground stem (not the root) of a plant.

Heartburn and stomachaches. Researchers in Taiwan gave 24 healthy people 1,200 mg of ginger and measured gastric emptying—the speed at which the stomach digests food. (Too-slow stomach emptying can produce heartburn, as well as bloating, belching, and flatulence right after eating.) Ginger cut gastric emptying time in half, compared to placebo. This effect "could possibly be beneficial" in people with heartburn and other types of digestive upset, concluded the researchers in the *European Journal of Gastroenterological Hepatology*.

Cholesterol problems. Researchers studied 95 people with blood fat problems (high "bad" LDL cholesterol, high total cholesterol, high triglycerides, and low "good" HDL cholesterol). They divided them into two groups: one group took 1,000 mg of ginger, three times a day; the other group took a placebo. After 45 days, those taking ginger had a greater drop in LDL and a greater increase in HDL.

Heart attacks and stroke. Researchers in Taiwan found that ginger decreased *platelet aggregation*—clumping of blood components that can trigger the artery-clogging blood clots that cause most heart attacks and strokes. Combining ginger with standard blood-thinning medication "could be valuable for cardiovascular [heart attack] and cerebrovascular [stroke] complication," they concluded in the *American Journal of Chinese Medicine*.

Getting to Know Ginger

Ginger was a favored spice for cooking and healing in ancient China and Rome. By the ninth century, ginger arrived in Europe—and after a couple of centuries it was so popular (especially in England) that it was used on the table like salt and pepper, and sprinkled on beer. (The origin of "ginger ale.") Henry VIII may not have always loved his wives, but he always loved ginger. And so did his daughter, Elizabeth I—who sometimes presented each guest at a state dinner with a "Gingerbread Man" shaped in his or her own image.

England is still famous for its gingerbread—nearly every town has its own recipe and unique mold for fashioning figures. And gingerbread figures are part of the November ritual called Guy Fawkes Day (also called Guy Fawkes Night and Bonfire Night) that celebrates the foiling of a plot to blow up the Houses of Parliament.

And speaking of houses: the gingerbread house is a German invention, and now a Christmas tradition that has spread throughout the world.

Ginger is a staple in the cuisines of India, China, Korea, Thailand, Indonesia, and Vietnam, where it's used more in savory foods than in desserts. (Ginger is to these cuisines what garlic and onions are to American cooking.) And since Asian and Indian cuisines are spreading in popularity, the savory use of the spice is enjoying an international revival.

But ginger is popular, well, *everywhere.*

In Germany, it's a Christmas eve tradition to eat carp cooked with gingerbread and gingersnaps. The Japanese are fond of *shoga,* a locally grown ginger, which they eat pickled. Ginger is a main ingredient in *kimchi,* the well-known Korean fermented salad. It's a key ingredient in many curries, especially those made in Thailand and Malaysia. And it's a popular addition to spice mixes, including Jamaica's hot jerk spice mix.

The people of Myanmar (Burma) discovered an unusual quality about ginger: when used in large quantities, it masks the odor of fish. Burmese freshwater fish dishes *always* include ginger.

Ginger is a big hit in beverages too. There is, of course, ginger ale and ginger tea. Jamaica produces a carbonated soft drink called ginger beer. Bermuda also produces a brand of ginger beer called Barritts (connoisseurs consider it superior), and drink it straight or mixed with rum in a drink called a Dark and Stormy. A Manhattan bar invented the Moscow Mule, which is ginger beer and vodka. The French make a ginger liqueur called Canton. In Thailand, you'll find *Khing sot,* a fresh ginger drink made with ginger oil. In Yemen, ginger flavors coffee.

How to Buy Ginger

Ginger is a knobby *rhizome*—the underground stem (not the root) of a plant. A ginger rhizome is called a *hand.* You can buy fresh ginger whole, sliced, diced, or preserved in brine. You can buy dried ginger sliced, ground, or crystallized. Because of ginger's popularity, you can usually find all these forms in most supermarkets.

When buying fresh ginger, look for hands that are firm and swollen-appearing, with smooth skin. (Wrinkled ginger is old.) Fresh ginger is light brown, with a slightly pink tinge, and knobs tinged yellow-green.

Ginger derives its intense flavor from its gingerols. But gingerol content varies, depending on where and how the plant was grown, and when it was harvested. So fresh ginger can be

Other recipes containing ginger:

Berbere (p. 267)

Caribbean Curry Paste (p. 287)

Chaat Masala (p. 256)

Chesapeake Bay Seafood Seasoning (p. 273)

Coconut Meatballs with Peanut Sauce (p. 101)

Garbanzo Beans with Mushrooms and Toasted Almonds (p. 29)

Jamaican Jerk Marinade (p. 269)

La Kama (p. 266)

Los Banos Low-Fat Brownies (p. 97)

Madras Curry Paste (p. 286)

Madras Curry Powder (p. 284)

Malaysian Curry Paste (p. 287)

Mulling Spice (p. 273)

Mussels with Thai Red Curry Sauce (p. 156)

Potato Cauliflower Curry (p. 252)

Ras-el-hanout (p. 266)

Sesame Seared Tuna with Pickled Ginger and Vanilla Slaw (p. 220)

Spiced Milk Tea (p. 66)

Spiced Mixed Nuts (p. 90)

Vindaloo Curry Paste (p. 286)

Ginger Carrot and Squash Soup

This light and tasty soup makes a nice first course for Thanksgiving or with spring lamb.

1½ teaspoons coriander seeds
½ teaspoon yellow mustard seeds
2 tablespoons canola or vegetable oil
2 cups diced onions
1 heaping tablespoon diced fresh ginger
½ teaspoon turmeric
½ teaspoon Madras Curry Powder (p. 284) or
  commercial curry powder
1 pound carrots, peeled and coarsely chopped
1 acorn squash, peeled, seeded, and coarsely
  chopped (1 pound)
1 teaspoon lime zest
6 cups chicken stock
½ cup light cream
1 tablespoon fresh lime juice
Salt and pepper to taste
½ cup fresh parsley

1. Dry roast the coriander and mustard seeds separately and cool. Place both spices in a spice mill and grind to a fine powder.

2. Heat the oil in a heavy-bottomed large Dutch oven and brown fry the onions for 10 minutes until they are golden brown. Add the ginger, turmeric, and toasted seeds, and the curry powder and stir for one minute. Add the carrots, acorn squash, and lime zest, cover, and cook for five minutes, stirring frequently.

2. Add the chicken stock and bring to a boil. Reduce the heat, cover, and simmer for 30 minutes or until the carrots and squash are soft. Cool slightly.

3. Working in batches, puree the soup in a blender or food processor until smooth. Return the soup to the pot. Stir in the cream and lime juice and season with salt and pepper. Sprinkle with parsley.

Makes 6 servings.

any degree of tangy, sweet, or spicy, with temperature ranging from mild to hot.

Half the world's ginger is produced on India's Malabar Coast, in the cities of Calicut and Cochin, with Cochin ginger considered the superior variety. According to ginger-savvy chefs, the best ginger in the world—with a mild flavor that's ideal for cooking—grows in Jamaica. Ginger from Nigeria and Sierra Leone is the most pungent. Most of the ginger shipped to the US is from Hawaii.

Peeled, sealed, and refrigerated, fresh young ginger keeps for about two weeks. You can also freeze it peeled and sliced; thaw before using.

You can keep older ginger unpeeled, in a cool dry place, just as you keep garlic and onions. You also can keep unpeeled ginger indefinitely by freezing it in a freezer bag. When using unpeeled frozen ginger, cut off as much as you think you'll use, and slice or grate it while still frozen.

Ground ginger lacks the aroma of fresh ginger, but the spicy fragrance and characteristic flavor are intact.

Preserved ginger and crystallized ginger are processed with sugar; needless to say, they're sweet. They also range in temperature. They keep in a cool, dry place for up to a year.

In the Kitchen with Ginger

Ginger is quite versatile—you can use it in almost anything. But keep in mind that fresh and dried ginger differ noticeably in their flavoring effects. Though you can often substitute one for the other, you won't get the same intense flavor from dried.

Both fresh and dried ginger are used in savory dishes, with dried ginger almost always called for in sweet dishes. In contemporary cuisine, the accent is on fresh ginger, especially if you're making Asian or Indian dishes.

Fresh ginger is easy to work with. Peel it with a paring knife or with a vegetable peeler. Then slice it. The ideal slice is the size of a quarter. In Indian cuisine it is ground with a mortar and pestle.

Fresh ginger is rather strong, but mellows in cooking.

Here are ideas for putting more ginger in your diet:

- Make a Chinese dipping sauce by combining ¾ cup of Japanese dark soy sauce with ¼ cup black Chinese vinegar, 2 tablespoons each of grated fresh ginger and garlic, and ½ tablespoon of sesame oil. If you can't find black Chinese vinegar (available in Asian markets), you can substitute balsamic.
- Fresh ginger goes great with shellfish. Grate fresh ginger and dried mint into melted butter and serve as a dipping sauce with steamed lobster or shrimp.
- Sprinkle ginger and brown sugar on acorn squash or sweet potatoes before baking.
- Rub into meat before grilling, to help tenderize and add flavor.
- Ginger works well in white sauces and dessert sauces.
- Finely grate fresh ginger over cooked tofu or noodles.
- Sprinkle ground ginger in applesauce or use it in fruit pie fillings.
- Grate fresh ginger into cheesecake batter.
- Grind crystallized ginger and sprinkle it on top of whipped cream or ice cream.
- Make ginger syrup by combining ¼ pound peeled and diced ginger with 1 cup of sugar and 1 cup of water, bring to a boil, and cook for 30 minutes. Strain and cool.

HORSERADISH *Potent Infection Fighter*

Horseradish is to spices what apples are to pies—very American. An estimated 85 percent of the world's horseradish is grown here and a lot of it stays here: Americans consume six million gallons of horseradish a year!

But horseradish isn't an American original. Native to the Mediterranean, by the 15th century it was growing in Britain, where it was described as *hoarse*, meaning "of coarse and strong quality."

Raw horseradish has no odor, but cut into its flesh and you'll sniff a waft of heat that can open the sinuses even on the worst day of allergy season. No wonder it was used as a medicine long before it was used as a food. Ye Olde physicians employed its mucous-moving abilities to help treat colds, coughs, kidney stones, urinary tract infections—and hoarseness, of course.

What gives horseradish its healing kick? The volatile oil *sinigrin*, which breaks down into *allyl isothiocyanate*, a powerful natural antibiotic.

Allyl isothiocyanate most likely accounts for the proven effectiveness of horseradish in treating upper respiratory problems. But it's not the only healing component in the spice. Ounce for ounce, horseradish contains more medicinally active compounds than most other spices. And they are *very* active—they can clear congestion, thin mucous, reduce inflammation, squelch cell-damaging oxidants, fight bacteria and viruses, relax muscles, stimulate the immune system—and even battle cancer. That makes the humble horseradish one special spice. As noted botanist and spice expert Dr. James A. Duke put it, "Horseradish is about as useful in the medicine chest as it is in the spice rack."

A Natural Antibiotic

Even though horseradish is loaded with healing phytonutrients, only a few scientific studies have been conducted to test its curative powers. However, the spice has been declared medically safe and effective for upper respiratory tract infections by the German *Commission E Monographs*, which helps guide physicians and other health professionals in Germany in the medical use of herbs.

One of that country's most popular infection-fighting natural medicines is a preparation called Angocin Anti-Infekt N, which contains horseradish root and the herb nasturtium. Since the preparation hit the German market, several laboratory and human studies have found that it is as effective as antibiotics in treating:

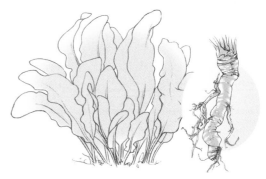

Horseradish is a coarse, colorless, odorless root.

- Bronchitis
- Ear infection
- Gastrointestinal illness caused by food contaminated with the *E. coli* bacteria
- Gastrointestinal illness caused by food contaminated by the bacteria *Staphylococcus aureus*
- Haemophilus influenza, which typically strikes children under age five
- Pneumonia
- Sinusitis
- Strep throat and other serious illness cause by the bacteria *Streptococcus pyogenes*, such as cellulitis, impetigo, and scarlet fever
- Urinary tract infection

One of those studies, involving 858 children and teenagers in 65 German treatment centers, compared the effectiveness of Angocin Anti-Infekt N to an antibiotic in the treatment of bronchitis and urinary tract infection (UTI). Effectiveness was measured by the degree of symptom relief and the speed at which infections cleared up—and the horseradish-containing medication was very effective! "The results prove that there is a rational basis for treatment of both UTIs and respiratory infections with this medicinal product," commented the researchers.

Another German study compared the effectiveness of the horseradish preparation to antibiotics in 536 people with sinusitis, 634 people with bronchitis, and 479 people with UTI. Again, the natural medicine worked just as well as the antibiotic.

The horseradish medication also has been shown to help *prevent* infection. In one study, researchers recruited 219 women and men ages 18 to 75 to test the effectiveness of the natural medicine in preventing recurrent UTI. All the patients were symptom-free at the beginning of the study. Half the participants took a daily dose of the horseradish-containing supplement and half took a placebo. After three months, the researchers found that the rate of recurrence was 50 percent lower in the people taking the horseradish remedy than in those taking the placebo. Another study involving children with recurrent urinary tract infections had similar results.

Better than Broccoli?

On the outside, horseradish isn't much to look at. It is a coarse, colorless, odorless, gangly root with no taste-appeal whatsoever—the ugly duckling of an attractive family of colorful vegetables called the crucifers. These crucifers (broccoli, watercress, mustard greens, kale, cabbage, and brussels sprouts, to name a few) are well known for producing the plant kingdom's largest supply of *isothiocyanates* (ITCs), compounds that have been found to protect against cancer.

But ITCs wouldn't exist if it weren't for another important compound: *glucosinolates*. When the flesh of a crucifer is broken—when it is torn, cut, or chewed—glucosinolates get into gear and produce ITCs. That's why horseradish stands out as more than just a homely spice in a family of lovely greens. When researchers at the University of Illinois put horseradish under the microscope, they found it contained more glucosinolates than broccoli, the king of all crucifers.

"Horseradish contains more than 10-fold higher glucosinolates than broccoli, so you don't need much horseradish to benefit," commented Dr. Mosbah Kushad, the study's lead researcher. "In fact, a little dab on your steak will go a long way to providing the same health benefits as broccoli." (Good news for you broccoli-haters out there!)

In one study on the ITCs in horseradish, researchers at Michigan State University tested their ability to inhibit the activity of colon and lung cancer cells. As the dosage of ITCs increased, the disease-promoting activity of the cancer cells became weaker—30 to 68 percent weaker for colon cancer, and 30 to 71 percent weaker for lung cells.

ITCs aren't the only cancer-fighting compound in horseradish—the spice contains more than two dozen anti-cancer compounds, and researchers in England are investigating one of them—*horseradish peroxidase* (HRP)—as a component in an anti-cancer medication. In one laboratory study, the experimental drug helped control the growth of breast and bladder cancer cells.

High Hopes for Low Cholesterol

The ITCs in cruciferous vegetables (broccoli in particular) promote heart health by helping control two major risk factors for heart disease: the blood fats cholesterol and triglycerides. A study reported in the journal *Nutrition Research* found that the ITCs in horseradish can do the same.

In the study, researchers fed mice a cholesterol-rich diet with and without horseradish. After three weeks, the mice eating the diet with cholesterol *and* horseradish had much lower cholesterol

levels. The researchers theorize that horseradish blocks the production of cholesterol.

The Unique Crucifer

Not only does horseradish contain higher concentrations of ITCs than other crucifers—it also contains *thiocyanate*, a rare substance that sends a pungent rush into the nasal cavity when the flesh is cut or chewed. Thiocyanate is only found in two other spices, mustard seed and wasabi, both members of the crucifer clan.

Thiocyanate delivers its zing by a different route than capsaicin, the chemical that torches your tongue when you eat chiles. When horseradish meets moisture in the mouth, thiocyanates are released into the air and up the nasal

FIRST PRODUCED IN PITTSBURGH IN 1869, HEINZ HORSERADISH WAS AMERICA'S ORIGINAL MASS-MARKETED CONVENIENCE FOOD.

passage, which is why a strong dose makes the nose run and the eyes water. The heat dissipates quickly, however, and you are left with the spice's distinctive taste—a white radish with the heat of a jalapeño.

Pure horseradish, however, is not a familiar taste—it's usually one ingredient in a sauce. That's why we don't recognize that the so-called "wasabi" served in sushi restaurants *is* pure horseradish, colored with spinach and spirulina. (To find out more about wasabi, please see page 256.)

Getting to Know Horseradish

Horseradish first came to the United States in the 1600s with the original settlers, but it really took off as a coveted condiment in the mid-1800s when German and Polish immigrants brought their love for the spice and their recipes to America. It was so popular as a topping for cold meats and fish that in 1869 a young entrepreneur by the name of Henry J. Heinz mixed it with the preservative vinegar, packed it in small glass jars to "display its purity," and peddled it in a hand basket in his hometown neighborhood in Pittsburgh, Pennsylvania. Heinz Horseradish went on to became America's first mass-marketed convenience food, and local legend has it that Heinz grated so much horseradish in his parent's home basement you could smell the potent vapors coming through the floorboards long after he moved the operation elsewhere.

Today, horseradish plays a leading culinary role in both the United States and Europe. We use it to turn ordinary ketchup into sinus-opening cocktail sauce, the ubiquitous dip traditionally served with boiled shrimp and raw shellfish. It's a popular addition to the tomato-juice-and-vodka cocktail Bloody Mary, and it is often found sitting on the bar in taverns and seafood houses next to a bowl of oyster crackers. It's the classic condiment found on tables in steakhouses and in the serving line at fast food places from coast to coast. Every June, Collinsville, Illinois, the self-proclaimed horseradish capital of the world, hosts the annual International Horseradish Festival, with every horseradish contest imaginable, including a Little Miss Horseradish beauty pageant.

But first prize for horseradish adoration goes to the Germans, who still follow the arduous custom of grating the tough, large root and serving it fresh. Germans are so fond of horseradish because its potent tang cuts the fatty flavor of sausages and the unusual cuts of meat that are the standard fare in their diet. German cuisine contains countless recipes for horseradish sauce. There's vinegar horseradish sauce, lemon horseradish sauce, horseradish bread sauce, horse-

Horseradish may help prevent and/or treat:

Bronchitis	Food poisoning
Cancer	Pneumonia, bacterial
Cholesterol problems (high total cholesterol)	Sinusitis
	Strep throat
Ear infection	Urinary tract infection
Flu	

Horseradish pairs well with these spices:

Basil	Parsley
Black pepper	Rosemary
Celery seed	Sesame seed
Fennel seed	Sun-dried tomato
Mustard seed	

and complements recipes featuring:

Apples	Eggs
Baked beans	Fresh and smoked fish
Beef roasts	Pork
Cheese	Potatoes
Cold cuts	Shellfish
Cured ham	

Substitute: Since most wasabi sold in the US is really horseradish, you can use the two interchangeably. True wasabi is stronger, however, so if using it as a substitute for horseradish in a recipe, start with half as much and add more until you get to the desired taste and consistency.

radish whipped cream sauce, beer horseradish sauce, and the most well known, *apfelmeerrettich*, which is made with sour green apples. It's not unusual to find *meerrettichkartoffeln*—potatoes baked in horseradish cream—sitting on the table, too.

Eastern Europeans and Scandinavians also have their horseradish traditions.

In Norway, the grated root is whipped with sweet-and-sour cream, sugar, and vinegar to create a sauce called *pepperrotsaus* that is served with cold salmon and other fish. The Danes freeze creamed horseradish and serve it like sherbet in a chilled sauceboat. The Poles grate beets into horseradish to make a purple-red condiment called *chrzan* that is served with spring ham. Horseradish soup is a Polish Christmas-day lunch tradition.

The French are not fond of fiery food, but horseradish is the exception. They feel the heavy red horseradish sauce preferred by Americans is too heavy for the delicate taste of raw oysters and instead serve a dipping sauce called *mignonette*, which combines the spice with vinegar and oil. In England, standing rib roast with horseradish cream sauce is a national tradition.

Horseradish is on the table at the Seder, the meal that celebrates the Jewish holiday of Passover—it's one of the *maror* (bitter herbs) that symbolize the suffering the Israelites endured as slaves in Egypt.

In the Kitchen with Horseradish

You'll get the most pungent horseradish by serving it the way the Germans prefer: freshly grated and undiluted. But grating horseradish is painstaking—even painful! The root is tough, coarse, and long (a foot or more), and grating it calls for strength and a sharp steel grating blade. The vapors hit your nostrils like a punch in the nose, so work outdoors if possible, or at least in a well-ventilated room by an open window. Also warn others to stay upwind from the fumes. And once grated, the flavor deteriorates quickly. All of which is why I highly recommend you take the easy route and purchase prepared horseradish preserved in vinegar, which is inexpensive and readily available. It won't give you the zing of fresh horseradish, but it's close, and its healing powers are the same.

You can find prepared horseradish in the dairy section of any supermarket, and it will last for months in the refrigerator at home. Just check the label to make sure you're getting the minimum ingredients—horseradish, distilled white vinegar, and salt. When using it in recipes, make sure to squeeze the vinegar out with the back of the fork, so you get the pure taste of horseradish. You can also purchase the spice as granules and flakes, which must be rehydrated.

Generally horseradish relishes and sauces aren't cooked—heat destroys the spice's pungency, and cooked horseradish is quite mild. So, when you see a horseradish-potato crusted fish on the menu (quite popular these days), there's no need to pass it up because you think the dish might be too hot.

Horseradish is versatile and easy to work with.

Bavarian Apple and Horseradish Sauce

This popular German specialty makes a great accompaniment to pork tenderloin or chops and spicy sausages. You can also serve it as a spread on cold beef sandwiches on thick crusty bread.

½ cup prepared horseradish, drained
1 large sour green apple, peeled, cored, and diced
¼ cup lemon juice
1 teaspoon sugar
½ teaspoon salt
⅓ cup sour cream
1 tablespoon dried parsley

In a medium mixing bowl mix the horseradish, apple, lemon juice, sugar, and salt. Cover and let the mixture stand at room temperature for 30 minutes. Stir in the sour cream, sprinkle with parsley, and serve. Or refrigerate until ready to use, stir, and bring to room temperature before serving.

Makes about 1½ cups.

Here are some of the many ways you can put more of the spice into your diet:

- Add a dollop of horseradish to potato salads, slaws, and dips.
- Use it to give applesauce a tasty zip.
- Add a tablespoon or two to spike barbecue sauce served with grilled meat.
- Mix a tablespoon of prepared horseradish with ⅓ cup of sour cream as a topping for smoked fish. Sprinkle it with chives.
- Mix horseradish with sour cream and whip it into mashed potatoes.
- To make a basic cocktail sauce, mix equal parts of ketchup and horseradish. Add a few splashes of Worcestershire sauce and lemon juice.
- Make a different dipping sauce for seafood by combining 2 tablespoons of mayonnaise, 1 tablespoon of sour cream, 1 tablespoon of prepared horseradish, and ¼ teaspoon each of mace and mint. Sprinkle with garlic salt.
- To make a traditional horseradish cream for roast beef, beat ½ cup of heavy cream until slightly stiff and fold in 2 tablespoons of prepared horseradish. Add 3 tablespoons of lemon juice and salt and pepper. Chill for at least an hour before serving.

JUNIPER BERRY   *The Natural Diuretic*

The juniper berry (not a real berry, but a tiny pinecone from the juniper tree and bush) is best-known as the spice that defines the flavor of gin. If at last night's party you had a martini, a gin and tonic, a Long Island iced tea, and a Tom Collins, and today (along with your hangover) you seem to be going to the bathroom more than usual—you are. Juniper berry is also a standout *diuretic*, a compound that increases the output of urine.

Kind to Your Kidneys

Many modern medicines aimed at healing the urinary tract include one or more compounds extracted from juniper berries. The compounds not only stimulate the kidneys to produce fluid, but also help kill bacteria, making them ideal for battling bladder and urinary tract infections. In fact, juniper berry is so kind to the kidneys that researchers at the University of California found it helped prevent organ rejection in test animals with kidney transplants.

Evergreen Healing

Other ways that juniper might help heal include:

Stomachache. The *Commission E Monographs*—scientific summaries used in Germany to guide physicians and other health practitioners in the use of natural remedies—approved the use of juniper berries for treating indigestion.

Heart problems. In an animal study reported in *Phytotherapy Research*, researchers found that preparations made from juniper berries had an action similar to amiloride HCl (Moduretic), a diuretic used to control high blood pressure and congestive heart failure.

Inflammation and infection. Juniper berries have been used to treat "various inflammatory and infectious diseases such as bronchitis, colds, cough, fungal infections, hemorrhoids, gynecological diseases, and wounds in Turkish folk medicine," wrote a team of Turkish researchers in the *Journal of Ethnopharmacology*. (They also note the juniper berry is used *worldwide* for many of those conditions, as well as for rheumatoid arthritis, and to regulate menstruation and relieve menstrual pain.) When they tested an extract of juniper berries in an animal experiment, they found it had "remarkable" anti-inflammatory and pain-relieving activity equal to

Juniper berry may help prevent and/or treat:

Arthritis, osteo- and rheumatoid	Hemorrhoids
Breast cancer	High blood pressure (hypertension)
Bronchitis	Indigestion
Cold sores	Kidney disease
Colds	Liver disease
Diabetes, type 2	Menstrual cramps
Flu	Pain
Fungal infection	Urinary tract infection
Heart failure	Wounds

Juniper berry pairs well with these spices:

Allspice	Onion
Bay leaf	Oregano
Black pepper	Parsley
Caraway seed	Rosemary
Marjoram	Sage
Nutmeg	Thyme

and complements recipes featuring:

Ham	Pork
Game	Sauerkraut
Marinades	Vodka
Pickled vegetables	

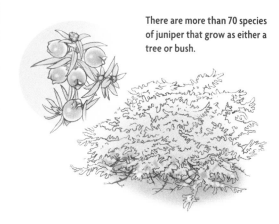

There are more than 70 species of juniper that grow as either a tree or bush.

Liver damage. In an animal study, researchers at the University of North Carolina at Chapel Hill found a juniper berry extract helped prevent the type of liver damage seen in alcoholism.

Cold sores. In test tube studies, compounds in juniper inhibited the virus that causes cold sores.

Getting to Know Juniper Berry

There are more than 70 species of juniper that grow as either a tree or bush. Juniper "berries" take three years to ripen, starting out green, turning to blue, and then to deep purple. Dried, they darken to blue-black.

Harvesting usually occurs in the fall, and it can *hurt*—sharp, stiff foliage enfolds the berries. If you plan to pick juniper berries, wear gloves. And make absolutely certain you're picking from an *edible* juniper bush. Some varieties are poisonous.

Juniper thrives in the northern hemisphere, so it's no surprise that this spice complements the meaty cuisines of northern Europe, especially those of Scandinavia and Germany. (Where there is game, there is juniper berry—it's used to mellow the gaminess of venison, goose, duck, and wild boar.) The Scandinavians used it to roast reindeer, and also put it in *gravlax*, a specialty smoked salmon cured with salt, sugar, and dill. The Germans put juniper berries in pot roasts, in fermented vegetable dishes such as

that of indomethacin (Indocin), a non-steroidal anti-inflammatory drug (NSAID) prescribed for arthritis and other pain problems.

Diabetes. Several animal studies have found that juniper berry is effective in lowering high blood sugar.

Breast cancer. In a laboratory study in *Oncology Reports*, juniper berry extracts "significantly decreased" the growth of human breast cancer cells. The extract "might be useful in cancer treatment," concluded the researchers.

Alsatian Pork and Sauerkraut

This is a classic dish in the German-inspired cuisine of the Alsace-Lorraine region of France. Juniper, caraway, and bay are common seasonings in German sauerkraut.

2 pounds sauerkraut, preferably German
1 cup white wine
1 four-pound bone-in pork roast or pork
    tenderloin
2 tablespoons canola or olive oil
1 cup diced onions
2 large apples, peeled, cored, and chopped
8 juniper berries
1 teaspoon caraway seeds
1 bay leaf

1. Drain the sauerkraut through a sieve into a large mixing bowl, pressing down to extract all the juice. Add the white wine to the sauerkraut juice and set aside.

2. Brown the pork in the oil in a large sauté pan until it is lightly browned on all sides. Set aside. Add the onions and apples to the oil and sauté until soft but not brown, about 10 minutes. Add the drained sauerkraut, stirring to mix well, and continue to cook for five minutes. Add the juniper berries and caraway seeds and mix.

3. Put the sauerkraut mixture in the bottom of a roasting pan. Place the roast on top. Cover with the sauerkraut liquid. Bury the bay leaf in the sauerkraut. Bake in a preheated 350°F oven for one and a half hours or until the roast is cooked to the desired temperature.

Makes 6 servings.

sauerkraut, and as a key flavoring in a popular white Schnapps liqueur. It's the main spice in the famed German-French dish Alsatian pork and sauerkraut. The French put juniper berries in pates and charcuterie.

Juniper's fragrance—pungent, with a scent of pine—is popular in perfumed toiletries and room deodorizers. At one time, the Swiss put juniper berries in heating fuel for schools, to sanitize classrooms.

How to Buy Juniper Berry

Dried juniper berries are available in most supermarkets. They should feel moist and pliable to the touch, and easily crush between your fingers.

You may find a cloudy bloom on the skin of some berries. It's mold, and it's commonplace, because the berries retain moisture. Avoid berries with excessive mold, however.

Juniper berries keep well in an airtight container away from heat or light. Hard berries have gone bad and should be thrown out.

In the Kitchen with Juniper Berry

Juniper berries are easy to work with in the kitchen. They should always be crushed rather than used whole. Because they're somewhat soft, you can do this with your fingers, or tap them slightly with a mortar and pestle. Crushing releases their oils, so don't crush or grind the berries until you're ready to use them.

Juniper berries are traditionally used in game dishes, but they can enhance any meat dish, including beef and chicken roasts. Some cooks even add them to seafood stews.

Here are ways to add more juniper berries to your diet:

- Use juniper berries in spice rubs for pheasant, duck, or squab along with cloves, bay leaf, rosemary, thyme, nutmeg, and garlic.
- Make a marinade for game steaks and kabobs by combining apple cider and olive oil with crushed juniper berries, black peppercorns, garlic, and bay leaf.

- Juniper goes well with purple fruits—plums, blackberries, and blueberries.
- Add it to roasting goose and duck to reduce the taste of congealed fat.
- Add ground juniper berries to bread stuffings.

- Add a few berries to the casserole when making *coq au vin*, the classic French chicken in wine.

KOKUM   *India's Exotic Weight-Loss Wonder*

Unless you've visited the Western coast of India or been a dinner guest in an Indian household, you have probably never tasted kokum. Once you've done so, however, it's likely you'll be eager to taste it again.

People who have been lucky enough to visit India's Western Ghats region in the summertime often talk about an unusually tasty and refreshing creamy pink drink unique to the area called *sol kadhi*. The drink gets its creaminess from coconut milk, but the pink comes from kokum, an exotic spice from a lush ornamental fruit tree native to Ghats.

The tiny fruit, which emerges red amid large green foliage and turns a deep purple when ripe, is harvested and dried in the spring, just in time to feature sol kadhi on the menu for the searing summer months. The drink is not only popular for its taste, but also because it helps the locals cool down in the humid, tropical air—a medicinal property of kokum that also helps prevent dehydration and sunstroke. And though many people may not realize it or even notice, kokum offers another benefit—it may help cut down on the urge to overeat!

Natural Weight-Loss Aid

Kokum is being investigated as a natural weight loss aid because it contains *hydroxycitric acid* (HCA), a compound found in the dried rind—the spice itself. HCA is a known appetite suppressant, and numerous studies show that ingesting HCA not only leads to weight loss, but *fat* loss.

In a study conducted in Thailand, researchers asked 50 obese women to go on a diet consisting of 1,000 calories a day, along with a daily diet "pill." Half got a pill containing HCA; the other half got a placebo. After the two months, the women taking the HCA had lost almost twice as much weight. The greater weight loss "was due to a loss of fat storage," reported the researchers.

In another study, reported in the journal *Nutrition*, researchers put lab animals on a three-week diet, during which they lost 20 percent of their body weight. For the next four weeks, they let the animals eat at will, just as humans often do after a calorie-restricted diet. But half the animals received food laced with HCA. The researchers found that the animals getting the HCA ate less and gained back less weight.

Weight loss is the latest addition to the many health benefits historically credited to kokum. Centuries before the spice became a staple in the area's famed Konkani cuisine, Ayurvedic

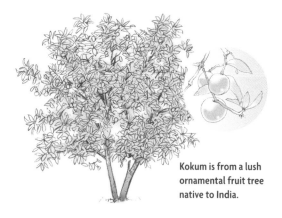

Kokum is from a lush ornamental fruit tree native to India.

physicians used it to treat sores and prevent infection, improve digestion, stop diarrhea and constipation, soothe the sore joints of rheumatoid arthritis, cure ear infections, and heal ulcers. It's also a folk remedy for fever and skin rashes.

Kokum gets this diverse combination of healing actions from its major active ingredient: *garcinol*, a substance with antioxidant and anti-inflammatory qualities. These qualities led me and other researchers to wonder whether this spice might have potential as a cancer fighter. Studies show it does . . .

Kokum Against Cancer

Human and animal studies at major cancer centers, including M.D. Anderson, have found that garcinol has the ability to track and kill renegade cells on two dozen different pathways to tumor progression. This is significant, because agents that have this ability can not only *prevent* cancer but also have potential as a *treatment* for the disease.

Researchers in Taiwan, for example, observed the compound's power when they induced cancer in laboratory animals with human cancer cells. A subsequent dose of garcinol annihilated those cells.

In another study, oral cancer specialists in Japan injected the tongues of lab animals with cancer cells. For the next eight months, half the animals were given daily doses of dietary garcinol from kokum. At the end of the study, the researchers found that the kokum-fed animals had developed less cancer and had smaller tumors.

Kokum also showed its strength as a cancer fighter when researchers in Taiwan tested it against curcumin, the well-studied active ingredient in the Indian spice turmeric that possesses potent anti-cancer activity. Kokum is structurally similar to turmeric. In the lab experiment, reported in the *Journal of Agriculture and Food Chemistry*, both curcumin and garcinol were effective at stopping the proliferation of leukemia cancer cells, but garcinol proved to be the more powerful of the pair.

Kokum may help prevent and/or treat:

Cancer	Rash
Indigestion	Ulcer
Overweight	

Kokum pairs well with these spices:

Cardamom	Galangal
Chile	Garlic
Cinnamon	Lemongrass
Clove	Mustard seed
Cumin	Star anise
Curry leaf	Tamarind
Fennel seed	

and complements recipes featuring:

Curries	Potatoes
Legumes	Vegetables
Lentils	

Substitute: Kokum is similar to tamarind and one can stand in for the other in recipes. One teaspoon of ground kokum is equal to one teaspoon of tamarind extract.

Help for Ulcers

For centuries, Ayurvedic physicians have used kokum successfully to treat and prevent stomach ulcers, and modern medicine is proving why it works—by killing *H. pylori*, the bacteria that are the chief cause of both gastric (stomach) and peptic (stomach, small intestine, or esophageal) ulcers.

Chronic ulcer problems can lead to stomach cancer. And although the incidence of stomach cancer in the US is low, it's also of growing concern, because *H. pylori* is becoming increasingly resistant to antibacterial medication. Garcinol's antibacterial, ulcer-targeting activity makes it a prime candidate to eradicate *H. pylori* naturally.

Early studies show promise. A study in lab animals, reported in the journal *Molecular Cell Biochemistry*, found that garcinol inhibited the growth of *H. pylori* and was "equivalent or better" than clarithromycin (Biaxin), a potent antibiotic, in treating the infection.

In Japan, which has the highest rate of stomach cancer in the world, researchers found dietary garcinol so effective at preventing ulcers in lab animals that they suggested it has potential to be the next anti-ulcer drug.

Protecting the Brain

Preliminary research suggests garcinol's antioxidant strength has the ability to promote brain health. Taiwanese scientists found that seven days of treatment with garcinol promoted the growth of neurons in test tubes, and stopped damage from substances that can oxidize neurons. The researchers concluded that garcinol may be "neuroprotective."

A Powerful Antioxidant

One of the reasons kokum is proving to be a stellar medicinal spice is because garcinol oper-ates in such diverse ways on the molecular level. For example, there is a type of cell-damaging molecule called a *reactive oxygen species* (ROS) that is produced by factors such as high-fat diets, air pollution, and stress. ROS play a leading role in cardiovascular disease, cancer, and many other chronic health problems. Garcinol's antioxidant power, which is stronger than vitamin E, has been shown to suppress production of ROS. And this is just *one* of the ways it protects your cells.

It's still too early to establish garcinol's true ability as a healing agent. To date, only a small number of studies have been conducted in animals, and none in humans. Until there are more studies, I suggest you benefit from garcinol by familiarizing yourself with kokum and kokum recipes, especially those that come from India.

Getting to Know Kokum

Kokum is not what you'd call attractive, especially when compared to other spices, but its taste defies its looks. Unlike the beautifully colored kokum fruit, the dried rind that is kokum spice is deep purple (in fact, almost black), with gnarly edges. It's also slightly sticky.

Spicy Hash Brown Potatoes

Spicy with a nip of sweetness, kokum potatoes are traditionally served over rice in India. They also go great as is, as a side to grilled meat or fish.

2 pounds Yukon gold potatoes
4 kokum rinds
½ teaspoon cumin seeds
4 cloves of garlic, chopped
1 teaspoon sugar
½ teaspoon cayenne powder
2 tablespoons olive or canola oil
½ cup water

1. Peel and boil the potatoes in salted water until just tender, about 10–15 minutes. Drain and cool.
2. Meanwhile, grind the kokum and cumin seeds in a spice grinder or mini food processor until the kokum resembles coarsely ground pepper. Place in a small bowl and add the garlic, sugar, and cayenne.
3. Cut and slice the potatoes into small cubes. Heat the oil in a large skillet over medium heat and add the spice mixture. Cook and stir until fragrant, about 30 seconds. Add the potatoes and stir well to coat the potatoes with the spices. Lower the heat, cover, and cook until the potatoes are soft, about 10 minutes. If potatoes are too dry in the pan, add the water before covering.

Makes 6 servings.

Sol Kadhi

This drink is traditionally made with coconut milk, but I prefer it made with yogurt. It's also less caloric that way.

5 kokum rinds
2 cups plain yogurt
4 cups water
2 cloves garlic, chopped
2 green chiles, crushed with salt and chopped
2 tablespoons vegetable oil
2 teaspoons yellow mustard seeds
2 sprigs curry leaves
Salt and sugar to taste
1 tablespoon finely chopped cilantro

1. Put the kokum in a small pot, cover with water, bring to a boil, and cook for five minutes. The water should be bright pink. Strain the water into a bowl and discard the rinds. Cool.

2. Combine the yogurt, water, garlic, chiles, and 2 tablespoons of the reserved kokum juice into a mixing bowl and stir until well blended. Strain the liquid from the mixture with a fine sieve and return the solids to the mixing bowl.

3. Heat the oil in a small sauté pan. When hot, add the mustard seeds, and immediately remove the pan from the heat. Add the curry leaves and stir.

4. Pour the seasoning over the sol kadhi, adding salt and sugar to taste. Pour into tall chilled glasses. Garnish with cilantro.

Makes 4 servings.

It's somewhat sour in taste, lending a sweet-and-sour contrast to (and enhancing the quality of) coconut-based curries. And while it doesn't have a heady perfume like other spices, if you get real close you can detect a slightly sweet aroma.

Kokum is not well known as a culinary spice outside of India. But it is one of the key ingredients in Konkani cuisine, which is an adventure in itself—as those who have tasted sol kadhi will no doubt agree!

When kokum travels beyond its borders, it mostly does so in the guise of kokum butter, an emollient used in cosmetics, much the same as shea and cocoa butters. In Europe, it's a common ingredient in lipstick, moisturizing creams, conditioners, and soap. And it is used extensively in products made for dry, chapped, irritated, and sunburned skin.

Kokum is also used as a souring agent, and you might come across it as an ingredient in imported chutneys and pickles.

Kokum goes by many names, including kokam, kokkum, fish tamarind, mangosteen, wild mangosteen, and red mango, though it bears no resemblance to mangosteen or mango. Mangosteen, the weight-loss product, does not contain kokum (but it does contain HCA, the same weight-loss chemical found in kokum).

How to Buy Kokum

With a little ingenuity, you can introduce kokum into your pantry and give your taste buds and health a boost. You'll be hard pressed to find kokum outside of an Indian market, but you can find mail order sources in the "Buyer's Guide" on page 309.

In the marketplace, look for rinds that are tinged with purple (as opposed to looking black). They should be soft and pliable. If they are too hard or are kept too long, they start to lose their flavor. If you notice a coating of white on some of the rinds, there is no need for concern—it's just salt left behind in the drying process. Wash it off with cold water before using.

Buy a small quantity of kokum and transfer it to a jar with an airtight lid. It should keep well for about a year. A small pack contains about a dozen rinds. Unfortunately, you won't know the quality of kokum until you submerge it in liquid. It should turn pink to purple in color. The deeper the color, the better the quality.

In the Kitchen with Kokum

Kokum is used three ways in the kitchen. It is ground whole and used as a dry spice, usually with other spices; it is submerged whole in liquid, where it softens and flavors dishes; and it is pulverized into a powder.

It is most popular in curries and in sol kadhi.

It goes well with potatoes, okra, beans, and lentils. It is also used in chutneys and pickles. Here are a few ways you can use it at home:

- Put a rind or two in curry pastes and tomato sauces.
- When cooking lentils, add a few pieces at the beginning.
- Grind and sprinkle on guava, pomegranate seeds, cooked vegetables, potatoes, and soups.
- Stir ground kokum into yogurt.

LEMONGRASS *The Calming Spice*

You know the saying: When life hands you lemons, make lemonade. Well, when life hands you lemongrass, make lemongrass tea. You'll feel a whole lot better.

Overwrought Brazilians drink *abafado*, a lemongrass tea believed to relieve tension and aid sleep. Nigerian folk healers use lemongrass tea to soothe sore throats, lower fevers, and control type 2 diabetes. In Thailand and Vietnam—where lemongrass is a much-used ingredient in the cuisine—folk healers also use it to improve circulation.

One reason these folk remedies might work is *citral*, an antioxidant oil in lemongrass that is anti-inflammatory, antibacterial, and antifungal. The oil is also rich in *plant sterols*, a cholesterol-like compound that cuts the absorption of dietary cholesterol.

Taming Tough-to-Lower Cholesterol

Researchers in the Department of Nutritional Sciences at the University of Wisconsin studied 22 people with high total cholesterol (an average of 315 mg/dL; 200 or less is normal). They gave them 140 milligrams (mg) a day of lemongrass oil. After three months, eight had big drops in total cholesterol, of up to 38 mg/dL.

In another study on lemongrass and cholesterol, researchers in Chile found that a compound in lemongrass stopped the oxidation of "bad" LDL cholesterol—the same process that forms artery-clogging plaque. "As oxidative damage to LDL is a key event in the formation of atherosclerotic lesions, the use of this natural antioxidant may be beneficial to prevent or attenuate atherosclerosis," concluded the researchers in the journal *Molecules*.

High cholesterol is common in people with type 2 diabetes, 75 percent of whom die of heart disease. Noting that lemongrass is used by the Yoruba healers of southwest Nigeria to treat type 2 diabetes (as well as fever, jaundice, throat and chest infections, moderate-to-severe pain, hypertension, and obesity), scientists in Nigeria tested an extract of the spice on laboratory animals. They found it lowered LDL, total cholesterol, and triglycerides, increased "good" HDL, and also lowered blood sugar levels, "confirming its folkloric use and safety in type 2 diabetic patients."

Keep on the Lemongrass

There are many other ways lemongrass might be good for you.

Cancer. In the laboratory, a team of researchers from the Indian Institute of Integrative Medicine studied the power of lemongrass oil against 12 types of human cancer cells. The more lemongrass oil, the worse it was for the cancer cells—with lemongrass destroying projectile-like structures on the surface of cancer cells, blocking the first stage of cancer cell division, and killing cancer cells. Lemongrass oil "has a promising anticancer activity and causes loss in tumor cell viability," concluded the researchers in the journal *Chemical and Biological Interactions*.

When Israeli researchers investigated "the anti-cancer potential" of citral—the amount found in a typical cup of lemongrass tea—they found it could kill human cancer cells.

Researchers from the Department of Dermatology at the UCLA School of Medicine found citral protected animals against skin cancer, and has a "possible role as an anti-tumor" agent. Japanese researchers also found that citral activated antioxidants in the skin that could protect against skin cancer.

Another team of Japanese researchers found that a lemongrass extract protected laboratory animals against chemical-induced liver cancer, publishing their results in the journal *Cancer Letter*. And writing in the journal *Carcinogenesis*, a group of Japanese researchers found lemongrass extract protected laboratory animals against colon cancer.

Researchers in India found that a lemongrass extract protected laboratory animals against DNA-damaging ionizing radiation—the same type of cancer-causing radiation we get from the sun and from medical devices such as CT scans and x-rays.

Anxiety. Noting that lemongrass tea is used in Brazilian folk medicine to reduce anxiety, Brazilian researchers tested an extract of lemongrass in mice. Using a standard maze device to measure the animals' level of anxiety, they found the tea significantly calmed the mice.

Insomnia. They also found that lemongrass extract reduced physical activity and induced sleep in mice as effectively as a sedative drug.

Epilepsy. The spice also reduced the number of chemically induced epileptic seizures in the mice.

Fungal and yeast infections. Doctors in South Africa found that lemongrass in lemon juice was an effective treatment for oral thrush (an infection on the inner cheeks and tongue with the fungus *Candida albicans*) in HIV/AIDS patients. The findings were in the journal *Phytomedicine*.

Researchers in Brazil also found that lemongrass oil and citral had "potent" activity against candida. Japanese researchers found the same, and said their results "provide experimental evidence suggesting the potential value of lemongrass oil for the treatment of oral or vaginal candidiasis."

Getting to Know Lemongrass

Lemongrass is, well, *grass*—tufted, razor-like blades with a central rib that are native to Southeast Asia. When the leaves are chopped and crushed they give off the lemony aroma that is characteristic of the cuisines of Thailand and Vietnam, where lemongrass is widely used in stews, and in soups such as hot-and-sour soup.

In Thailand, the tender stalks are also added fresh to salads and pounded into spice pastes for curries. (Sometimes the leaves are tied in a knot

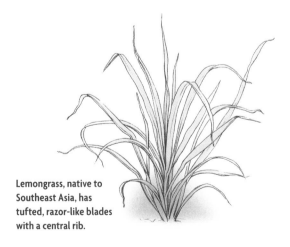

Lemongrass, native to Southeast Asia, has tufted, razor-like blades with a central rib.

and simmered in a curry.) In fact, lemongrass is used to flavor spice pastes and blends throughout Southeast Asia. It's a key ingredient in hot condiments called *sambals*, and in an Indonesian spice called *bumbu*, which is popular at roadside food stands.

Lemongrass is cultivated in Southeast Asia, Sri Lanka, India, the Caribbean, Australia, and Florida. However, Florida lemongrass is not grown for culinary purposes. The oil is extracted for use in cosmetics, soaps, bath salts, perfumes, and furniture polish.

LEMONGRASS WAS USED

TO SCENT BATHS IN

ANCIENT ROME.

Lemongrass oil is often called citronella—the name of the scented oil and candles used as bug repellents. But bug-repelling citronella oil is derived from two varieties of lemongrass that are inedible.

How to Buy Lemongrass

You can often find lemongrass fresh in large or high-end markets in areas where there is a large Asian population. Even though the entire plant is aromatic, you'll usually find only the lower white stalk—the only part of the plant tender enough to eat.

Fresh lemongrass stalks are usually sold in bunches. Choose stalks that are firm and don't look dried or wrinkled. They should be white with a greenish tinge. However, if lemongrass is native to your cuisine, you're more likely to

Lemongrass may help prevent and/or treat:

Anxiety	Diabetes, type 2
Cancer	Epilepsy
Cholesterol problems (high total cholesterol, high "bad" LDL cholesterol, low "good" HDL cholesterol)	Insomnia
	Thrush (oral candida infection)
	Triglycerides, high
	Vaginal yeast infection

Lemongrass pairs well with these spices:

Black cumin seed	Coconut	Galangal
	Coriander	Garlic
Cardamom	Cumin	Ginger
Chile	Fennel seed	Onion
Cinnamon	Fenugreek seed	Tamarind
Clove		Turmeric

and complements recipes featuring:

Asian stir-fries	Poultry
Curries	Shrimp
Marinades for meat and poultry	Soft-shell crabs
	Tomatoes

Other recipes containing lemongrass:

Malaysian Curry Paste (p. 287)	Thai Red Curry Paste (p. 286)
Thai Coconut Chicken Soup (p. 126)	

purchase the whole plant, including the root and leaves, using the leaves to make lemongrass tea. Lemongrass enthusiasts also fold the leaves to release the aromatic flavor, and add them to foods cooked in a liquid. The leaves are discarded before eating, like a bay leaf. Asian and Latin markets usually carry the whole plant. But

Mussels with Thai Red Curry Sauce

With the make-ahead curry paste as an ingredient, this is an easy dish that is special enough to serve company. Serve it with a loaf of crusty bread to enjoy the sauce. To complete the meal, add a green salad made with Mediterranean Vinaigrette (p. 160).

3 pounds mussels, cleaned and debearded
1 tablespoon olive oil
2 tablespoons Thai Red Curry Paste (p. 286)
4 large red ripe tomatoes
3 garlic bulbs, peeled and diced
2 tablespoons chopped fresh ginger
1 fourteen-ounce can unsweetened coconut milk
1½ cups seafood stock
1 tablespoon Asian fish sauce
½ teaspoon salt
Freshly ground black pepper
½ cup fresh basil, coarsely chopped

1. Pick over the mussels and discard any that are open.

2. Heat the olive oil in a heavy large pot over medium-high heat. Add the red curry paste and fry until fragrant, stirring constantly, about one minute. Add the tomatoes, garlic, and ginger and continue to fry, stirring, until garlic is soft, about three minutes.
3. Stir in the coconut milk, stock, fish sauce, salt, and pepper to taste. Lower the heat and simmer 10 minutes. Add the mussels, turn up the heat, cover and cook, shaking the pot occasionally, until the mussels open, about 5–10 minutes. Transfer the mussels to four bowls and pour the sauce over them. Sprinkle with basil and serve.

Makes 4 servings.

be careful: the blades are sharp. (Whole lemongrass is also sold frozen.)

Lemongrass is also sold preserved in jars, with lemon juice or vinegar. It's the next best thing to fresh.

You can purchase dried lemongrass in Asian markets, sometimes sold under the Indonesian name *sereh*. It's also available online. (For a list of online resources, please see page 309.) You can find dried lemongrass whole, shredded, or ground. Reconstitute in warm water before using.

Ground lemongrass is available at most supermarkets with a well-stocked spice aisle.

All forms of dried lemongrass lack the characteristic intense lemony flavor of fresh, however. You'll get the best flavor from fresh lemongrass. If you can't find fresh, preserved is better than all forms of the dried.

You also can find dried lemongrass leaves for making tea in Asian and Latin markets. But don't use them for cooking: they contribute little to the taste of a dish.

Fresh lemongrass can be kept refrigerated in plastic wrap for about two weeks. It can also be frozen in an airtight freezer bag for six months. Dried lemongrass should be stored in an airtight container in a dry, dark place. It will keep for about a year.

In the Kitchen with Lemongrass
Because of its robust flavor, lemongrass can withstand long cooking without losing its flavor. It is best used in long-simmering dishes, such as a stew or curry. But to get the best results from its strong lemony taste, you need to prepare it properly.

If you've bought a stalk, cut it into thin rings. Or cut it into large pieces, and crush it with the back of a knife, as you would garlic, and add it to the dish. (Use it the same way you use scallions.)

If you've bought an entire plant, leaves and all, trim it to get to the edible part. Cut off the root end with a knife, and pull off the outer leaves right down to the white stalk. (It's a good idea to wear plastic gloves to protect your fingers from cuts.) Slice or chop the stalk.

Lemongrass Iced Tea

In Thailand, people drink lemongrass tea iced and slightly sweetened, as a cooling counterbalance to the hot cuisine. It is served at both lunch and dinner.

1 cup lemongrass pieces, about ½" each
½ cup sugar
8 cups water

1. Bring the lemongrass pieces, sugar, and 2 cups water to a boil in medium-size saucepan, stirring until sugar is dissolved. Remove from heat and steep, partially covered, until cool.

2. Put the steeped tea with the lemongrass pieces in a blender or food processor and process until finely chopped. Pour the tea through a fine-mesh sieve into a pitcher, pressing to get out all of the liquid. Discard the solids. Add ice, fill the pitcher with the rest of the water, and stir. Serve over ice.

You can use the entire stalk by tying the full length in a knot and dropping it into the pot. The bruising will release the lemon flavor. Again, be careful that you don't cut your fingers on the sharp leaf edges. The whole stalk isn't meant to be eaten—discard it at the end of cooking. (It will leave behind its intense aroma!)

You can use the fresh leaves to make a tea. Place the leaves in a large pot and pour a quart of hot water on top of them. Steep for 10 minutes. Strain the tea and discard the leaves.

Here are some ways to put more lemongrass in your diet:

- Cut the stalks coarsely and add them to the water when steaming seafood.
- Put stalks in foil when you barbecue fish.
- Use whole stalks as stirrers to put a touch of lemon in drinks or to intensify lemonade.
- You can use lemongrass to tenderize and aromatize meat. Break 2 stalks of lemongrass in pieces and put them in a spice grinder with a garlic clove and 1 tablespoon of coriander seeds. Combine the ground spices with 2 tablespoons of brown sugar and ¼ cup of Asian fish sauce, and rub the mixture into steaks or beef kabobs before grilling.
- Combine lemongrass (sweet) with copious amounts of garlic and shallots to make a sweet-and-sour sauce like they do in Malaysia.

MARJORAM   *The Mediterranean Miracle*

There's no doubt the Mediterranean diet is good for you. Study after study links it to improved health—those who consistently eat the diet have less heart disease, less high blood pressure and stroke, less cancer, less prediabetes and type 2 diabetes, less Alzheimer's, less obesity, even less depression. But there's still a lot of scientific debate about *which* elements in the Mediterranean diet bestow the greatest degree of health. Is it the olive oil, rich in monounsaturated fat? The antioxidant-rich fruits and vegetables? The red wine and its resveratrol? The blood-thinning garlic? Or is the diet so healthful because of what's *not* in it, such as the saturated fat in red meat?

Well, one study shows a *spice* might play

a big role in the health-giving power of the Mediterranean diet—marjoram.

Double the Protection

For the study, Italian researchers created several versions of the typical Mediterranean-style salad—leafy greens, crunchy fresh vegetables, and a spicy olive oil-based dressing. Their purpose: calculate the antioxidant power of each salad, as measured by its ability to stop cell-damaging, cell-destroying oxidation. (It's an accepted scientific fact that oxidation is a key process underlying most chronic diseases and aging itself.) To do this, the researchers used a test that measured antioxidant activity in terms of units of *oxygen radical absorbance capacity* (ORAC)—the capacity of antioxidants to absorb and disarm the "radical oxygen species" that do oxidative damage.

Each salad contained standard Mediterranean goodies: locally grown Romaine lettuce, tomatoes, cucumbers, onions, and carrots; a salad dressing of olive oil and red wine vinegar, infused with either basil, parsley, or a combination of garlic, rosemary, sage, and red chile; and—the important part—a *varying* combination of one or more of 30 other vegetables and spices. Each salad was tested four times for ORAC.

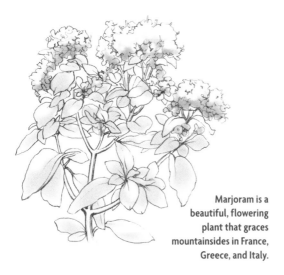

Marjoram is a beautiful, flowering plant that graces mountainsides in France, Greece, and Italy.

Marjoram Alert!

When the researchers sprinkled one of the salads with marjoram, ORAC units *doubled*. And sprinkled means *sprinkled*—the researchers added only three grams of the spice, about a teaspoon.

Why is marjoram so powerful? *Ursolic acid, carvacrol,* and *thymol*, said the researchers.

Marjoram may help prevent and/or treat:

Alzheimer's disease	Indigestion
Blood clots	Infection, bacterial
Cancer	Pollution side-effects
Fungal infection	Stroke
Heart disease	Ulcer

Marjoram pairs well with these spices:

Basil	Parsley
Celery seed	Rosemary
Cumin	Sage
Garlic	Sun-dried tomato
Oregano	Thyme

and complements recipes featuring:

Beans	Salad dressings
Bell peppers	Sausage
Cabbage	Tomato sauces
Eggs	Venison
Lamb	White sauces

Other recipes containing marjoram:

Bouquet Garni (p. 271)	Pizza Spice Blend (p. 272)
Hungarian Goulash (p. 61)	Spice de Provence (p. 271)
Penne and Sausage with Fennel Tomato Sauce (p. 117)	

These and other antioxidants in marjoram can protect the body in many ways.

Marvelous Marjoram

Many animal and cellular studies show that marjoram may help defeat some of the same diseases as the Mediterranean diet—and others, as well.

Helping slow Alzheimer's disease. The drugs used to slow the progress of Alzheimer's disease do so by boosting levels of *acetylcholine,* a neurotransmitter that speeds communication between brain cells. In an animal study, Korean researchers found that ursolic acid was nearly as powerful as an acetylcholine-increasing drug. Ursolic acid "could slow down the decline of cognitive function and memory in some patients with mild or moderate" Alzheimer's disease, and "might be a therapeutic treatment for the disease."

Fighting cancer. In the laboratory, researchers in Lebanon found that marjoram extracts stopped the growth of human leukemia cells. The extract is a "potential therapeutic agent," they concluded in *Leukemia Research.*

Stopping heart attacks and strokes. Marjoram is used as a blood thinner in Iranian folk medicine, noted a team of researchers from the University of Tehran. When they tested the spice in the laboratory, they found it cut platelet aggregation (the clumping of blood components that form artery-clogging blood clots) by 40 percent. This observation provides "the basis for the traditional use" of marjoram "in treatments of cardiovascular diseases and thrombosis [blood clots]," wrote the researchers in the journal *Vascular Pharmacology.*

Better digestion. Noting the "high consumption of marjoram in the Iranian population," another team of Iranian doctors tested the spice's ability to trigger the release of *pepsin,* a protein-digesting enzyme. Marjoram increased pepsin production in laboratory animals by 30 percent.

Pollution protection. In a study by Egyptian researchers, marjoram extracts protected laboratory animals against liver and kidney damage

Antioxidant Superstars

The vegetables in the list were tested for antioxidant activity in the Italian study discussed earlier in the chapter. They're listed in order of antioxidant power, from top to bottom (though they all scored high!).

1. Artichoke
2. Garlic
3. Beetroot
4. Radish
5. Red chicory
6. Broccoli
7. Leek
8. Spinach
9. Beet greens
10. Cabbage
11. Onion
12. Eggplant
13. Butternut squash
14. Yellow pepper
15. Cauliflower
16. Romaine lettuce
17. Red bell pepper
18. Green bell pepper
19. Tomato
20. Zucchini
21. Celery
22. Cucumber

from lead toxicity, probably because of its antioxidant power. "Populations with low-level lead exposure should use" marjoram extracts, the researchers concluded.

Preventing ulcers. Researchers in Saudi Arabia found that marjoram protected laboratory animals against chemically induced ulcers. In another study from the Middle East, marjoram extracts protected experimental animals from chemically induced damage to the liver, kidney, and testes.

Infection protection. Indian researchers found that a marjoram extract effectively killed a range of disease-causing fungi and bacteria, including *Candida albicans* (vaginal yeast infections), *Escherichia coli* (food poisoning), and *Staphylococcus aureus* (staph infections).

Getting to Know Marjoram

Marjoram is a beautiful, flowering plant that graces mountainsides in France, Greece, and Italy, and also graces Mediterranean kitchens with its aroma. (It's also a kissing cousin to

MARJORAM WREATHS
ARE ANCIENT SYMBOLS
OF LOVE AND JOY.

oregano—its Latin name is *Origanum marjorana*—and many cooks find them hard to tell apart.)

In ancient Greece, brides and grooms wore marjoram wreaths as a symbol of love and joy. Today's Greeks are still in love with marjoram—the scent of marjoram in meats and vegetable dishes cooked on open grills is a fixture of Greek life. (And it's a key ingredient in the *gyro*, a Greek dish that's become popular in the US and worldwide.)

The French also use a lot of marjoram. It's particularly popular in France's southern Provence region, and a key ingredient in the spice mix *bouquet garni*. The French use both fresh and dried marjoram to flavor chicken, lamb, fish, and butter sauces.

Germans call marjoram the "sausage herb" and often pair it with thyme when making homemade sausage.

Italians use it much the same way they do oregano: to the typical Italian cook, if something tastes good with oregano, then it tastes good with marjoram.

In the kitchen, Americans favor oregano over marjoram, but it's a commonly used commercial preservative in liverwurst, bologna, cheeses, soups, and salad dressings. It's also a key spice in commercial poultry seasoning.

How to Buy Marjoram

Marjoram is often called *sweet marjoram*, to distinguish it from oregano (which also is called *wild marjoram*, to make matters even more confusing). Worldwide, most commercial marjoram

---

Mediterranean Vinaigrette

Make a large batch and keep it on hand in the refrigerator. For salad fixings, favor the antioxidant-rich vegetables listed in the box on page 159.

1 teaspoon Dijon mustard
¾ cup extra-virgin olive oil
¼ cup red wine vinegar
1 clove garlic, diced
1 teaspoon dried marjoram
¼ teaspoon crushed rosemary
Salt and freshly ground pepper to taste

1. Put the mustard in a small mixing bowl and whisk in the olive oil. Add the vinegar, garlic, marjoram, rosemary, salt, and pepper. Put in a dressing jar with a firmly fitting lid. Shake well before using.

is grown in the Mediterranean region. Most of the marjoram sold in the United States is from Egypt.

Marjoram is available fresh, dried (whole or broken), and ground. It is sold dried in the spice section of most supermarkets. Kept in an airtight container in a cool, dry place, it maintains freshness for about a year.

In the Kitchen with Marjoram

Marjoram has a slightly bittersweet taste that is more like thyme than oregano. You can't go wrong putting it in any dish, but it works best with Mediterranean-style dishes and flavors.

Compared to oregano (as it often is), marjoram is mild. As a rule of thumb, use marjoram to flavor more delicate foods, such as eggs, and oregano to flavor stronger foods, such as eggplant. Being mild also makes it quite versatile.

There is really only one mistake you can make cooking with marjoram, and that's cooking it too long. Because it's delicate, it has a tendency to turn bitter, so always add it toward the end of a recipe with long-cooking foods.

MINT   *The Essence of Freshness*

"Mint" is a name like "Smith"—*very* common. There's field mint, forest mint, marsh mint, and mountain mint; Egyptian mint, Vietnamese mint, and Corsican mint; curly mint, thorn mint, and slender mint. And, of course, there are the famous twins, spearmint and peppermint. In all, about 600 plants answer to the name "mint." (There's even a Smith's mint.) And thousands of products contain it.

Mint is one of the most popular and recognizable flavors in the world. It's an ingredient in (among other things) soft drinks, candies, cocktails and liqueurs, jellies, syrups, cakes, ice teas, and ice creams. However, the mint that flavors these tasty treats is *one* mint: Peppermint. The *sweet* mint.

When you go to the grocery store to buy a jar of mint for recipes that call for the spice, you also are buying *one* mint: Spearmint. The *savory* mint.

But sweet or savory, refreshing mint is a potent healer. Starting with your digestive tract.

Keep Your Digestive Tract in Mint Condition

Studies show peppermint can help ease the symptoms of irritable bowel syndrome (IBS), a digestive problem that strikes an estimated one out of every seven Americans, many of them women. Medical scientists call IBS a "functional" health problem—they can't find any structural abnormality in the bowel, but they do know that it's not functioning normally, as intestinal muscles contract slower or faster than normal. The result: a range of symptoms that can include abdominal pain, cramping, and bloating; excess gas; diarrhea and constipation (sometimes one, and sometimes both, alternating).

Peppermint relaxes the muscles of the GI tract, helping to normalize those contractions and ease symptoms.

In a study by Italian researchers, 54 people with IBS took enteric-coated peppermint oil for four weeks. (The coating ensures the pill dissolves in the intestines rather than the stomach.) At the start and end of the study, the researchers measured the severity of abdominal bloating, abdominal pain or discomfort, diarrhea, constipation, feeling of incomplete evacuation, pain at defecation, passing of gas or mucus, and urgency of defecation. Seventy-five percent of people taking the remedy had at least a 50 percent reduction in symptoms.

In another study, 110 people with IBS were divided into two groups: one group took a placebo, and one group took an enteric-coated peppermint oil capsule 15 to 30 minutes before each meal. Of those taking peppermint, 79 percent reported relief from abdominal pain and discomfort, and 29 were pain-free. Bloating was reduced in 83 percent. Flatulence was eased in 79 percent. And 83 percent reported having to take fewer trips to the bathroom. There was little improvement in the placebo group.

Researchers in Canada found that peppermint oil can help clear up bacterial overgrowth in the small intestine, a suspected cause of IBS. "The results in this case suggest one of the mechanisms by which enteric-coated peppermint oil improves IBS symptoms," they concluded in *Alternative Medicine Review*.

And when researchers in the Gastroenterology Division of McMaster University in Canada evaluated 38 studies on treatments for IBS, they found three treatments were effective: more fiber in the diet, anti-spasmodic drugs—and peppermint oil.

But IBS isn't the only digestive problem that mint can help solve.

Indigestion. Researchers in the UK evaluated 17 studies using a natural remedy combining peppermint and caraway oil, and found it effectively reduced stomachache and other post-meal digestive symptoms 60 to 95 percent of the time.

A study of 96 people in Germany found that a peppermint-containing remedy offered significant relief from what doctors call "dyspepsia" (and you call indigestion). After four weeks of use, there was a 40 percent reduction in symptoms.

Colonoscopy. Japanese researchers found that using peppermint oil during a colonoscopy reduced GI spasms in 86 percent of 409 people, with "no adverse affects"—making it a "convenient alternative" to anti-spasmodic drugs that "sometimes cause side effects."

Upper endoscopy. During this medical test, a tube is inserted into the esophagus, stomach, and small intestine. The same team of Japanese researchers found that peppermint oil had "superior efficacy" compared to an anti-spasmodic drug in easing the procedure. Peppermint also

---

Mint may help prevent and/or treat:

Allergies	Indigestion
Anxiety	Irritable bowel
Breastfeeding	syndrome
problems	Menopause problems
Cancer	Menstrual cramps
Chronic obstructive	Nasal congestion
pulmonary disease	Nausea, postoperative
(COPD)	Polycystic ovarian
Cough	syndrome (PCOS)
Fatigue, mental	Postherpetic neuralgia
Gum disease (gingivitis)	Stress
Hirsutism (unwanted	Tooth decay
hair growth in women)	

---

produced "no significant side effects," whereas the drug produced dry mouth, blurred vision, and urinary retention.

Caution: Peppermint isn't perfect for all digestive problems. Some medical experts urge caution for those with heartburn, hiatal hernia, and kidney stones, because peppermint's ability to relax the GI tract might make those problems worse.

Breathing Easier

Peppermint is rich in the compound *menthol*—the rush of coolness you feel from peppermint-containing foods, beverages, and self-care products is menthol stimulating coldness receptors in the mucous membranes or the skin.

In a study by Germany researchers investigating how menthol works to ease nasal congestion, they reached the same conclusion as enthusiastic buyers of mentholated lozenges: it produces "the subjective feeling of a clear and wide nose."

Researchers in Wales agree. They studied 62 people with a cold, dividing them into two groups: half received a lozenge containing 11 milligrams (mg) of menthol and half a placebo lozenge. There was a "significant change" in "nasal sensation of airflow" in those sucking on menthol.

In the UK, researchers asked 20 people to repeatedly inhale a substance that would make them cough. Five minutes before each "cough challenge," the people inhaled either menthol, a pine scent, or air. Only "menthol inhalation caused a reduction in cough," wrote the researchers in the medical journal *Thorax*.

And when Japanese researchers impaired the breathing of 11 people, they found that breathing menthol produced a "significant reduction in sensations of respiratory discomfort."

Minting More Relief

There are many other ways that peppermint and spearmint can refresh your health.

Postherpetic neuralgia. As mentioned a moment ago, menthol triggers cold-sensitive receptors in cells, producing a cooling sensation so intense that the compound is an ingredient in pain-relieving topical products such as Icy Hot and Bengay. Well, that rush of cold sensation is also why menthol might work in relieving the intense pain of postherpetic neuralgia—nerve pain after a bout of shingles, a blistering viral rash that typically afflicts people in middle and old age.

In a report in the *Clinical Journal of Pain*, researchers at the Pain Management Center of University College found that applying peppermint oil containing 10 percent menthol "resulted in an almost immediate improvement of pain" in a patient with postherpetic neuralgia, with the relief lasting four to six hours.

Work performance. Menthol also seems to refresh the mind. Researchers at Wheeling Jesuit University in the US found that sniffing peppermint oil improved performance on two clerical tasks: typing (speed and accuracy) and alphabetical filing. "Peppermint oil may promote a general arousal of attention" so people "stay focused on their task and increase performance," concluded the researchers in the journal *Perceptual and Motor Skills*.

Polycystic ovarian syndrome (PCOS). This con-

Mint pairs well with these spices:

Allspice	Coriander	Rosemary
Basil	Cumin	Sage
Cardamom	Fennel seed	Sesame seed
Chile	Lemongrass	Thyme
Cinnamon	Onion	

and complements recipes featuring:

Chutney	Curries	Papaya
Crabmeat	Lamb	Peas
Cranberries	Mango	Yogurt

Other recipes containing mint:

Chaat Masala (p. 265)	Shellfish in Saffron
Dukkah (p. 268)	Broth (p. 211)
Roasted Tomato Soup with Fennel and Mint (p. 231)	

---

dition of abnormally high testosterone levels afflicts one out of 10 American women. One feature of the syndrome is unwanted facial and body hair (hirsutism). Researchers in the UK found that drinking spearmint tea twice a day for one month reduced abnormally high levels of testosterone in women with PCOS. "Spearmint has the potential for use as a helpful and natural treatment for hirsutism in PCOS," they concluded in *Phytotherapy Research*.

Stress and anxiety. Korean researchers found that nursing students who inhaled peppermint and other essential oils had less stress and anxiety. Inhalation of peppermint and the other essential oils "could be a very effective stress management method," concluded the researchers.

Postoperative nausea. US researchers studied 33 surgery patients and found that inhaling peppermint oil decreased postoperative nausea (a common problem) by 29 percent.

Breastfeeding. "Nipple pain and damage in breastfeeding mothers are common causes of premature breastfeeding cessation," noted a team of researchers, writing in the *International Journal of Breastfeeding*. They studied 196 breastfeeding women, and found that those who used a topical treatment of peppermint water on their nipples were three times less likely to develop a cracked nipple and five times less likely to suffer from nipple pain.

Tuberculosis. Russian researchers found that adding peppermint oil to combined multidrug therapy for tuberculosis helped kill bacteria and improve symptoms. "This procedure may be used to prevent recurrences and exacerbations of pulmonary tuberculosis," they concluded.

Chemotherapy-induced hot flashes. In a study by researchers in the UK, some women found a spray containing peppermint oil "extremely helpful" in lessening hot flashes induced by treatment for breast cancer.

Cancer. There are dozens of test tube and animal studies showing mint can battle cancer. Peppermint, spearmint, and compounds in them have been effective in slowing, stopping, or killing lung, prostate, liver, skin, stomach, bladder, brain, oral, and blood cancers.

Chronic obstructive pulmonary disease (COPD). A combination of emphysema and chronic bronchitis, this lung disease is the fourth leading cause of death in the US. Researchers in China found that spearmint oil decreased inflammation in the lungs of rats with experimentally induced COPD.

Cavities and gum disease. Researchers in the Middle East found that peppermint oil killed the bacteria that cause tooth decay and helped stopped plaque buildup.

MINT IS A COMMON

FLAVORING IN TOOTHPASTES

AND MOUTHWASHS.

Hay fever. In the laboratory, researchers in Japan found that mint extracts stop the release of histamine, the chemical that causes allergic symptoms such as watery eyes, itching, and nasal congestion. "These results suggest that extracts [of mint] may be clinically effective in alleviating the nasal symptoms of allergic rhinitis [hayfever]," concluded the researchers.

Getting to Know Mint
Spearmint and peppermint have been used as an ingredient in toiletries and cosmetics for centuries, and today they're a common flavoring in toothpaste and mouthwash. But mint didn't flavor food until the 17th century.

The English were the first to eat mint and they're still big fans—no English cook would serve lamb without the traditional mint sauce. Americans also favor mint with lamb, preferring mint jelly.

Countries in the eastern Mediterranean (Greece, Turkey, and the Mediterranean coun-

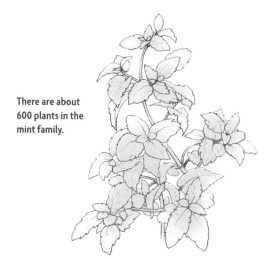

There are about 600 plants in the mint family.

Grilled Lamb Patty Pockets with Cucumber Mint Sauce

This Middle-Eastern dish, perfect for a picnic, gives a spicy twist on the traditional cucumber mint sauce called tzatziki.

For the sauce:
1 cup plain yogurt
1 cup peeled and seeded cucumber, coarsely chopped
¼ cup fresh mint, tightly packed
1 tablespoon lime juice
½ teaspoon salt
¼ teaspoon ground cumin
¼ teaspoon sweet paprika
¼ teaspoon chili powder
¼ teaspoon sugar
Freshly ground white pepper to taste

For the patties:
1 pound lean ground lamb
½ cup fresh breadcrumbs
½ cup diced onions
1 large egg, beaten lightly
1 large garlic clove, minced
2 teaspoons olive oil
1 tablespoon dried mint leaves, crumbled
1 teaspoon ground allspice
½ teaspoon ground cinnamon
¼ cup white sesame seeds, toasted
Salt and freshly ground black pepper to taste
4 large pita breads

Toppings:
1 green bell pepper, sliced
1 red bell pepper, sliced
1 small red onion, thinly sliced
1 cup pepperoncini peppers, sliced

1. *To make the sauce:* Place the yogurt in a fine mesh strainer set over a bowl and let it drain for about five minutes. Discard any liquid that drains from the yogurt.
2. Combine the cucumber, mint, lime juice, salt, cumin, paprika, chili powder, sugar, pepper, and drained yogurt in a food processor and blend until smooth. Refrigerate until ready to use.
3. *To make the lamb patties:* Combine the ground lamb, breadcrumbs, onions, egg, garlic, olive oil, mint, allspice, cinnamon, sesame seeds, salt, and pepper and mix well.
4. Wet your hands and form into eight patties. Spray the grate of a grill with non-stick spray and heat to high. Grill the patties for two minutes on each side or until desired doneness. Place two patties on a pita, ladle with the sauce, and serve with the toppings.

Makes 4 servings.

tries of the Middle East) and Southeast Asia use a *lot* of mint, as does India—fresh or dried, in sweet and savory dishes. (And, of course, in tea: black tea brewed with spearmint is a favored beverage in the Middle East and Africa.)

In India, mint *raita*, made with cucumber and yogurt, is a popular condiment; it's a cooling contrast with hot curries. Mint is a key spice in the Indian meatballs known as *kofta*, and in the spice mix *chaat masala*. Spearmint is ground with coconut, chiles, onion, and green mango for chutney. It is also added to spicy rice dishes called *biryanis*.

In North Africa, mint is always around when *harissa*, one of the world's hottest condiments, is served. It is a popular spice in Moroccan stews called *tagines*, and in stuffed vine leaves, a Middle Eastern specialty popular in the US. It is an ingredient in the Egyptian spice mix *dukkah*. It is also an important spice in Iranian and Turkish cuisines. Mint is the spice that defines the popular Greek yogurt and cucumber sauce called *tzatziki*.

In Malaysia, mint is combined with turmeric, galangal, lemongrass, and shrimp paste to flavor spicy noodle broths called *laksas*. Mint is in Thai green curry paste. It's used in Asian stir-fries.

Mint is also one of a bartender's best friends. There are about five dozen drinks in the bartender's repertoire that include mint leaves or mint-flavored alcohol, such as the liqueur crème de menthe, used to make stingers and grasshoppers. The most popular mint cocktail these days is a mojito, which includes citrus juice and tequila. And, of course, there is the German favorite peppermint Schnapps. On the first Saturday in May, when Churchill Downs hosts the Kentucky Derby, 1,000 pounds of fresh mint are mulled to make Mint Juleps, the classic derby drink, made with bourbon, simple syrup, bitters—and lots of mint.

How to Buy Mint

As already mentioned, the generic mint you get from the grocer is dried spearmint, but you can get dried peppermint from specialty spice shops or online. (You'll find a list of spice retailers in the "Buyer's Guide" on page 309.)

Dried mint (spearmint) is sometimes referred to as rubbed mint, because the leaves break into tiny pieces when the dried leaves are rubbed off the stems. It darkens when dried, becoming almost black. But the color doesn't affect quality or freshness.

For freshness, check the aroma. Spearmint should smell warm and slightly pungent; peppermint, cool and slightly peppery.

In the Kitchen with Mint

Unless you're into making specialty cakes and confections, there is little use for peppermint in the kitchen other than making tea. There are, however, many uses for spearmint.

Mint is a dominant flavor. For this reason, many cooks think mint doesn't marry well with other spices. But chefs adept at Indian and Asian cuisine blend it with other strong spices with success.

Here are ideas to put more mint in your diet:

- Break mint sprigs in small pieces and freeze them with water in ice cube trays. Use the ice in iced tea, lemonade, and tonics.
- Sprinkle mint in butter spread for corn on the cob.
- Grind fresh or dried mint with a pinch of salt in a mortar and pestle and add it to olive oil and vinegar dressing.
- Add mint to cream-based soups and sauces.
- Add mint to pea soup and dishes featuring peas.
- Add mint to cold cucumber soup.
- Substitute mint for basil in a mint pesto.
- Make an untraditional chimichurri sauce (p. 190) by substituting mint for the parsley.
- For a change of taste, use mint instead of oregano or marjoram in eggplant and tomato dishes.

MUSTARD SEED *Faithful to Good Health*

Because it's so small—about 1/10 inch in diameter—the mustard seed has played a big role in religion. Jesus Christ said that those with faith even as small as a mustard seed could move mountains. Gautama the Buddha used the mustard seed as a measure of eternity, comparing the endless time in a "world cycle" to the time it would take to move an enormous pile of mustard seeds if one seed were moved every one hundred years. The Koran says that even the equivalent of a mustard seed will be accounted for on the Day of Judgment.

Well, nowadays even scientists are starting to have faith in the tiny mustard seed. The source of the seed—the mustard plant—is a *crucifer*, the cancer-fighting plant family that includes broccoli, brussels sprouts, kale, and cabbage. The mustard seed, it turns out, contains concentrated amounts of the same anti-cancer compounds found in those greens.

The Anti-Cancer Connection

The main compounds: *glucosinolates*, released from crucifers when they're chewed and from mustard seed when it's broken or soaked. An oily, fiery byproduct of the glucosinolates—*allyl isothiocyanates* (AITC)—gives mustard seeds (and its cruciferous cousins, horseradish and wasabi) their distinctive bite and a lot of their healing power.

The mustard seeds we're talking about, however, are not from the mustard greens you'll find in a supermarket. They're seeds from three mustard plants venerable enough to have made it into ancient religious texts. The seeds are:

- *White, or yellow, mustard seeds.* Popular in the United States for the American-style yellow mustard they produce, they are the largest of the three seeds, with the mildest flavor.
- *Brown mustard seeds.* Popular in Europe and Asia, they also go by the name Chinese mustard and are medium-sized and pungent.
- *Black mustard seeds.* Indigenous to India, they are the smallest and most potent of the three—about 30 percent hotter than brown.

Significant Protection

More than two hundred test tube and animal studies show that the AITC in cruciferous vegetables and plants can help prevent and slow the growth of a number of cancers, including colon, lung, prostate, bladder, and ovarian. A recent scientific review of research on AITC, from the Roswell Park Cancer Institute in Buffalo, New York, concluded that the compound shows "anti-cancer activity" and "exhibits many desirable attributes of a cancer chemopreventive agent" (a natural substance that fights cancer).

A few of those studies have tested AITC and other anti-cancer compounds in mustard seeds:

The omega-3 fatty acids found in fatty fish such as salmon can protect against the development of colon cancer. Researchers at South Dakota State University found that mustard seed oil—rich in *alpha-linolenic acid* (ALA), a plant-based omega-3—was *more* protective against colon cancer in experimental animals than fish oil.

Indian researchers found that brown mustard seeds reduced the level of tumors in animals with chemically induced colon cancer. The inclusion of mustard seeds "in a daily diet plays a significant role in the protection of the colon against chemical carcinogenesis," concluded the researchers.

Canadian researchers found that an extract of white or yellow mustard seeds reduced colon cancer up to 50 percent in experimental animals fed a high-fat diet, and that the extract might help defeat "obesity-associated colon cancer" in people.

Another team of Indian researchers (noting that mustard seed oil "is extensively used as a cooking medium in several countries because of a characteristic pungent and acrid flavor, and as a condiment" and that mustard seeds are "widely utilized in the preparation of edible sauces, pastes and pickles") found that mustard seed oils protected laboratory animals against chemically induced cancer. They theorized it works by detoxifying cancer-causing chemicals and as an antioxidant that protects cells from damaging oxidation. The findings were in *Cancer Letter.*

In Healing, Mustard Cuts the Mustard

Researchers have found many other ways mustard seed might protect health:

Heart disease. Researchers from the Harvard School of Public Health analyzed data on diet and heart disease from more than 1,000 people living in India and found those who cooked with mustard seed oil—rich in heart-protecting ALA—had a 51 percent lower risk of heart disease than those who cooked with sunflower seed oil. The findings were in the *American Journal of Clinical Nutrition*.

Researchers in India fed experimental animals brown mustard seeds, lowering their total and "bad" LDL cholesterol, and increasing "good" HDL cholesterol. The findings were in the journal *Plant Foods for Human Nutrition*.

Prediabetes. More than 50 million Americans suffer from this health-defeating condition, in which cells no longer respond to the glucose-controlling hormone insulin (a condition also called *insulin resistance*), and glucose (blood sugar) levels stay high. Uncontrolled, prediabetes can turn into type 2 diabetes—and type 2 diabetes can turn into heart disease, stroke, blindness, nerve pain, and kidney failure.

Indian researchers fed animals a high-sugar diet and their glucose and insulin levels skyrocketed. But when they also fed the animals brown mustard seeds, glucose and insulin levels normalized. Mustard seed "can play a role in the management of the prediabetes state of insulin resistance and should be promoted for use in patients prone to diabetes," concluded the researchers in the *Journal of Ethnopharmacology*.

Prostate problems. An enlarged prostate—the medical condition called *benign prostatic hypertrophy* (BPH)—is a common problem in older men, causing urinary difficulties. Chinese researchers found that two compounds in white mustard seeds helped prevent induced BPH in experimental animals.

Chronic obstructive pulmonary disease (COPD). Doctors in China used the traditional folk remedy of a "mustard plaster"—a cloth (poultice) saturated with mustard seed powder, put inside a protective dressing, and applied to the chest—to treat 59 people with chronic bronchitis (a form of chronic obstructive pulmonary disease, or COPD). Twenty-five other people with COPD didn't receive the treatment. After one year, those using the mustard plaster had a higher improve-

ment rate—in symptoms of the disease (such as coughing and breathlessness) and in levels of disease-fighting immune factors.

Brain health. Astrocytes are star-shaped cells in the brain and spinal cord with many important functions: they help neurotransmitters relay signals from neuron to neuron; they help control healthy blood flow in the brain; they supply neurons with key nutrients; they regulate potassium in the brain, a nutrient critical to normal neural functioning; and when nerve cells are injured (such as in spinal cord injury), they remove debris and help repair the area. Essential fatty acids are crucial to the health of brain cells, and researchers in India conducted laboratory studies on the fatty acids from several cooking oils, to see how they affected astrocyte growth and development. They found the ALA in mustard seed oil "was more effective than other oils" in sparking the growth and development of the cells. The role of mustard seed oil in "facilitating astrocyte development . . . can have potential impact on human health," concluded the researchers in the journal *Cell Molecular Neurobiology*.

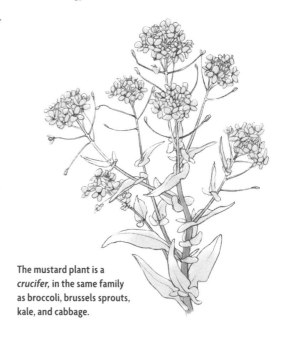

The mustard plant is a *crucifer*, in the same family as broccoli, brussels sprouts, kale, and cabbage.

Getting to Know Mustard Seed

Mustard seeds have no aroma or flavor. But when the seed coat is broken and comes into contact with cold (not hot!) water, an enzyme called *myrosinase* goes into action, setting off the process that produces the distinctive flavor of the condiment mustard.

It takes 10 minutes for the seeds to reach their full flavor, after which it starts to dissipate. And that's the secret to good mustard-making: bring the seeds to the flavor level you desire, then add an acid such as vinegar to kill the enzyme, then add your favorite combination of flavorings.

The ancient Romans were the first to develop the technique of mustard-making. They spread the practice throughout their empire, introducing white and black mustard seeds to England, where the condiment is now a favorite (perhaps because the sharp taste gives a heady lift to the country's notoriously bland food).

The Romans also took mustard seeds to Dijon, France, and in the 14th century that city became home to the first commercial mustard business. (If you find yourself in Dijon, consider a visit to the Mustard Museum.) Today, the French produce more than 3,500 varieties of prepared mustard.

In the 18th century, the English invented a way to mill the oily seeds into a dry powder. In the 19th century Colman's Mustard was founded, now the world's most famous dry mustard. Initially, dry mustard was manufactured by mixing white and black mustard seeds with turmeric, the bright yellow Indian spice, to give the mustard color and with wheat flour to give it texture. Today, only white mustard seeds are used.

Mustard didn't hit the American culinary scene until the late 19th century, when the brothers Robert and George French bought a processing mill in Fairport, New York. Robert invented the bright yellow French's mustard, which made its debut in 1904 on a hotdog at the St. Louis World's Fair.

Today, mustard powder and seeds are among the world's most popular spices. Both the powder

Mustard seed may help prevent and/or treat:

Benign prostatic hypertrophy (BPH)	Chronic obstructive pulmonary disease (COPD)
Cancer	Diabetes, type 2
Cholesterol problems (high total cholesterol, high "bad" LDL cholesterol, low "good" HDL cholesterol)	Heart disease
	Insulin resistance (prediabetes)

Mustard seed pairs well with these spices:

Allspice	Cinnamon	Galangal
Black cumin seed	Clove	Ginger
	Coriander	Star anise
Cardamom	Cumin	Tamarind
Chile	Fennel seed	Turmeric

and complements recipes featuring:

Ale and beer	Fish
Beef	Meats, especially cold or boiled
Brussels sprouts	
Cabbage	Pickles
Cauliflower	Sauerkraut
Curries	Sausage

and seeds are used to make prepared mustards, which come in a wide range of temperatures, from mild to tongue-scorching, with a seemingly infinite number of flavorings.

The English favor strong mustards made from brown seeds or a combination of brown and white. Germany boasts a vast array of mustards, and bottles of both mild and strong mustards are a mainstay on tables in German households and restaurants. Dusseldorf, made from black seeds, is Germany's most famous brand. Both the English and Germans use prepared mustard generously on meats, sausages, and cold cuts.

Derby Day Mustard

This mustard can be served with grilled sausages, meats, and cold cuts, on sandwiches, or as a spread for smoked fish. Or combine equal parts of mustard and mayonnaise to making a dipping sauce for vegetables. The recipe gets its name in honor of the annual Radnor Hunt Races in Radnor, Pennsylvania.

1 cup dry mustard
1 cup cider vinegar
⅓ cup yellow mustard seeds
2 eggs, beaten
1 cup sugar

1. Blend the dry mustard and vinegar together in a small bowl. Cover and let stand overnight at room temperature.

2. The next day, soak the mustard seeds in enough cold water to cover, for 10 minutes. Strain. Combine the mustard seeds, beaten eggs, and sugar in the top of a double boiler. Scrape in the mustard and vinegar mixture. Cook, stirring occasionally, for 15 minutes, or until it thickens. Store in a sealed container.

Makes about 2 cups.

Dijon mustard is also made from black seeds, and it is an ingredient in two famous French sauces—sauce Robert and sauce verte—which are used on grilled meats.

World-famous Chinese mustard is made from powdered brown mustard seeds and water. The Chinese make a dipping sauce by combining dry mustard with sesame oil and chile oil.

Mustard is considered indispensible to Argentina's famed beef.

Indian cooks use brown or black mustard seeds, frying them in hot oil at the beginning of cooking until they pop. The process takes away the heat and leaves behind a nutty flavor. In South Indian cooking, brown mustard seeds are fried in oil with cumin seeds, curry leaf, and asafoetida (a process called tempering), and added to food at the end of cooking.

Indians also add whole seeds to countless numbers of chutneys, curries, pickles, and legume dishes called *dals*. Mustards seeds are also used to flavor many curry blends, pastes, and spice blends.

Mustard oil, made from brown seeds, is a popular cooking oil in India. Though pungent smelling and bitter tasting in the raw, it takes on a sweet, pleasant aroma when it meets heat.

In the United States, a ballpark frank would be unthinkable without yellow mustard. It's the perfect condiment for deviled eggs and potato salads, and on grilled meats, sausages, corned beef, and cold cuts. It is a custom in the Carolinas and other parts of the South to slather mustard-based "mop sauce" rather than red barbecue sauce on ribs and slow pit-roasted pork.

How to Buy Mustard Seed

Here's the rule of thumb when it comes to mustard seeds: the smaller and darker, the hotter. Black seeds taste sharp with a nutty aftertaste. Brown seeds are sweeter and mellower than black. White seeds have a subtle flavor.

White mustard seeds and dry mustard are readily available in any well-stocked market. The seeds are sold whole, crushed, or ground.

Brown mustard seeds are harder to come by, but you can find them in Indian and Asian markets and online.

Black mustard seeds are hard to find because they're not in wide-scale production. (Black seeds are difficult to harvest because they're so small.)

Even culinary experts have trouble distinguishing black from brown seeds, because brown seeds are a very dark brown, with a subtle deep red tinge. But it doesn't matter: brown seeds are a suitable substitute for black in any recipe.

Other recipes containing mustard seed:

Whole mustard seeds are quite stable and will keep for three years. It's not essential to keep them away from heat, but do keep them dry.

Prepared mustards come in a seemingly infinite variety, with a wide range of heat. When buying prepared mustard, avoid bottles that show signs of separation (a film of vinegar floating on top). For the best flavor, keep prepared mustard at room temperature.

In the Kitchen with Mustard Seed

Even though there are thousands of styles of prepared mustards, it's also fun to make your own. (And it's a great way to impress guests.)

Prepared mustard is made by first combining ground mustard seeds with water (or another liquid) to draw out the heat, then using vinegar or another acidic liquid to hold the heat in, and then adding flavorings to give it individuality. Almost anything goes when adding flavorings—exotic spices, edible flowers, wines, chiles, and honey are among the many options. Using dry mustard, of course, makes the whole process easier.

The acid doesn't add flavor, but stops the action of the enzyme and extends the blend's penetrating odor. When vinegar is added at the outset, it prevents the enzyme from acting, producing a mild flavor.

The initial soaking liquid is what develops the flavor. Cold water, milk, wine, and beer are among the popular choices. Water will give mustard a sharp taste, milk will give it a spicier and pungent flavor, and beer will make it very hot.

The seeds should sit in the liquid for 10 minutes to develop the full flavor. Vinegar or hot water can be added at any time within the 10 minutes to stop heat from developing. However, if you go over 10 minutes, the flavor will start to dissipate. White seeds produce the mildest mustard. Brown seeds produce a hot mustard. (If you've ever tasted Chinese mustard, you know how hot it can be!) Black seeds produce even more heat.

Making mustard is only one of the many uses for mustard seeds. Mustard seeds don't have to be toasted like other seeds, but doing so will give your dishes more texture and flavor. Here are some ideas for using them:

- Add whole seeds to marinades for grilled food, barbecue sauces, and rubs.
- Toast mustard seeds and grated coconut, and sprinkle over steamed beans.
- Mustard seeds go naturally with all the cruciferous vegetables. Fry seeds in oil until they pop, and sprinkle them over cooked cabbage, cauliflower, broccoli, brussels sprouts, collards, or mustard greens.
- Combine mustard seeds with 1 tablespoon each paprika and oregano for a coating on red meats.
- Mix ¼ cup ground mustard seeds with ¼ cup Worcestershire Sauce and the juice of one lime, and smear it over leg of lamb or other lamb roast about an hour before roasting.
- Make a Memphis mop sauce by combining ½ cup of ballpark-style mustard

with 2 cups of cider vinegar and 1 teaspoon of salt. Use as you would barbecue sauce.

- Make mustard vinaigrette by combining 2 teaspoons of mustard seeds, 1 teaspoon Dijon mustard, 1 tablespoon of lemon juice, and 2 tablespoons of apple cider vinegar. Slowly whisk in ⅓ cup of extra-virgin olive oil.
- Add prepared mustard to potato salad and powdered mustard to chicken salad.

NUTMEG *A Sprinkle of Healing*

When nutmeg was first imported into Connecticut in the 18th century, it quickly became the rage among young, wealthy gentlemen to carry nutmeg and a silver grater with them, so they could sprinkle the spice on food whenever and wherever they dined. But fraud followed fashion, as it often does: merchants whittled tree bark into nutmeg look-alikes and sold the fake "spice" for the same steep price as the authentic version. Imagine the chagrin when a young gentleman intent on impressing a young lady pulled out his shiny grater and began to try to shred a wooden "nutmeg" over a piece of pie! The widespread practice of this deception, say some historians, led to Connecticut's unofficial moniker: *The Nutmeg State.*

Now, it's more like Nutmeg Nation—Americans enjoy nutmeg as a flavoring in baked goods, and in classic beverages such as hot chocolate, mulled cider, and eggnog. And when nutmeg is sprinkled in your drink, you might be toasting to your own good health.

The Healing Promise of Myristicin
Nutmeg is unlike any other taste in the world. That intense, sweet flavor is from *myristicin*, a volatile oil found in many plants (including carrots, celery, and parsley) but most abundant in nutmeg. And while there aren't any human studies on myristicin, scientists have conducted test tube and animal studies on its healing powers (as well as that of other compounds in nutmeg).

High cholesterol. Two animal studies by researchers in India found that nutmeg reduced total cholesterol and "bad" LDL cholesterol.

Cancer. Researchers in Thailand found that extract of nutmeg killed human leukemia cells.

Wrinkles. Researchers in South Korea tested 150 plants to find compounds that could inhibit *elastase*, an enzyme that breaks down *elastin*, the protein fibers that keep skin youthfully taut and flexible. (When elastin is broken down, skin sags.) Nutmeg was one of six plants with the ability. Added to a cosmetic, nutmeg could have "anti-aging effects on human skin," the researchers concluded in the *International Journal of Cosmetic Science.* In another study from Korean researchers, a compound in nutmeg protected skin from the sun's skin-damaging UVB rays.

Anxiety. In an animal study in India, nutmeg was similar to common anti-anxiety drugs in alleviating anxiety-like symptoms.

Depression. In an animal study in the *Journal of Medicinal Food*, treatment with nutmeg was as effective as antidepressants in producing "significant antidepressant-like effects."

Memory. In an animal study, Indian researchers found nutmeg "significantly improved" learning and memory.

Low sexual desire. Nutmeg is a central nervous system stimulant, and is considered an aphrodisiac in Unani medicine (a healing system from ancient Greece, now widely taught in India and Pakistan). To test this use, researchers in India gave experimental animals nutmeg—and they went nuts. "The resultant significant and sus-

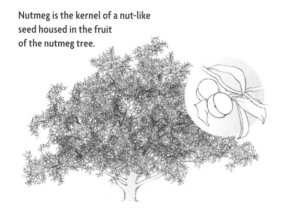

Nutmeg is the kernel of a nut-like seed housed in the fruit of the nutmeg tree.

Getting to Know Nutmeg

Take a trip to the Caribbean island of Grenada—where nutmeg trees are prolific, the spice scents the salty sea air, and a nutmeg fruit is pictured on the national flag—and you're as likely to come across someone massaging nutmeg butter into an arthritic joint as you are to encounter someone sprinkling the spice on rum punch. Nutmeg is an enduring folk medicine. Traditional healers use it to ease stomach cramps, diarrhea, and other digestive disorders, relieve headaches, calm troubled emotions, stimulate menstruation, and soothe hemorrhoids.

Nutmeg also has a long political and economic tradition: it was at the center of the world's spice trade for many centuries, with the source of the spice (the Maluku Islands in Indonesia, formerly known as the Moluccas and as the "spice islands") kept a closely guarded secret by spice traders. From the 14th to the 18th centuries, the Dutch, Portuguese, French, and English warred over the islands, until the English began to grow nutmeg trees elsewhere—including Grenada.

Today, nutmeg still thrives in the Maluku Islands and on Grenada, with these two areas providing most of the world's supply.

The spice is the kernel of a nut-like seed housed in the fruit of the nutmeg tree. The tree actually produces two culinary spices: nutmeg, the kernel, and mace, the *aril* or sheath that surrounds the seed like a net. Nutmeg is sweet, while mace is tart and strong.

tained increase in sexual activity indicated that extract of nutmeg possesses aphrodisiac activity, increasing libido," the researchers concluded in the journal *BMC Complementary and Alternative Medicine.*

Epilepsy. In an animal study, researchers in Pakistan found nutmeg "possesses significant anticonvulsant activity," preventing seizures. The findings were in *Phytotherapy Research.*

Diarrhea. In a study by Brazilian researchers, myristicin killed 90 percent of rotaviruses, the most common viral cause of diarrhea. Nutmeg "can be useful in the treatment of human diarrhea if the etiologic agent is a rotavirus," concluded the researchers in the *Journal of Ethnopharmacology.* Another study found that Medbarid, an Ayurvedic remedy containing nutmeg, is an effective natural medication for diarrhea.

Is Nutmeg a Narcotic?

Nutmeg has a reputation as an inexpensive narcotic—and that's not an urban legend. Ayurveda, the Indian system of natural medicine, calls nutmeg *madashaunda,* meaning "narcotic fruit." Many scientific studies conducted on nutmeg have examined it for its intoxicating effects—and found them. However, these studies also confirm that you have to ingest a *lot* of nutmeg—about two ounces—to produce intoxication, an amount impossible to consume in a normal culinary context, where a teaspoon can flavor an entire cheesecake.

That's why the Drug Enforcement Administration isn't conducting raids on the spice cabinets of Americans: the FDA considers nutmeg GRAS (generally recognized as safe) when used as a culinary spice. (Needless to say, never experiment with nutmeg as an intoxicant. There is more than one case of fatal nutmeg poisoning in people who did just that.)

Nutmeg's use varies from country to country. In the US and England, it's mostly used to flavor sweet dishes and beverages, both alcoholic (eggnog, hot rum, mulled wine, Kahlùa and cream) and non-alcoholic (cocoa and milkshakes). In England of old, it gave a spicy lift to pease porridge, the food of nursery-rhyme fame that is served hot, cold, or nine days old.

In the Caribbean, nutmeg is used in a variety of dishes, including jerked meats, curries, and spice mixes. In Grenada—where nutmeg syrup, made with sugar and rum, is a popular condiment—nutmeg goes in just about *everything*, including ice cream, soup, sweet potato pie, chicken, and a medley of rum cocktails.

France's fondness for nutmeg goes back centuries, when trees smuggled from the "spice islands" were planted on French soil. Nutmeg helps cut the richness in the French white sauce called *béchamel*, and in potatoes au gratin. Nutmeg is also one of the four spices in the blend *quatre épices*.

Nutmeg is a standard spice in Germany, where it is used to cut the richness in potatoes, puddings, and dumplings. Germans also sprinkle it in chicken soup.

India grows its own variety of nutmeg, which contains more oil and is therefore slightly stronger than Grenadian or Indonesian nutmeg. It is used in Moghul and Kashmiri cuisines to flavor vegetables and some desserts. It is a key ingredient in the spice mix *garam masala*.

Nutmeg also is an ingredient in Indian betel leaves that are rolled tightly and chewed (like chewing tobacco) for their digestive and stimulant effects.

How to Buy Nutmeg

Nutmeg is available whole or powdered, but it is most flavorful purchased whole and used freshly ground. Whole nutmegs are about 1 to 1¼ inches long, with a rough, light-brown shell. Quality can vary. Look for nutmegs that are unbroken and that show no signs of worms (such as worm-

---

Nutmeg may help prevent and/or treat:

Anxiety	Depression
Cancer	Diarrhea
Cholesterol problems (high total cholesterol, high "bad" LDL cholesterol)	Epilepsy
	Memory loss
	Sexual desire, low
	Wrinkles

Nutmeg pairs well with these spices:

Allspice	Clove	Coriander
Amchur	Cocoa	Ginger
Cinnamon	Coconut	Lemongrass

and complements recipes featuring:

Avocado	Soups
Bananas	Tomatoes
Biscuits and breads	Vegetables
Lobster	White sauces
Scallops	

Other recipes containing nutmeg:

Apple Pie Spice (p. 271)	Mulling Spice (p. 273)
Banana Cinnamon French Toast (p. 86)	Quatre Épices (p. 271)
Baharat (p. 268)	Ras-el-hanout (p. 266)
Garam Masala (p. 264)	Spiced Mixed Nuts (p. 90)
Jamaican Jerk Marinade (p. 269)	Spicy Vanilla Rice Pudding (p. 256)
La Kama (p. 266)	

---

holes), which can infest them. Whole nutmegs will keep in a tightly sealed jar in a dark and dry place for a few years. Whole nutmegs that have been stored too long dry out and lose their volatile oils.

Because it is high in oil, ground nutmeg retains

its flavor well and keeps for a year or more under the same conditions as whole. Unless you are heavily into baking, buy ground nutmeg in the smallest container possible, as a little goes a long way.

Nutmeg's flavor can vary from sweetly spicy to strong and slightly bitter, depending on its place of origin. The major exporters are Indonesia (the Maluku Islands), Grenada, France, and India. Indonesia is by far the largest supplier, and most of the nutmeg imported into the US is from Indonesia, but Grenada's nutmeg is considered by many to be the best. You can purchase Grenadian nutmeg (as well as French and stronger-flavored Indian nutmeg) from a specialty spice dealer or online. (See the "Buyer's Guide" on page 309 for a list of top specialty spice dealers.)

Whole nutmeg seeds are hard and require a grater to extract the spice. Nutmeg graters are small, cylindrical, handheld gadgets that you can find in any kitchen store or kitchen section of a department store. Once an expensive specialty item, nutmeg graters are now widely available and relatively inexpensive, ranging in price from $3 to $15. They are usually either acrylic or stainless steel. (You might come across an English silver grater in an antique shop.) Nutmeg graters are nice because they contain a small compartment to store nutmeg, but an all-purpose stainless steel kitchen grater will also do the trick.

In the Kitchen with Nutmeg

Nutmeg's flavor is richest the moment you grate it, so grate it directly over the food when it's time to add it to a dish. It retains its flavor best when added toward the end of cooking.

Nutmeg is a favorite for flavoring cakes, pie fillings, and piecrusts, but it's also great in savory dishes. A tiny bit sprinkled at the end of cooking in a braise or slow-cooking casserole, for example, imparts a sweet spiciness and a new layer of flavor.

Grenada Nutmeg Syrup

Drizzle this over ice cream, cocoa, or fruit desserts. It stores well in the refrigerator.

½ cup water
½ cup sugar
¼ cup dark rum
4 teaspoons freshly grated nutmeg

1. Put the water and sugar in a small saucepan and stir until dissolved. Add the rum and nutmeg and simmer until slightly thick, about 10 minutes.

Makes about 1½ cups.

Nutmeg and dairy make a perfect marriage. Nutmeg cuts through the fat of milk, cream, eggs, cheese, and custards. It goes especially well in rich, flour-thickened white sauces. It's a natural in potato dishes, and with strong vegetables, such as cauliflower, eggplant, brussels sprouts, and spinach.

Here are some other ways to put more nutmeg in your diet:

- Sprinkle nutmeg in thick soups, such as split pea, lentil, and black bean.
- Add a sprinkle of nutmeg to mask the sulfurous taste of cabbage.
- Add nutmeg to quiche.
- Grind a little nutmeg over slow-cooked stews and braises.
- Sprinkle nutmeg over creamed vegetables. It goes especially well in creamed spinach and potato casseroles.
- Sprinkle nutmeg over onions in an onion tart.
- Sprinkle it in hot cocoa, or over ice cream, milkshakes, or smoothies.
- Sprinkle it in thick stews and in curries made with a coconut milk base.

ONION *Too Strong for Cancer*

It's not surprising that the only vegetable powerful enough to make you cry is also powerful enough to make you well. Onions are rich in *quercetin*, a powerful type of antioxidant called a *flavonoid* that may reduce the risk of cancer. Onions are a member of the same botanical family as garlic, and like garlic they contain *allicin*, which transforms into *organosulfurs*—which can lower cholesterol, thin your blood, keep arteries flexible, and kill cancer cells. Red and purple onions deliver *anthocyanins*, the same antioxidants that make berries a nutritional superstar. Altogether, these nutrients (and many other compounds) add up to a uniquely healing spice.

Onions Are Anti-Cancer

Quercetin and cancer don't mix. Research shows that quercetin can: slow the growth of cancer cells; stop cancer cells from migrating to other parts of the body (metastasis); and force cancer cells to die in a variety of ways, such as cutting off their blood supply or activating cancer-killing genes. The organosulfur compounds in onions have many of the same effects. And all that cellular activity has a real impact on a daily activity—staying alive! Study after study links a higher intake of onions with lower rates of deadly cancers.

In a study in the *American Journal of Clinical Nutrition*, Italian researchers analyzed diet and health data from thousands of people. They found a consistent pattern of protection—the more onions in the diet, the less cancer. Specifically, they found that, compared to those who ate the fewest onions, those who ate the most onions had lower risks for developing:

- *Colon cancer:* 56 percent lower risk
- *Breast cancer:* 25 percent lower risk
- *Prostate cancer:* 71 percent lower risk
- *Ovarian cancer:* 73 percent lower risk
- *Esophageal cancer:* 82 percent lower risk

- *Oral cancer:* 84 percent lower risk
- *Kidney cancer:* 38 percent lower risk

"Our findings confirm a protective role of onions on the risk of several common cancers," the researchers concluded.

Endometrial cancer. Italian researchers found that women who ate two or more servings of onions a week had a 60 percent lower risk of developing endometrial cancer.

Pancreatic cancer. Researchers at the University of California, San Francisco analyzed health and diet data from more than 2,000 people and found that those who ate the most onions (and garlic) had a 54 percent lower risk of pancreatic cancer, compared to those who ate the least.

Stomach cancer. Researchers from the University of Southern California analyzed diet and health data from more than 1,900 people from China and found the more onions people ate, the lower their risk of stomach cancer.

The Outstanding Onion

There are many other ways that onions protect your health.

Heart attacks. Italian researchers analyzed diet and health data from more than 1,400 people. Those who ate one or more serving of onions per week were 22 percent less likely to have a heart attack than people who hardly ever ate onions. "A diet rich in onions may have a favorable effect on the risk of acute myocardial infarction [heart attack]," concluded the researchers in the *European Journal of Nutrition*.

High cholesterol. Japanese women have much lower rates of heart disease. Why? To find out, researchers analyzed the diets of 115 Japanese women. They found that the more flavonoids they ate (principally from onions), the lower their level of total cholesterol and LDL cholesterol, two risk factors for heart disease. The fact that Japanese women have such a high consumption of flavonoids—mainly quercetin, and mainly from onions—"may contribute to their low incidence of coronary heart disease, compared with women in other countries," the researchers concluded in the *Journal of Nutrition*.

Heart disease. In another study, Dutch researchers measured the flavonoid intake—mainly from tea, onions, and apples—in 805 men. Those who had the highest flavonoid intake had a 58 percent lower risk of heart disease, compared to those with the lowest. The results were in the journal *Lancet*.

High blood pressure. Researchers from the University of Utah treated 41 people with high blood pressure, dividing them into two groups. One group took 730 mg of quercetin a day and one group didn't. After one month, those taking the supplement had a drop in blood pressure of 7 points systolic (the upper reading) and 5 points diastolic (the lower reading).

Osteoporosis. Researchers from the Medical University of South Carolina analyzed data from the nationwide National Health and Nutrition Examination Survey, involving more than 35 million women. They found that perimenopausal and postmenopausal women who ate one or more onions a day had a bone density 5 percent greater than women who ate onions once a month or less. "Onion consumption seems to have a beneficial effect on bone density," concluded the researcher. And those denser bones meant fewer fractures: "Older women who consume onions most frequently may decrease their risk of hip fracture by more than 20 percent versus those who never consume onions," wrote the researchers in the journal *Menopause*.

Surgical scars. Researchers found that people who used onion extract gel on surgical scars had scars that were softer, less red, with a smoother texture, and an overall better appearance. The findings were in the *Journal of Cosmetic Dermatology*.

Allergies. In an article on allergies, researchers at the Boston University School of Medicine point out that quercetin blocks the release of his-

tamine—the immune factor that causes allergic symptoms such as watery eyes and runny nose. Quercetin is a "safe, natural therapy" for allergies that can be used either as a "primary therapy or in conjunction with conventional methods," wrote the researchers.

Benign prostatic hypertrophy. This condition—commonly called "swollen" or "enlarged" prostate—affects tens of millions of middle-aged men, causing urinary difficulties. Italian researchers analyzed diet and health data from more than 1,800 men and found that those who ate the most onions had a 59 percent lower risk of developing the problem.

Diabetes. There have been so many studies on onions lowering blood sugar in experimental animals with type 2 diabetes that one team of scientists from Korea conducted a "meta-analysis"—they combined the data from *all* the studies to see if there was one big result. And there was: onions lower blood sugar. The findings were in the *Journal of Medicinal Food*.

Getting to Know Onion

Onions are cultivated everywhere, including the backyard vegetable garden.

They come in hundreds of varieties of colors, shapes, textures, and strengths. There are yellow,

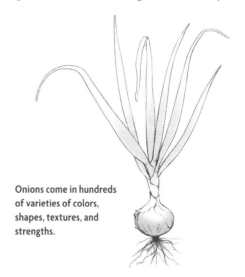

Onions come in hundreds of varieties of colors, shapes, textures, and strengths.

Shallots: The Healthiest Onion of Them All

Don't underestimate the healing power of the little shallot. When researchers at Cornell University measured the nutritional content of 13 varieties of onions sold in the United States, they found that, ounce for ounce, shallots have more antioxidant activity than the strongest yellow onions and contain six times more antioxidant phenols than the mildest Vidalia onions.

Shallots can be used both cooked and raw. The flavor of shallots is like a strong onion with a hint of garlic. They are strong, so when using them raw make sure to dice them finely.

Store shallots in a cool place where they have room to breathe. Do not buy shallots that are bruised and do not use shallots that are sprouted. Not only will they taste bitter, but they'll spoil the other shallots.

Roasted shallots are a nice accompaniment to vegetables, especially when serving beef, pork, duck, or chicken. To make roasted shallots, simmer them in their skins, covered in milk, for about 10 minutes. Drain the milk and roast in a small covered casserole until they are tender, about 20 minutes. Season with Mediterranean Vinaigrette (p. 160).

---

red, purple, green, white, and brown onions. They range in size from that of a fingernail (cocktail onion) to a baseball (storage onion). There are Italian onions, Bermuda onions, pearl onions, leeks, scallions, and shallots.

Onions flavor more dishes than any other spice. They are the foundation of virtually every base for soups, sauces, meat, fish, and vegetable dishes. They are also a prominent spice in virtually every cuisine, where they are eaten raw, fried, batter-fried, baked, creamed, roasted, broiled, boiled, and pickled.

In China, cooks are partial to sweet and mild scallions. They chop or slice them raw, and put them in soups, stir-fries, and pickled dishes. Onions are put on top of cooked noodles called *laksas*, stirred into rices, mixed into condiments, and crumbled into sauces.

In Indonesia, onions are sliced and mixed raw into hot condiments called *sambals* and served alongside marinated meat kabobs called *satays*. They are pounded and added to spice blends and condiments, and cooked in sauces. They are fried in oil for their crunch and caramelized taste, and added as toppings to stir-fried noodles and fried rice.

In India, pungent, brown-skinned globe onions are used in virtually every dish, and are savored not only for their flavor, but for the texture and consistency they lend to curries. They

are eaten raw in a popular onion relish called *kache piaz* and a tomato-based relish called *kachoomar*. Indians enjoy eating brown onions just so (they are drier than the brown onions found in the United States) with lemon, especially when they feel a cold coming on.

In Turkey, whole shallots traditionally accompany lamb on the kabob. In Tunisia, cooks favor couscous with a fermented onion paste call *hrous*.

The French are partial to delicate and strong-flavored shallots, which are used as a base in many sauces, such as *béarnaise*. The French are known the world over for their French onion soup and the Provencal specialty *pissaldière*, which is a thick layer of caramelized onions on a thick, crusty dough, resembling pizza. Onion tart is a specialty in the Alsace-Lorraine region, where the food influence is both French and German.

Germans are fonder of onions than the French, and sauté them in fat as a topping on many meat and potato dishes. They are also served on their own, creamed or fried, as a vegetable.

The Spanish enjoy a caramelized onion and tomato sauce called *sofregit*. The British eat stuffed onions. Russians often grate onions into marinades and other dishes rather than chop them to make their flavor stronger.

In the United States, onions are a staple top-

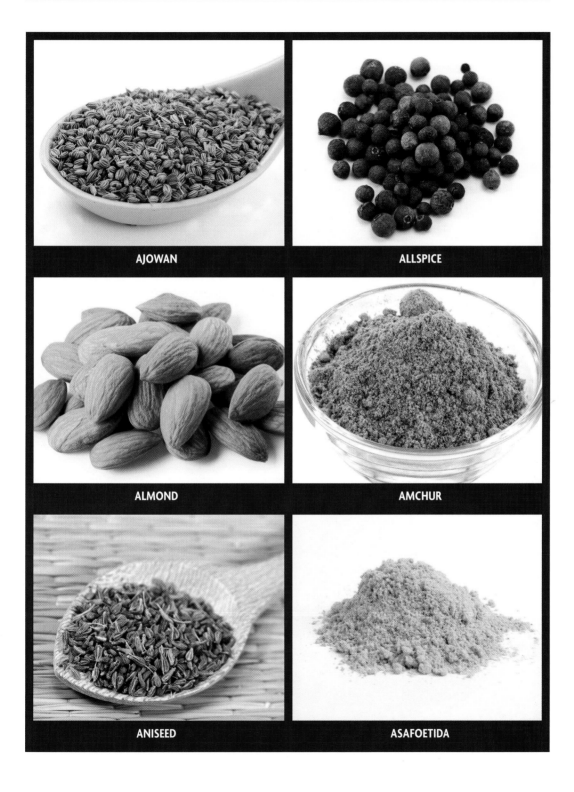

AJOWAN

ALLSPICE

ALMOND

AMCHUR

ANISEED

ASAFOETIDA

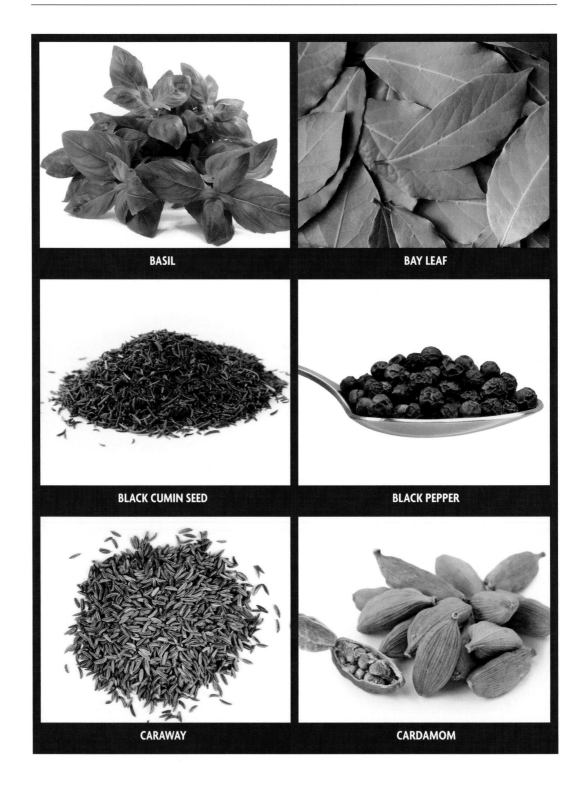

BASIL

BAY LEAF

BLACK CUMIN SEED

BLACK PEPPER

CARAWAY

CARDAMOM

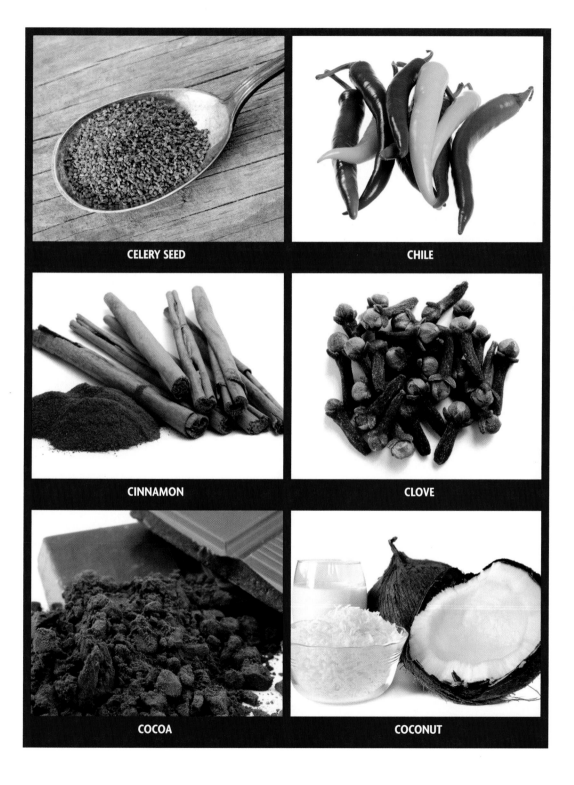

CELERY SEED

CHILE

CINNAMON

CLOVE

COCOA

COCONUT

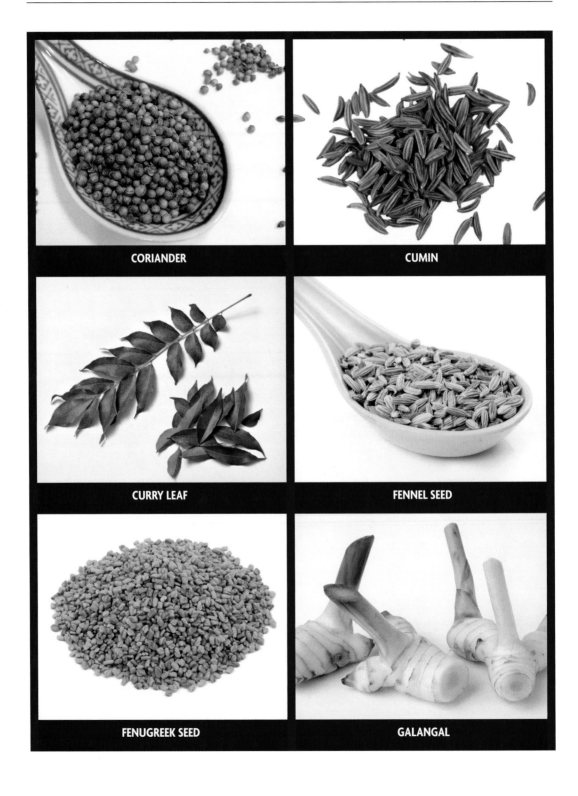

CORIANDER

CUMIN

CURRY LEAF

FENNEL SEED

FENUGREEK SEED

GALANGAL

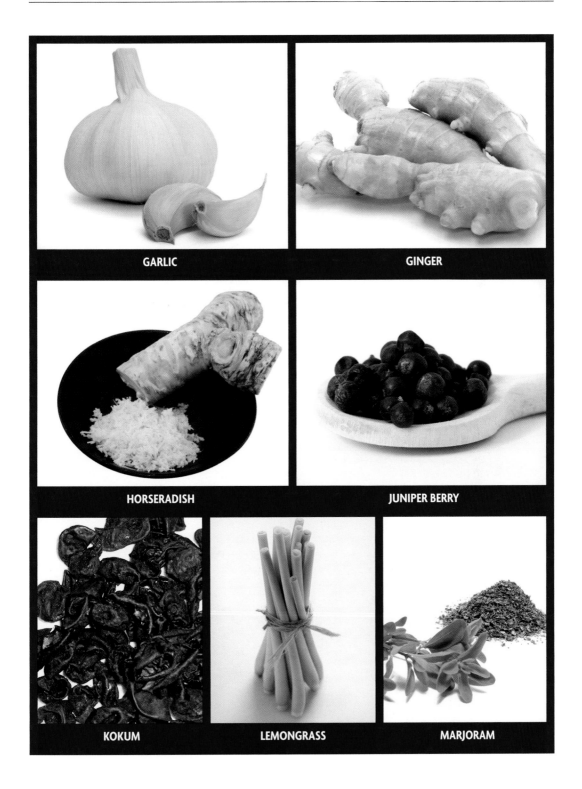

GARLIC

GINGER

HORSERADISH

JUNIPER BERRY

KOKUM

LEMONGRASS

MARJORAM

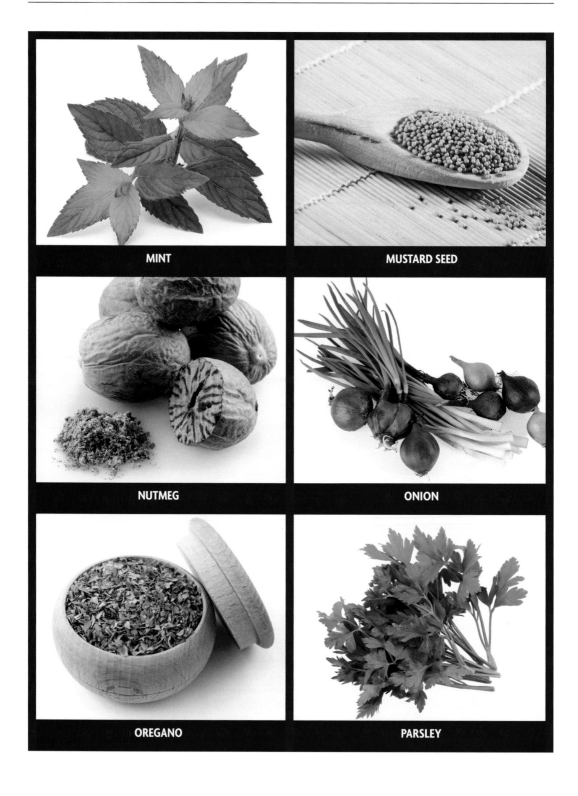

MINT

MUSTARD SEED

NUTMEG

ONION

OREGANO

PARSLEY

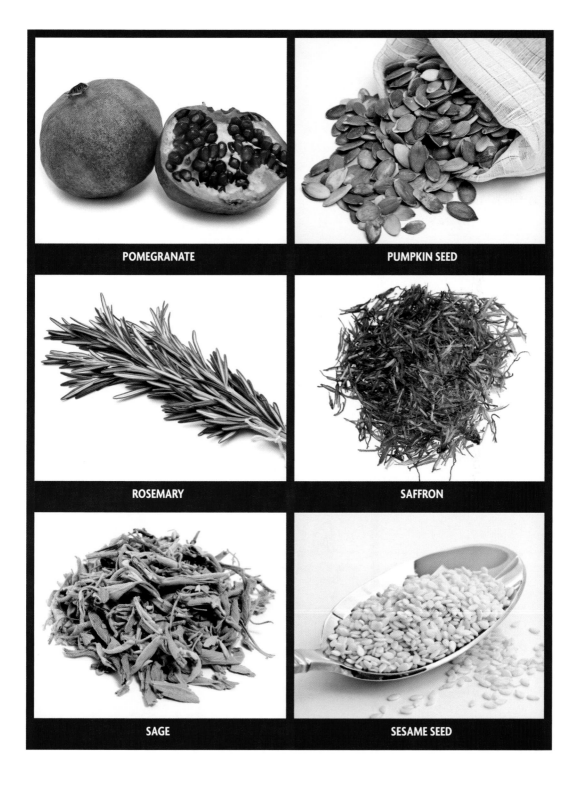

POMEGRANATE

PUMPKIN SEED

ROSEMARY

SAFFRON

SAGE

SESAME SEED

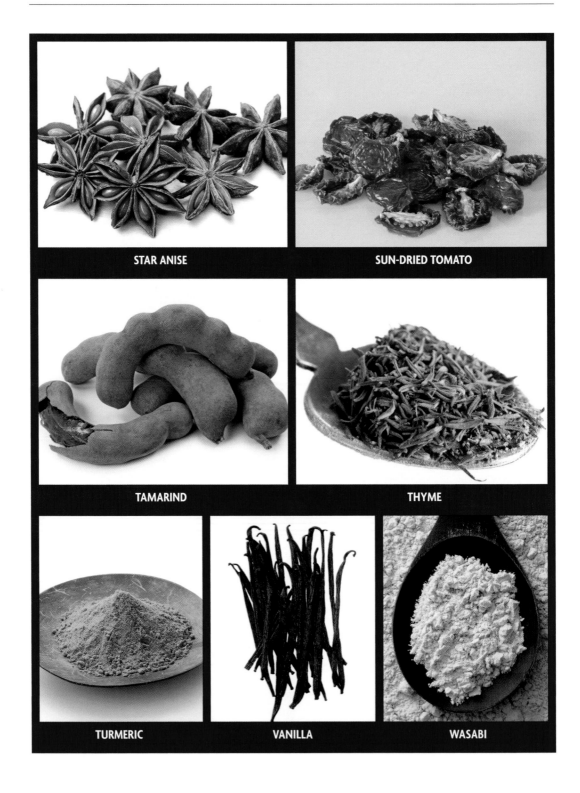

STAR ANISE

SUN-DRIED TOMATO

TAMARIND

THYME

TURMERIC

VANILLA

WASABI

Onion may help prevent and/or treat:

Allergies	Diabetes, type 2
Benign prostatic hypertrophy (BPH)	Heart attack
	Heart disease
Cancer	High blood pressure (hypertension)
Cholesterol problems (high total cholesterol, high "bad" LDL cholesterol)	Osteoporosis
	Scars

Onion pairs well with virtually *all* spices, but particularly well with:

Caraway	Marjoram
Coconut	Oregano
Cumin	Rosemary
Garlic	Sun-dried tomato
Ginger	Thyme
Kokum	Turmeric

and goes with virtually *all* savory dishes, including:

Apples	Relishes
Curries	Salads
Grilled meats	Sandwiches
Pizza	

ping, either raw or fried, on hot dogs, hamburgers, ballpark franks, and fast foods. The US has made the batter-fried onion ring world famous.

In the US market, onions fall into two classes defined by season and harvest: spring onions, which are mild, moist, and perishable; and storage onions, which are pungent, dry, and enduring.

Spring onions are also called green onions, scallions, or Welsh onions. They are literally baby onions that haven't had a chance to grow. Some are picked before the bulb starts to blossom, and there are varieties that never form bulbs. They are sweet and moist and can be eaten raw. (In generations past, spring onions were dipped in salt and eaten as a snack.)

Storage onions grow through the summer and are harvested in the fall. All storage onions are strong, meaning they are rich in sulfur compounds. Because they don't have the moisture that is in spring onions, they are stronger and more durable. The strongest and most pungent onions are yellow onions, commonly referred to as globe or Spanish onions. They are followed in pungency by white onions, which are often called Texas or Vidalia onions (from a town in Georgia of the same name).

Storage onions are categorized as follows:

- Spanish onions are the large onions seen at market. These are actually globe onions, but somewhat milder than the globe onions fancied in India.
- Bermuda onions are also mild, and come as red Bermuda, white Bermuda, and yellow Bermuda onions.
- Vidalia onions (Georgia) and Maui onions (from the Hawaiian island) are white onions that are hybrids. They are the sweetest storage onions.

When it comes to onions and health, there is only one thing you need to know: the stronger the onion, the richer it is in sulfur compounds, and the better it is for you.

How to Buy Onion
You'll do your health and your taste buds a favor by buying fresh onions and using them liberally—daily, whenever possible. Onions, however, also come dried in these forms: granulate, powdered, ground, minced, chopped, and toasted. Both fresh and dried can be found in all green grocers and supermarkets.

When buying storage onions, look for bulbs that are firm and uniform in color and have a lot of layers of thick, papery skin. They should be crisp and dry. Avoid onions that have dark blemishes, are open at the neck, show moisture, have soft spots, or show signs of sprouting or decay. (Dark patches are signs of decay.)

Scallions should have rich, green, fresh-looking tops that are crisp rather than limp.

The best place to keep storage onions is in a root cellar, where the temperature is cool. Next best is to store them at room temperature in an open container, such as a wire mesh basket, which gives them good ventilation. Keep onions away from potatoes: they will absorb their moisture and gases, and spoil.

Fresh onions shouldn't be refrigerated. Once you cut them, however, wrap them tightly and store them in the refrigerator, where they will keep sliced for about a week (or chopped for a few days). Try to avoid cutting them in advance of using them; otherwise, they start to lose their nutrients.

Because scallions are perishable, they should be refrigerated in a plastic bag. They will keep for about a week.

Storage onions can keep from a few weeks up to a few months, depending on the type of onion and its age when you bought it. Generally speaking, the more pungent the onion, the longer the storage life.

Dried onions will keep for about a year in an air-tight container in a cool, dark place.

In the Kitchen with Onion

Onions are synonymous with home cooking and are as indispensible as salt and pepper. Onions give dishes flavor, color, and texture.

Yellow onions are best for stews, soups, and sauces that require long cooking. Sweet onions, such as Vidalia, are best for baked whole onions and battered, deep fried onion rings. Red onions are best for serving raw in sandwiches and salads, and in pickled dishes. Use pearl onions to make glazed onions or pickled onions.

To minimize watery eyes when you cut them, refrigerate onions for at least an hour before cut-

Other recipes containing onion:

All-American Chili con Carne (p. 110)

Alsatian Pork and Sauerkraut (p. 148)

Berbere (p. 267)

Black Pepper Rice with Almonds (p. 57)

Bloody Mary Soup with Jumbo Lump Crabmeat (p. 70)

Boeuf Bourguignon (p. 240)

Brussels Sprouts Kulambu (p. 123)

By-the-Bay Fisherman's Chowder (p. 46)

Caribbean Curry Paste (p. 287)

Garbanzo Beans with Mushrooms and Toasted Almonds (p. 29)

Ginger Carrot and Squash Soup (p. 140)

Green Pumpkin Seed Sauce (p. 200)

Grilled Lamb Patty Pockets with Cucumber Mint Sauce (p. 165)

Hungarian Goulash (p. 61)

Jamaican Jerk Marinade (p. 269)

Madras Beef Curry (p. 106)

Malaysian Curry Paste (p. 287)

Onion and Tomato Chutney (p. 113)

Pomegranate Guacamole (p. 197)

Potato Cauliflower Curry (p. 252)

Sage Sausage and Apricot Stuffing (p. 215)

Sesame Seared Tuna with Pickled Ginger and Vanilla Slaw (p. 220)

Shellfish in Saffron Broth (p. 211)

Spaghettini with Basil-Tomato Sauce (p. 42)

Tamarind Sauce (p. 236)

Thai Red Curry Paste (p. 286)

Wasabi Orange Chicken with Toasted Almonds (p. 260)

Yucatan Pickled Red Onions (p. 21)

ting. The chill will slow down the volatility when allicin is released into the air. Cutting onions under cool running water also can help avoid tears, but washes away allicin, which you don't want.

French Onion Soup

This is the classic soupe à l'oignon from Le Pied au Cochon (Foot of the Pig), the 24-hour bistro where Parisians would stop on their way home after a night of partying to eat a soup famed for preventing hangovers. If you don't have a homemade stock, the brand Kitchen Basics, available in most supermarkets, is an excellent substitute. The soup benefits from being made a day or two in advance. It also freezes well.

2 tablespoons butter
2 tablespoons vegetable oil
2½ pounds yellow onions, thinly sliced
½ teaspoon sugar
3 tablespoons flour
8 cups beef stock
½ cup dry vermouth
Bouquet garni (p. 271)
½ teaspoon salt
¼ cup cognac or brandy (optional)
1 small French baguette
1 clove garlic, cut in half
½ teaspoon olive oil
1 cup shredded Gruyère cheese

1. Heat the butter and oil in a large heavy-bottomed Dutch oven over medium-high heat. Reduce the heat to low, add the onions, and stir to coat them with the fat. Cover and sweat the onions slowly for 15 minutes, stirring once or twice in-between.

2. Uncover, raise the heat to moderate, and stir in the sugar. Cook for 30 minutes, stirring frequently, to soften. The onions should turn a golden color. Do not let them burn. Sprinkle the onions with the flour and stir continuously for five minutes.

3. Pour in the stock and vermouth, and add the bouquet garni and salt. Bring to a simmer, cover partially, and cook for 40 minutes. Add the cognac or brandy, if desired. Let the soup cool for at least a half hour.

The soup up to this point can be made in advance then continue as follows when you are ready to serve.

4. Cut four thick slices of bread from the baguette and put them on a cookie sheet. Smear the garlic clove on top of each slice and brush lightly with the olive oil. Bake in a 400°F oven for seven minutes.

5. Reduce the oven heat to 350°F. Ladle the soup into individual oven-proof onion soup bowls or gratins almost to the top. Place a slice of bread on top of each and cover the entire top with the cheese, including the rim. Put the bowl on a cookie sheet on the top shelf and bake for 15 minutes or until hot and bubbly. Run the bowls under the broiler for 30 seconds to brown the cheese. Serve with the rest of the baguette on the side.

Serves 4 as a dinner entree.

To get the smell of onions out of your hands after peeling and chopping, rinse your hands under cool water. Or rub some salt between your palms, then wash your hands with soap and warm water.

Here are some ways to put more onions into your diet:

- Think sautéed onions when serving meat. Onions supply moisture that is missing in meat, especially cuts with little fat.

- Onions make an excellent marinade for tough cuts of meat that need tenderizing. Chop onions and put them on top of the meat. Pour the marinade over the onions and around the meat. Turn every few hours, spooning the onion topping on the other side.

- If you don't like eating raw onions because they taste too strong, cut the pungency by soaking them in cool water overnight.

- Add chopped raw red or Vidalia onions to

green salads, chicken, and tuna salads.

- Add sliced red onions or scallions to salads and put them in sandwiches.
- Add diced shallots to salad dressings.
- Sauté onions and serve them atop grilled burgers. One study found that serving grilled hamburgers with sautéed onions can neutralize the carcinogenic compound HCA that forms on grilled meats, especially ground beef.
- Do not peel onions when combining them with other aromatic vegetables to make stock. The skin helps add color to the stock without adding bitterness.
- When cooking onions, forget the butter and sauté them in a little olive or canola oil. To prevent onions from soaking up too much oil, and adding unwanted calories, lower the heat and cover them with

a tight lid. You'll end up with crunch, but not greasy onions.

- If you don't like your onions too strong, chop or dice them just before adding them to your recipe. Onions get stronger the longer they are in contact with air.
- You can keep fresh chives inexpensively all year round by growing them on your windowsill. Keep snipping them so they continue to grow.
- Make Nicaraguan pickled onions called *cebollita* by combining 1 cup of distilled white vinegar with 2 teaspoons of salt and 1 teaspoon of sugar, and pour over 1 onion and 3 red chiles, both thinly sliced. Let the onions sit at room temperature for an hour or two and refrigerate at least a day before eating.

OREGANO *Infection Protection*

You can't find a pizza parlor or Italian restaurant anywhere in the US that doesn't have canisters filled with the pungent dry leaves of oregano. The spice is synonymous with Italy and Italian food. Lasagna, pizza, and even garlic bread wouldn't

EVERY PIZZA PARLOR IN THE US HAS CANISTERS FILLED WITH THE PUNGENT DRY LEAVES OF OREGANO.

be considered Italian without it.

However, Oregano Nation #1 is *not* Italy. It's *Turkey*, which annually exports 20 tons of oregano—with Turks using 1,000 tons a year themselves. And not just because they like the taste. The Turkish people are firm believers in the *healing* power of oregano.

Household kitchens are often equipped with distillation stills for making oregano water, which families drink to keep digestion running smoothly. The stills are constructed so they can sit safely on the stove, dispersing the vapors of oregano oil that are thought to relax nerves and maintain good health. Turks rub the condensed oil vapors of oregano on limbs when muscles ache or rheumatism sets in. And oregano is Turkey's favorite tea.

Visit a scientific database, enter the keyword "oregano," and you'll find study after study supporting the Turkish tradition of using oregano as medicine.

Fighting Intestinal Infection

Modern gastrointestinal research points a finger at various bacteria, fungi, and parasites as common causes of intestinal troubles, from ulcers to irritable bowel syndrome. (In fact, microbial disturbances in the gut are now thought to cause or complicate many conditions, from allergies to arthritis.) The major components of oregano oil—*carvacrol* and *thymol*—are powerfully antibacterial, antiviral, anti-fungal—and anti-parasitic.

Putting parasites in their place. There are many different types of intestinal parasites, from one-celled organisms to full-grown worms. You can pick them up from food, water, a pet—or a passport (travelers to developing countries sometimes end up with a "souvenir" they wish they could have left behind).

Intestinal parasites can cause intestinal symptoms, of course. Chronic diarrhea is the most common, but bloating, gas, constipation, and bloody stools (as well as non-digestive symptoms such as fever and fatigue) are among other unpleasant possibilities.

Anti-parasitic medications are the best way to eradicate parasites, but they don't always work. Doctors in the southwest US decided to try oregano oil on 34 people with persistent parasites. The treatment ended the reign of the invaders in most cases, and decreased the number of parasites in the rest.

Foiling food poisoning. Researchers have found that compounds in oregano can kill many of the bacteria that cause food poisoning, such as *E. coli*, *Salmonella*, *Listeria*, and *Shigella*. In a study from the US Department of Agriculture, oregano outperformed garlic and allspice in stopping those four nasty germs from multiplying.

Healing ulcers. Researchers in the Department of Food Science at the University of Massachusetts found that a combination of oregano and cranberry extracts could kill *H. pylori* bacteria, the cause of stomach ulcers.

Calming colitis. Slovakian researchers found that a combination or oregano and thyme

---

Oregano may help prevent and/or treat:

Age spots	Infection, parasitic
Alzheimer's disease	Insulin resistance
Cancer	(prediabetes)
Candida infection (systemic fungal infection)	Liver disease
	Metabolic syndrome
Cholesterol problems (high "bad" LDL cholesterol)	Overweight
	Staph infection
	Thrush (oral candida infection)
Colitis (inflammatory bowel disease)	Triglycerides, high
Food poisoning	Ulcer
Heart disease	Vaginal yeast infection
High blood pressure	

---

reduced inflammation in the colons of animals with chemically induced colitis, a type of inflammatory bowel disease that strikes more than a million Americans.

More life for the liver. Several animal studies show that oregano oil can strengthen and heal the liver—good news for the tens of millions of Americans with non-alcoholic fatty liver disease, hepatitis C, cirrhosis, and other liver diseases.

Fighting Vaginal Infections, Too

Infections aren't limited to the digestive tract, of course. A vaginal yeast infection—what doctors call *vulvovaginal candiasis*—bothers three out of four women at least once in their life. About 45 percent have a second infection, and 5 to 8 percent have recurrent infections, returning four to five times a year. These itchy, sometimes painful infections are almost always caused by the yeast-like fungus *Candida albicans*.

And some clinicians—led by William C. Crook, MD, author of *The Yeast Connection*, published in 1987—think whole-body infection with *C. albicans* is a common problem, causing a wide range of symptoms that include fatigue, headache, and digestive upsets.

When *C. albicans* is bothering you, call oregano.

Researchers from Georgetown University Medical Center found that oregano oil could "completely inhibit" the growth of *C. albicans* in the test tube and killed 80 percent of the fungus in experimental animals. The oil stops the yeast from growing and also blunts the limb-like "filaments" it uses to burrow into tissue. They also note it works as well as powerful antifungal antibiotics such as nystatin. (When a team of Italian researchers tested oregano and nystatin together, they found the spice boosted the fungus-killing power of the drug.)

"It is interesting to note," write the researchers in *Molecular and Clinical Biochemistry*, "that infections due to *C. albicans* in debilitated individuals such as those having diabetes and HIV infection may be prophylactically controlled by the daily intake of small amounts of oregano oil, either alone or added to a food."

"Daily oral administration of origanum oil may be highly effective in the prevention and treatment of candidiasis," they concluded.

Other researchers found that carvacrol and thymol could "significantly reduce" infection with *oral candidiasis*—a fungal infection of the tissues of the mouth—in animals.

More from Oregano

There is provocative research on oregano's possible role in alleviating other diseases.

Metabolic syndrome. This condition is a combination of overweight, high blood sugar, high blood pressure, and high triglycerides, a blood fat (lipid). Researchers in Italy found that oregano extracts worked in the same way as drugs used for metabolic syndrome. Their study, said the researchers, showed the extracts could help with "weight reduction" (overweight), "prevent atherosclerosis" (from high blood pressure), and "ameliorate the lipid profile" (high triglycerides).

Making Sense of "Mexican Oregano"

So-called "Mexican oregano" isn't oregano. It's not even in the same botanical family. When dried, however, it *looks* like oregano and *tastes* like oregano, except it's stronger. And that makes a big difference when you add it to tacos or empanadas.

Like "real" oregano, it's rich in carvacrol and thymol.

And like "real" oregano, it's used in folk medicine throughout Mexico and South America for digestive and respiratory complaints, and research shows it's a bacterial fighter, antioxidant, and anti-tumor agent.

"The results warrant further investigation of oregano extract for its potential to prevent and ameliorate metabolic syndrome and its complications," concluded the researchers in the *Journal of Agricultural and Food Chemistry*.

High cholesterol. Turkish researchers studied 48 people with mildly elevated cholesterol, dividing them into two groups. One group took oregano extract after every meal, and one group didn't. Three months later, the oregano group had greater decreases in "bad" LDL cholesterol and in C-reactive protein, a biomarker of artery-damaging inflammation. They also had greater increases in arterial blood flow. The findings were in the *Journal of International Medical Research*.

When researchers in Turkey tested spices in the laboratory for their ability to stop the oxidation of LDL cholesterol (the key step in the formation of artery-clogging plaque) they found oregano had "the most pronounced effect."

Researchers in Spain took the process a step further: they measured the ability of oregano extract to stop the process that occurs after oxidation of cholesterol—the activation of immune components called *cytokines* that attack the oxidized cholesterol as if it were a foreign invader, sparking the inflammation that worsens heart disease. The extracts stopped the release of three of those cytokines (TNF-alpha, IL-1beta, and IL-6).

"These results may suggest an anti-inflammatory effect of oregano extracts . . . in a cellular model of atherosclerosis [heart disease]," concluded the researchers in *Food and Chemical Toxicology*.

Colon cancer. "Oregano spice is widely used in the Mediterranean diet, which is associated with a low risk for colon cancer," said Italian researchers in the journal *Nutrition and Cancer*. When they mixed oregano extract in a test tube with colon cancer cells, the spice stopped cellular growth and killed the cells, an effect the researchers labeled "oregano-triggered death."

"Our findings suggest that oregano in the amounts found in the Mediterranean diet" can kill cancer cells, said the researchers.

Additional test tube and animal research on carvacrol and other compounds in oregano show they can slow or kill cancers of the lung, colon, blood, and uterus.

Alzheimer's disease. Researchers screened 139 spices for their ability to possibly boost the brain chemical acetylcholine, the same action as drugs that slow Alzheimer's disease—and only an oregano extract was as "potent" as the drugs.

Age spots. Researchers in Taiwan found that a compound in oregano can reverse the "hyperpigmentation" that causes age spots (solar lentigos) and "may be useful in skin-whitening agents." The findings were in *Journal of Dermatological Science*.

Staph infections. Infections with *Staphylococcus aureus* usually start in the hospital and are sometimes fatal. Researchers at Georgetown University Medical Center found oregano oil was "the most potent" killer of *S. aureus* among several compounds tested. Giving it daily to animals injected with the bacteria quadrupled their expected lifespan. Oregano oil "may prove to be useful" for the "prevention and therapy" of *Staphylococcus aureus* infections, concluded the researchers.

Getting to Know Oregano

Hippocrates, the "father of medicine" from ancient Greece, knew about oregano's antiseptic properties, and used it to treat digestive and respiratory diseases. The ancient Egyptians also used it as a healing disinfectant. The Romans favored it for stimulating hair growth. In Turkish folk medicine, oregano oil is used for pain relief from tooth decay, as an antiseptic for wounds,

Oregano pairs well with these spices:

Ajowan	Garlic	Sage
Basil	Marjoram	Sun-dried
Bay	Onion	tomato
Chile	Pumpkin seed	Thyme
Cumin	Rosemary	

and complements recipes featuring:

Black beans	Pizza
Cheese	Poultry
Chowders and soups	Provolone cheese
Eggplant	Rabbit
Game	Salsa
Grilled meat	Seafood
Ground beef	Tomato sauces and
Mushrooms	dishes
Pastas	

Other recipes containing oregano:

Adobo (p. 270)	Grilled Pork Chile
All-American Chili con	Adobo (p. 78)
Carne (p. 110)	Pizza Spice Blend
By-the-Bay Fisherman's	(p. 272)
Chowder (p. 46)	Roasted Tomato Soup
Chimichurri Sauce	with Fennel and Mint
(p. 190)	(p. 231)
Green Pumpkin Seed	Yucatan Pickled Red
Sauce (p. 200)	Onions (p. 21)

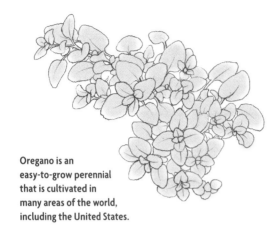

Oregano is an easy-to-grow perennial that is cultivated in many areas of the world, including the United States.

flavoring in Mexican restaurants in the United States, where it's used in soups, chili blends, salsas, and refried beans.

In Mexico, however, "Mexican oregano" is used—it's not botanically related to European oregano, but has a similar (though stronger) taste.

How to Buy Oregano

Oregano is an easy-to-grow perennial that is cultivated in many areas of the world, including the United States. Spice-lovers say the best oregano comes from Turkey. The US is a major importer of Turkish oregano, so chances are that when you buy oregano, this is the type you're buying. But Greek oregano is also imported into the US. The only way to know for sure where your oregano originated is to purchase the spice from a specialty retailer, who will know the country of origin.

You can purchase oregano fresh, dried, or ground. The flavor of the dried oregano is more robust than fresh. (And dried is preferred over ground because it's more flavorful.) Dried oregano keeps for about a year in a dark, dry place, in an airtight container.

The flavor of oregano is pungent and bal-

and as a remedy for inflammation of all kinds—psoriasis, tonsillitis, mouth ulcers, and inflamed gums, to name a few.

Oregano oil is a popular dietary supplement in the US, used for digestive upset, yeast infections, and as preventive therapy during cold and flu season.

Oregano is just as popular in American kitchens as it is everywhere else. Aside from being a staple in American pizzerias and Italian restaurants, it is a popular spice in Tex-Mex and Southwest cuisines. It is also popular as a

Chicken Oreganata

The name says it's Italian, but Turkey claims to have developed it first. Whatever its origin, this classic is enjoyed in many parts of the world.

2 boned chicken breasts, split
1 cup lemon juice
3 tablespoons olive oil
2 garlic cloves, minced
1 tablespoon dried oregano
½ teaspoon freshly ground black pepper
Salt to taste

1. Wash and pat dry the chicken. Combine the lemon juice, olive oil, garlic, oregano and pepper in a small mixing bowl. Put the mixture in a plastic ziplock bag, add the chicken, and seal. Shake the bag to make sure the chicken is evenly coated with the marinade. Refrigerate overnight.

2. Remove chicken from the marinade. Discard the marinade. Place the chicken in a shallow baking dish coated with non-stick spray. Bake the chicken in a 375°F oven for 30 minutes, turning once mid-way through.

Makes 4 servings.

samic, and comes from carvacrol and thymol oils, which vary in strength depending on where the plant was grown. The strongest oregano is from Turkey. Oregano grown and dried in backyard herb gardens in the US is delicate in comparison.

Oregano is also referred to as wild marjoram, and is often mistaken for marjoram (which is also called sweet marjoram). Though they both come from the same botanical family, and are often used interchangeably in the kitchen, there is only a vague resemblance in taste.

In the Kitchen with Oregano

Chefs prefer dried oregano to fresh because its flavor is more intense. You can intensify the flavor of fresh oregano, however, by rubbing the leaves between your palms and letting it drop in the dish.

Oregano is an easy spice to work with because it goes with just about everything. When experimenting, keep in mind that oregano is strong and can overpower a dish; it marries best with stronger flavors. It's typically used in garlic-based and tomato-based dishes, rich meat and game dishes, chilies and salsas, and pasta dishes.

A few ideas to put more oregano in your diet:

- Use it in marinades.
- Use it as a rub for grilled meat. Combine 1 teaspoon of oregano with ½ teaspoon each of red pepper flakes, salt, and freshly ground pepper, and rub the mixture into a thick steak before grilling.
- Put it in salad dressing.
- Add it to olive- and vinegar-based recipes.

PARSLEY *Antioxidant Enhancer*

Parsley is much more than a throw-away garnish on the *plat du jour* or an after-dinner breath freshener. It can hold its own against any green as a worthy supplier of cell-protecting antioxidants—especially the antioxidants known as *flavonoids*, which research shows play a role in fighting heart disease and cancer.

And parsley is uniquely rich in *apigenin*—an antioxidant that helps other antioxidants work better.

In a study by Danish researchers, 14 people ate a diet with almost no antioxidants or flavones for two weeks. The activity of two of the body's most powerful self-generated antioxidants—superoxide dismutase (SOD) and glutathione—was dramatically decreased, and there was a corresponding increase in cell-damaging oxidation. Until, that is, the volunteers ate apigenin-rich parsley. "The intervention with parsley seemed to overcome this decrease," said the researchers in the *British Journal of*

Nutrition, "and resulted in increased levels of SOD and glutathione."

Apigenin isn't all that parsley has going for it. It also delivers plenty of vitamins A and C, as well as *lutein*, an antioxidant that helps prevent age-related macular degeneration, the leading cause of blindness. It's also a good source of B vitamins and the minerals calcium and iron.

Parsley's Healing Power

Traditional healers have used parsley as a diuretic, to cleanse the kidneys and bladder, and to reduce high blood pressure. But parsley may have many other healing powers, as scientists are discovering.

Cancer. Researchers at Harvard Medical School analyzed the flavonoid content of the diets of 1,140 women with ovarian cancer and 1,180 women without the disease, and found that *only* apigenin intake was linked to a lower incidence of ovarian cancer—21 percent lower. There have been dozens of test tube and animal studies on apigenin and cancer. In a recent review of the research, scientists at Case Western University in Cleveland concluded that apigenin has "considerable potential to be developed as a cancer chemopreventive agent" (a natural substance that fights cancer). And they say that because apigenin is such a powerful antioxidant and anti-inflammatory, it may also have the potential to fight heart disease and Alzheimer's disease.

Heart disease. Noting that parsley is used in Morocco as a traditional medicine for heart disease, a team of Moroccan researchers tested its effectiveness in reducing *platelet aggregation*, the blood thickening that triggers the artery-plugging blood clots that cause most heart attacks and strokes. Parsley reduced platelet aggregation by up to 65 percent. "The dietary intake of parsley may benefit . . . the nutritional prevention of cardiovascular diseases," concluded the researchers in the *Journal of Ethnopharmacology*.

Diabetes. Parsley is used in Turkey as a natural medicine to treat type 2 diabetes. When a team of Turkish researchers tested the spice on animals with chemically induced diabetes, they found it significantly lowered blood sugar. Another team of Turkish researchers found parsley protected diabetic animals from a type of liver damage caused by the disease.

Constipation. "Parsley has been claimed in folk medicine to possess laxative properties," wrote a team of Lebanese researchers in the journal *Phytomedicine*. When they analyzed parsley, they found it contained properties similar to laxative drugs.

Ulcers. Researchers in Saudi Arabia reviewed the history of parsley's use as a folk medicine for many problems—for flushing the urinary tract and preventing kidney stones; for treating diarrhea, indigestion, gallstones, and flatulence; and for menstrual difficulties. When they tested the spice's healing action in animals, they found it had the power to prevent experimentally induced stomach ulcers. The findings were in *The American Journal of Chinese Medicine*.

Parsley may help prevent and/or treat:

Bad breath	Diabetes, type 2
Cancer	Heart disease
Constipation	Ulcer

Parsley pairs well with virtually *all* spices, but particularly well with:

Basil	Marjoram	Rosemary
Bay leaf	Mint	Sage
Fennel seed	Onion	Thyme
Garlic	Oregano	

and complements *all* recipes, especially those featuring:

Beans	Fish	Vegetables
Cheese	Legumes	
Eggs	Lentils	

Caution: Pregnant women should not eat parsley in large amounts as it can cause uterine contractions.

Other recipes containing parsley:

Bavarian Apple and Horseradish Sauce (p. 145)	Roast Chicken with 40 Cloves of Garlic (p. 134)
Boeuf Bourguignon (p. 240)	Roasted Tomato Soup with Fennel and Mint (p. 231)
Bouquet Garni (p. 271)	Sage Sausage and Apricot Stuffing (p. 215)
By-the-Bay Fisherman's Chowder (p. 46)	Shellfish in Saffron Broth (p. 211)
Ginger Carrot and Squash Soup (p. 140)	Spice de Provence (p. 271)

There are two common varieties of parsley:
curly parsley and flat leaf parsley.

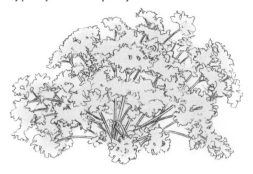

Getting to Know Parsley

Americans use a *lot* of parsley—it's third only to salt and pepper as the most heavily consumed spice. But Americans don't use anywhere near as much as people in the Middle East, who consume it by the cupful.

Virtually every nation in the Middle East and the eastern Mediterranean has its own version of tabbouleh, a salad containing equal parts parsley and cracked wheat (bulgur), mixed with olive oil, scallions, and mint. In Lebanon, where tabbouleh originated, cooks prefer to use much more parsley than cracked wheat, and spike the salad with cinnamon and allspice. *Baba ghanoush* is another Middle Eastern dish heavily enriched with parsley. (Like tabbouleh, it's also popular in the US.)

In fact, parsley forms the core of many popular dishes in many parts of the world.

Gremolata, a condiment made from parsley, garlic, and lemon zest, is the classic accompaniment to Italy's *osso buco*, a specialty from Milan.

In France, parsley and garlic form the cook's *mise en place* (meaning "everything in its place")—the base for many dishes. It is the foundation of *persillade* (which also includes garlic, oil, and vinegar), a sauce and seasoning mixture used in French and Greek cooking (and in Louisiana's Cajun and Creole cuisines). Germans prefer a variety called Hamburg parsley or turnip root parsley, which is strong and thick like celery. (It tastes a lot like celery heavily spiced with parsley.) Hamburg parsley enjoyed a brief period of popularity in the US, but is now almost unheard of. In Britain, parsley has been a favorite since the reign of Henry VIII, who enjoyed the taste it gave to white sauces.

Argentine cuisine is famous for *chimichurri*, an intense green sauce that tops grilled meat. It is also used as a marinade. Parsley is put in Cuba's version of *sofrito*, a popular Latin hot sauce, to mellow the flavor.

You'll rarely find parsley used in Asian cuisines, where the much stronger-tasting cilantro is preferred.

How to Buy Parsley

There are two common varieties of parsley: curly parsley, which is preferred in the US and Great Britain, and flat leaf parsley (also called Italian parsley), which is preferred everywhere else.

Flat leaf parsley is more richly flavored than curly parsley and is used exclusively in making tabbouleh and other Middle Eastern parsley dishes. It resembles cilantro, but a close whiff confirms that it's not. The curly variety is more popular in the US because it makes a prettier garnish. You can find both in just about any supermarket.

Parsley is sold fresh and dried. When buying fresh, choose bunches that aren't wilted and have springy, erect stems. Rinse parsley thoroughly in cold water to remove grit, especially curly varieties. It is best kept in the refrigerator in a glass of cold water. To freeze, wrap sprigs in foil. It will also freeze well finely chopped.

Choose dried parsley that is deep green and free of pieces of stalk or yellow leaves. Check it in the store: it can lose its color and flavor sitting on the supermarket shelf.

It's easy (and less expensive) to dry your own. Preheat the oven to 250°F. Lay parsley sprigs out flat on a baking sheet. Put the sheet in the oven and turn off the heat. "Bake" for 15 or 20 minutes until they get crisp. Turn them at least once while they are drying.

Chimichurri Sauce

This parsley sauce from Argentina is popular throughout South America, where it's used as a marinade and a sauce for grilled meats and poultry. This recipe makes enough to use as a marinade for steaks, and a sauce for eight people.

2 cups fresh flat leaf parsley, stems removed
　and tightly packed
5 large garlic cloves
2 dried red chiles, seeds removed
2 tablespoons white wine vinegar
½ cup extra-virgin olive oil
1 teaspoon dried oregano
½ teaspoon freshly ground black pepper

1. Combine the parsley, garlic, and chiles in a food processor and process until very fine. With the processor running add the vinegar, then olive oil. Transfer to a glass bowl. Stir in the oregano and black pepper. Refrigerate for a few hours before using.

Makes about 2 cups.

In the Kitchen with Parsley

Parsley can go in virtually any dish. When used as a spice, it is distinctive yet mild, and it will never dominate a recipe. It is also quite hardy. If you drop it in a deep fryer, it emerges with its shape and color intact.

The stalks have a stronger flavor than the leaves, so make sure to use them. The stalks (not the leaves) are best for adding to stocks and soups.

You can use fresh parsley whole, flaked, chopped, minced, or pureed, and it's best used toward the end of cooking, to enhance the flavor of other ingredients. Cook chopped parsley within an hour of cutting, as its pungency dissipates.

In long cooking, it's best to use dried parsley.

You'll get a richer aroma from dried parsley if you steep it in a little hot water before using.

Here are other ways to add more parsley to your diet:

- Parsley takes well to "wet" foods. Add it to omelets, mashed potatoes, pastas, and soup.
- Parsley can counteract the assertiveness of cilantro or other strong flavors, should you go too heavy on them in a dish.
- Mince fresh parsley and garlic and add to fried potatoes a few minutes before they are done, for *potatoes persillade*.
- Make gremolata by combining ½ cup of minced parsley and 3 minced garlic cloves with the juice of 1 lemon.

POMEGRANATE　*"A Pharmacy unto Itself"*

The slippery, garnet-red seeds of the pomegranate (dried and used in India as a spice) started to attain notoriety as a gourmet health food back in the '90s, when studies first linked them to heart and prostate health. These days, pomegranate is mega-trendy, and you can find it flavoring everything from water to popsicles to cocktails. It is also mega-healthy. Every bit of it. The seeds, pulp, skin, root, flower—even the bark from the pomegranate tree—are all brimming with *polyphenols*, disease-fighting antioxidants found in plants. (Pomegranate seed extracts and juice have two to three times the antioxidant activity of red wine and green tea, those antioxidant superstars.)

But while many foods and spices are rich in polyphenols, pomegranate is one of the few that is a top source of *several* varieties—flavonoids, anthocyanins, ellagic acid, punicic acid, and many others. Hundreds of scientific studies confirm that this natural pharmacy of polyphenols may help prevent or treat a variety of diseases, including the three leading killers of Americans: heart disease, cancer, and stroke.

Those scientific findings wouldn't surprise an Ayurvedic physician using India's ancient system of natural healing—an Ayurvedic text calls the pomegranate "a pharmacy unto itself."

Smooth Sailing for Blood Vessels

Heart attacks and strokes combined kill more Americans than any other health problem. The cause: arteries leading to the heart and brain become clogged with *plaque*, a deadly stew of cholesterol and ruined cells, thickened by inflammation and oxidation. The medical name for this circulatory disaster: *atherosclerosis*. The name of a plant so powerful it can prevent *and* reverse the problem? Pomegranate.

Reversing arterial plaque. Israeli researchers studied 20 people with atherosclerosis in the *carotid artery*—the artery in the neck that supplies blood to the brain. (A blockage in this artery produces a stroke.) Ten drank pomegranate juice and 10 didn't. After one year, those drinking the juice had a 30 percent *decrease* in arterial plaque, while those not drinking the juice had a 9 percent *increase*. The results were reported in *Clinical Nutrition*.

Researchers at the University of Chicago studied 189 people (ages 45 to 74) with one or more risk factors for heart disease, such as high cholesterol and high blood pressure. They divided them into two groups: one group drank eight ounces of pomegranate juice a day and the other didn't. After one year, those in the study with the highest risk for heart disease—with the highest total cholesterol, highest LDL cholesterol, highest triglycerides, and highest level of several other risk factors—had a much slower growth rate of arterial plaque *if* they were in the group drinking pomegranate juice. The findings were in the *American Journal of Cardiology*.

Reviving damaged hearts. Doctors from the University of California, San Francisco (UCSF) studied 45 people (average age, 69) with heart disease. Nearly half had suffered heart attacks, most had high blood pressure, and nearly all had high cholesterol. They were all taking several drugs to battle heart disease, including cholesterol-lowering statins, blood thinners, and blood pressure drugs.

The researchers divided them into two groups. For three months, one group drank eight ounces a day of pomegranate juice, while the other group drank a placebo juice.

At the beginning and end of the three months, the doctors gave both groups a *myocardial perfusion test*—a type of "stress test" that uses a CAT scan to measure blood flow (ischemia) to the heart during exercise.

After three months, the group drinking pomegranate juice had a 17 percent *increase* in blood flow to the heart, while the placebo group had a *decrease* of 18 percent.

And those are important test results: a study shows that the best predictor of whether or not a person with heart disease will have a heart attack is the amount of blood flow to the heart as measured by a myocardial perfusion test!

Less angina. The UCSF researchers also found that episodes of angina (intense chest pain) decreased by 50 percent in the pomegranate group, while increasing by 38 percent in the non-pomegranate group.

The findings were reported in the *American Journal of Cardiology*.

Increasing nitric oxide. The delicate lining of the arteries is called the *endothelium*. There, a thin layer of *endothelial cells* pump out *nitric oxide* (NO), a compound that fights oxidation and inflammation, keeping arteries flexible and young. Some experts think that a low level of nitric oxide is *the* primary cause of atherosclerosis.

Researchers from the University of Naples in Italy and UCLA conducted several studies testing the effect of pomegranate on nitric oxide. They found:

- Pomegranate juice was far more potent than Concord grape juice, blueberry juice, red wine, vitamin C, and vitamin E (all powerful antioxidants) at protecting nitric oxide against oxidative destruction. "Pomegranate juice possesses potent antioxidant activity that results in marked protection of NO against oxidative destruction," concluded the researchers in the journal *Nitric Oxide*.
- In the laboratory, pomegranate juice decreased the activity of genes that make endothelial cells more prone to oxidation, and it increased the production of an enzyme (endothelial NO synthase) that plays a key role in NO production. Pomegranate, the researchers concluded in the *Proceedings of the National Academy of Sciences*, may have a role in the "prevention and treatment of atherosclerosis."

Lowering high blood pressure. Israeli researchers asked people with high blood pressure to drink a small amount of pomegranate juice every day. After two weeks, they had a 5 percent drop in systolic blood pressure (the upper reading). They also had a 31 percent decrease in the activity of the enzyme (angiotensin-converting enzyme, or ACE) targeted by the pressure-lowering, ACE-inhibiting medications. "Pomegranate juice can offer…protection" against cardiovascular disease, they concluded in the journal *Atherosclerosis*.

Circulatory Protection for Diabetes
Diabetes, a blood sugar disorder, also damages blood vessels—75 percent of people with diabetes die from atherosclerosis. And almost all the so-called "complications" of diabetes (which

are more like diseases themselves) are caused by circulatory problems—blindness from damaged circulation to the retina of the eye, kidney failure from damage to blood vessels in kidneys, the burning and numbness of nerve problems from reduced blood flow to nerves, amputations (diabetes is the most common cause of non-trauma amputations) from poor circulation to the legs and feet. Pomegranate can protect blood vessels in people with diabetes.

Protecting HDL from oxidation. "Good" HDL cholesterol decreases artery-clogging plaque. Israeli researchers gave 10 people with diabetes either pomegranate juice or pomegranate extract. After one month, there was a 40 percent increase in enzymes that protect HDL from oxidation. "These beneficial effects . . . could lead to retardation of atherosclerosis development in diabetic patients," concluded the researchers in the *Journal of Agricultural and Food Chemistry*.

Lowering cholesterol. Researchers in Iran gave concentrated pomegranate juice to 22 people with diabetes. After one month, they saw significant decreases in total cholesterol and LDL cholesterol. Pomegranate consumption "could modify heart disease risk factors" in people with diabetes, wrote the researchers in the *International Journal of Vitamin and Nutrition Research*.

Stopping oxidation in arteries. Another team of Israeli researchers gave pomegranate juice for three months to 10 people with diabetes, measuring levels of oxidation in their bloodstream. The level of oxidized blood fats was decreased 58 percent and the overall level of cellular oxidation was decreased by 71 percent. "Pomegranate juice consumption . . . could contribute to attenuation of atherosclerosis" in people with diabetes, they concluded in the journal *Atherosclerosis*.

Controlling diabetes. And in animal studies from the US, Australia, and India, pomegranate (pomegranate flower and pomegranate seed oil) controlled or reversed diabetes itself.

Stopping Incurable Prostate Cancer

Prostate cancer kills more men than any other cancer, except for lung. In the last five years, there's been an explosion of research showing that pomegranate can battle the disease.

First, researchers in Germany and at the University of Wisconsin found that pomegranate extracts could stop prostate cancer cells from growing and then kill them, and also prevent prostate cancer from growing and spreading in experimental animals. "Pomegranate consumption may retard prostate cancer progression, which may prolong the survival and quality of life" of prostate cancer patients, concluded the US researchers in the journal *Cell Cycle*.

Then, researchers at UCLA gave eight ounces of pomegranate juice a day to men with prostate cancer who had been treated with either radiation or surgery (removal of the prostate, or radical prostatectomy) but still had rising levels of prostate-specific antigen (PSA), a biomarker of tumor growth.

Before the treatment, the men's average PSA "doubling time" (for example, the time it takes for PSA to rise from 2 to 4) was 15 months. After the treatment, it was 54 months!

Other tests showed a 12 percent decrease in the growth of cancer cells, a 17 percent increase in the death of cancer cells, and a 23 percent increase in blood levels of nitric oxide (which battles cancer).

"There are limited treatment options for prostate cancer patients who have undergone primary therapy such as radical prostatectomy but have progressive elevation of their PSA," wrote David Heber, MD, one of the study researchers, in the journal *Cancer Letters*. "Our data on pomegranate juice given daily for two years to 40 prostate cancer patients with rising PSA provides a non-toxic option for prevention or delay of prostate carcinogenesis. It is remarkable that 85 percent of patients responded to pomegranate juice in this study."

Since their study, the UCLA researchers have conducted several more, with the goal of discovering the main mechanism whereby pomegranate beats cancer. Their conclusion: it blocks the activity of *nuclear factor-kappa B*, a protein complex found in the nucleus of cells that fuels prostate cancer.

Test tube and animal studies show pomegranate may fight other types of cancer. A few examples of the more than 80 studies on pomegranate and cancer:

Breast cancer. Pomegranate reduced the growth of human breast cancer cells in test animals by up to 87 percent, in a study reported in *Breast Cancer Research and Treatment*.

Colon cancer. An extract of pomegranate seed oil cut colon cancer rates by 44 percent in experimental animals, reported Japanese researchers in *Cancer Science*.

Lung cancer. Pomegranate extract reduced lung cancer by 61 percent in experimental animals, in a study in *Cancer Research*.

Skin cancer. Pomegranate used as a topical lotion significantly decreased tumors and inhibited skin cancer from spreading in animals, in a study in *International Journal of Cancer*.

Leukemia. Pomegranate extract stopped the growth of leukemia cells, in test tube research from Japan, reported in the *Journal of Medicinal Food*.

The Promise of Pomegranate

Pomegranate shows promise in preventing and treating several other conditions.

Dental problems. Brazilian researchers studied 60 people and found that rinsing the mouth with an extract containing pomegranate reduced bacteria-causing dental plaque 84 percent *more* than a commercial mouthwash.

When researchers in Thailand treated gum disease (periodontal disease) with pomegranate extract, they found it decreased gum erosion and plaque.

And a pomegranate formula helped clear up *denture stomatitis*, a fungal infection in people wearing dentures.

Erectile dysfunction. A study at the Male Clinic

in Beverly Hills found that men who drank pomegranate juice for two weeks had improvements in erectile difficulties. The results were reported in the *International Journal of Impotence Research.*

Wrinkles and aging skin. Women who took pomegranate extract daily for four weeks experienced less skin damage from ultraviolet radiation—the same type of damage that causes wrinkles. In another study, ellagic acid prevented collagen destruction from ultraviolet radiation. Ellagic acid "may be a promising treatment" for wrinkles, said the researchers in *Experimental Dermatology.*

Sports recovery. Exercisers who took a pomegranate extract recovered their strength faster after a difficult weight-lifting routine compared to exercisers who didn't take the extract. The study was conducted by researchers at the University of Texas and appeared in *Medicine & Science in Sports & Exercise.*

Arthritis. In animal research, scientists from Case Western University in Cleveland, Ohio, found that a pomegranate extract slowed the development and reduced the severity (inflammation and bone destruction) of chemically induced rheumatoid arthritis. The extract "may be a useful approach for the prevention of the onset and severity of inflammatory arthritis," concluded the researchers in *Nutrition.*

Researchers in Iran found that pomegranate juice protected cartilage, reducing damage from chemically induced osteoarthritis in experimental animals. Their findings were in *Phytotherapy Research.*

Alzheimer's disease. Researchers from Loma Linda University in California fed experimental animals pomegranate extract from birth and found they were more alert as they aged and had 50 percent less amyloid-A in their brains, a protein linked to Alzheimer's disease.

Overweight. Obese animals fed pomegranate extract ate less, and lost weight and fat. The results were in the *International Journal of Obesity.*

Male infertility. Male animals treated with pomegranate had better sperm quality (normal shape and movement), more sperm, and higher testosterone levels.

Flu. Researchers from the University of Texas Health Science Center found that pomegranate extract killed flu viruses. "Pomegranate extracts should be further studied for therapeutic and prophylactic [preventive] potential . . . for influenza epidemics and pandemics," wrote the researchers in *Phytomedicine.*

Ulcerative colitis. In an animal experiment, researchers in India found that pomegranate reduced colon inflammation in this digestive disease.

Getting to Know Pomegranate

They grew in the Hanging Gardens of Babylon, one of the original "Wonders of the World." They are celebrated in the Old Testament, and were beloved by the ancient Egyptians and Greeks. They have been a symbol of health, luck, fertility, and immortality. The city of Granada (Spanish for pomegranate) bears their name, and the fruit is featured on the city's heraldic crest. The pomegranate, says an article in *Alternative Medicine Review*, is an "ancient, mystical, and highly distinctive fruit."

So distinctive, it's not edible! When you break it open, however, you find hundreds of

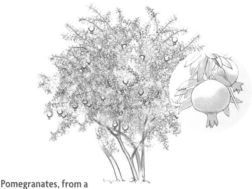

Pomegranates, from a
12- to 16-foot, gray-barked tree, have been
a symbol of health, luck, fertility, and immortality.

deep red seeds, suspended in a jelly-like honeycomb casing, glistening like garnets. One pomegranate contains about 500 seeds. They don't have much aroma, but you'll experience a juicy, thirst-quenching, cranberry-tart and rosewater-sweet flavor when you put them in your mouth.

Pomegranates first grew from the Himalayas of northern India to Iran, and are now cultivated throughout the Mediterranean, and also in Southeast Asia, the East Indies, and tropical Africa.

You can even find the 12- to 16-foot, gray-barked tree in Arizona and California, where they were first introduced by the Spanish in the 18th century. The fruit was slow to gain popularity in America, because it's so daunting to remove and eat the seeds. In fact, *very* slow. Pomegranate first hit the market a decade or so ago, and it was considered a health fad. But now its science-proven health benefits have made it one of the superheroes of the supermarket. Yet, when it comes to the fruit itself, people still wonder: What the heck am I supposed to *do* with it?

(If you don't know what you're doing, eating the seeds can create a scene that looks like it came out of a horror movie, with the seeds leaving their blood-red color on everything they contact—your skin, your clothes, and maybe even your hair!)

In India, where pomegranate is very popular, the seeds are dried and used as a spice called *anardana*, which has a deliciously fruity and tangy flavor. Indians use anardana whole or ground. It is found in curries and chutneys, in fillings for savory fried snacks called *pakoras*, and in flatbreads called *parathas*. Anardana is used as a flavoring in much the same way as Indians use the green mango souring spice called amchur. Anardana is often preferred to amchur, because it delivers a sweet-and-sour rather than just a sour flavor.

In Turkey and parts of the Middle East, the fresh seeds and their juice are considered an

Pomegranate may help prevent and/or treat:

Alzheimer's disease	Erectile dysfunction
Angina	Fatigue, physical
Arthritis, osteo- and rheumatoid	Flu
Atherosclerosis	Gum disease (periodontal disease)
Cancer	High blood pressure (hypertension)
Colitis (inflammatory bowel disease)	Infertility, male
Denture problems	Overweight
Diabetes, type 2	Wrinkles

Pomegranate pairs well with these spices:

Ajowan	Fenugreek seed
Allspice	Garlic
Cardamom	Ginger
Chile	Mint
Cinnamon	Mustard seed
Cumin	Onion
Fennel seed	Turmeric

and complements recipes featuring:

Chicken	Salads
Game	Sweet desserts
Pork	

essential flavoring to give a fruity, sweet-and-sour taste to meats and vegetables. They are used in marinades, sauces, and desserts. Dried or fresh seeds are sprinkled over salads and hummus (ground chickpeas). They are a key ingredient in the well-known Persian dish called *fesenjan*, a tart chicken or game stew thickened with pomegranate juice and walnuts.

Pomegranate molasses is popular in the Middle East. It's made by crushing the seeds into juice and cooking it until it reaches an almost black, thick molasses-like texture. The molasses has a berry-like taste with a citrus tang. It is somewhat similar to grenadine—made by mixing pomegranate juice with hot sugar syrup—a non-alcoholic flavoring used in many cocktail recipes. (Today, not all "grenadine" is true grenadine.)

Pomegranate seeds are very popular in Mexican cuisine. The Mexican town of Puebla is the birthplace of *chile en nogada*, an elaborately made stuffed poblano chile covered in a walnut sauce and sprinkled with pomegranate seeds.

Pomegranate is also popular in Russia. *Kupati* is sausage made with pomegranate as well as other spices (including allspice and coriander).

In the United States, pomegranate is most widely found as juice. It is also used to flavor water, teas, energy drinks, soda, and mixed drinks. One of the most popular among today's "fashion martinis" is the pomegranate martini—Oprah's favorite!

How to Buy Pomegranate

The only time to enjoy fresh pomegranate seeds is when the fruit is in season, from October to January. The fruit is picked ripe and can range in size from an apple to a large orange. The largest and heaviest should give you the juiciest seeds. Look for fruit that is free of cracks and soft spots, with a bright skin color (which can vary from pink to red).

Pomegranates will stay fresh at room temperature for several weeks before drying out, but will retain their moisture better and longer in the refrigerator. They should stay fresh in the refrigerator for a month or longer. The seeds can be frozen and will keep for six to nine months. You can find fresh seeds in season, but they're hard to come by out of season.

You can only find anardana in an Indian market or perhaps a specialty spice shop. Anardana is available dried or ground. The dried seeds are dark red with a black tinge. They will keep indefinitely. Soak them in water to soften them. Ground seeds keep for a year or longer if stored in an airtight container away from moisture and heat.

You can usually find pomegranate molasses in Middle Eastern, Armenian, or Indian markets. The molasses is easy to keep and doesn't need refrigeration. If it gets too thick, sit the bottle in hot water for a few minutes.

In the Kitchen with Pomegranate

The inside of a pomegranate is mostly all seeds, which are layered in two chambers. The key to getting delicious seeds is to avoid the pulpy and bitter pith and connecting membranes.

The traditional way to eat pomegranate was to pick each seed from the opened fruit with a pin, but no one does it that way anymore. The easiest way to open the fruit and remove the seeds—and avoid stains—is to do it underwater at the kitchen sink. The first step is to put on an apron. Then start by placing the fruit on a paper towel. Make a single cut around the circumference using a sharp knife. Be careful not to cut deeper than the skin. Place the scored fruit in a large bowl filled with water and break it open while holding it underwater. Rub your fingers across the seeds to separate them from the yellow membrane. As they separate, the seeds will float to the top. Use a strainer to retrieve them and transfer them to a bowl.

Seeds should be ground only in a mortar and pestle, as they will clog a spice mill.

To make juice, put the seeds in a food processor or blender and process until smooth. Press the liquid through a strainer to remove the fiber.

One medium pomegranate will provide about 1 cup of seeds and ½ cup of juice.

Making pomegranate molasses is simple. Put the seeds in a pot and boil down until the seeds turn liquid and develop a thick consistency.

You can sprinkle pomegranate seeds on almost any prepared food that would benefit from sweet flavor and crunchy texture.

Here are some other ways to enjoy pomegranate seeds:

Pomegranate Guacamole

A twist on this popular Mexican dip. It goes nicely with a pomegranate martini!

2 ripe avocados
1 lime
1 cup sliced scallions
4 garlic cloves, diced
2–3 serrano or jalapeño chiles, diced
¼ cup chopped cilantro
2 tablespoons pomegranate juice
¼ cup pomegranate seeds

1. Peel and pit the avocados and place them in a medium bowl. Sprinkle with the lime juice. Mash until it forms a coarse pulp.
2. Add the scallions, garlic, chiles, cilantro, and pomegranate juice. Continue to mash until well blended but still a little chunky. Fold in the pomegranate seeds.

Makes about 2 cups.

- The juice is a great tenderizer and a good addition to a marinade.
- Add a little pomegranate fruit or molasses to gravies and meat sauces as they cook.
- Before cooking, brush pomegranate molasses on chicken and pork like a marinade.
- Add a little pomegranate molasses to vinaigrette dressing.
- Put the seeds and the molasses over ice cream or frozen yogurt.
- Sprinkle seeds over salad greens or fold into fruit salads.
- Mix a little pomegranate molasses in the glass with club soda for a refreshing beverage.
- Sprinkle ground anardana on cooked vegetables or add it to soups or stews.
- Drip pomegranate molasses over beef and lamb kabobs when they are hot off the grill.
- Toss fresh seeds over lentils and other vegetarian dishes.
- To make a pomegranate martini combine 2 ounces of vodka with ½ ounce of lemon juice, ¼ ounce of pomegranate juice, and a dash of simple syrup.

PUMPKIN SEED *Shielding the Prostate*

When carving the pulp from a pumpkin for your Halloween jack-o'-lantern, don't throw out the seeds—they're a treat for your health.

Pumpkin seeds are rich in cell-protecting antioxidants, nerve-calming magnesium, blood-nourishing iron, muscle-building protein, immune-strengthening zinc, and heart-helping polyunsaturated fatty acids. They're also rich in *phytosterols*—plant compounds that are very good for the prostate.

The Prostate Loves You, Pumpkin

The size of the prostate gland is often compared to that of a walnut—maybe because the prostate can drive middle-aged men nuts.

By age 50, four out of five men have *benign prostatic hypertrophy* (BPH)—a "swollen" or enlarged prostate. Unfortunately, the gland is wrapped around the urethra, the tube that carries urine from the bladder out of the body. So by the age of 60, half of all men have urinary symptoms caused by their enlarged prostate. And those symptoms are really annoying, interfering with what scientific studies call "quality of life." You have to go more urgently. You have to go more frequently, sometimes waking up several times a night. The urinary flow is harder to start, weaker when it does start, and incomplete when it stops, with dribbling and a feeling of incomplete emptying.

Time to feed the prostate some pumpkin seeds.

Korean researchers gave 320 milligrams (mg) a day of pumpkin seed oil to men with BPH. After a year, their overall symptoms improved by 58 percent, their "maximal urinary flow rate" increased by 13 percent, and their score on a "quality of life" questionnaire improved by 41 percent.

"Pumpkin seed oil," concluded the researchers in *Nutrition Research and Practice*, can be a "clinically safe and effective complementary and alternative medicine for BPH."

In a Swedish study, researchers gave 53 men with BPH a supplement combining extracts from pumpkin seeds and a phytosterol-rich herb. After three months, all their symptoms improved: urination was less frequent, their urinary flow was stronger and faster, there was less dribbling—and the men felt a whole lot better.

How do pumpkin seeds work? The same way prescription drugs for BPH work, explain the Korean researchers. The phytosterols in the seeds block the action of *5-alpha-reductase*, an enzyme that converts the hormone testosterone to dihydrotestosterone (DHT), the compound that fuels prostate swelling in middle-aged men.

More Protection from Pumpkin Seeds

Animal studies (and a few in people) show pumpkin seeds may help prevent or treat several other health problems.

Heart disease. Feeding animals a mixture of pumpkin and flax seeds protected them from increases in cholesterol when they were fed a high-cholesterol diet. In fact, the seed mixture *lowered* heart-threatening total cholesterol, LDL, and triglycerides, and increased heart-helping HDL. The researchers theorize that the fiber and polyunsaturated fatty acids in the seeds produced the positive effect.

In another study, researchers found that giving pumpkin seeds to animals with high cholesterol enhanced the effects of the anti-cholesterol drug simvastatin (Zocor).

And when researchers gave pumpkin seed oil to animals with chemically induced menopause, they found the animals had lower blood pressure, lower total cholesterol, lower LDL, lower triglycerides, and higher HDL compared to animals that weren't fed pumpkin seed oil. "It's conceivable that adding pumpkin seed oil or the seeds to the diet of menopausal women may reduce the risk of cardiovascular complications associated with lack of estrogen," the researchers concluded in *Phytotherapy Research*.

Iron-deficiency anemia. Feeding women with iron-deficiency anemia an iron-fortified breakfast cereal along with an ounce a day of pumpkin seeds helped clear up the problem, according to a study in the medical journal *BioFactors*.

Arthritis. When researchers gave pumpkin seed oil to animals with chemically induced rheumatoid arthritis, they saw a "remarkable" reduction in swelling. The findings were in *Pharmacological Research*.

Getting to Know Pumpkin Seed

Pumpkins and other squashes are native to North and Central America; pumpkin seeds are

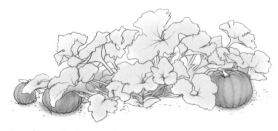

Pumpkins and other squashes are native to North and Central America.

one of the few spices the New World introduced to the Old.

Native Americans used pumpkin pulp for food, but valued the seeds for medicine. They ate the seeds to get rid of tapeworms, roundworms, and other intestinal infections, and to treat bladder and urinary tract problems. They also made a poultice with pumpkin seeds and put it on the skin to relieve burns, headaches, and arthritis.

Pumpkin seeds are eaten as a snack everywhere pumpkins are grown, but the seeds are popular as a spice in the cuisines of West Africa, Spain, Central America, and Mexico.

Pumpkin seeds—*pepitas*—are a popular snack in Mexico, but also an important spice. They're added to salads and are ground to thicken soups and sauces. They're a popular ingredient in Mexico's famous *moles*—hot and nutty sauces served over chicken and seafood. Genuine moles are time-consuming and painstaking to make and are considered the signature sauces of Mexican regional cuisine. The best-known moles come from Oaxaca, which is sometimes called the "land of seven moles." Among them is the popular *mole verde de pepitas*, a pumpkin seed sauce that is traditionally served with chicken.

In West Africa, where pumpkins are plentiful, the seeds are cooked, ground, and fermented, and used as a spice to enhance the flavor of gravies and soups.

Pumpkin seed oil is popular in India, Germany, and Austria for spicing sauces, pastas, salad dressings, and vegetables.

How to Buy Pumpkin Seed

You can purchase pumpkin seeds as a snack—raw or roasted, salted or unsalted. You can also purchase them hulled or in the shell. But to use them as a spice, you should buy them raw. They are available in many well-stocked markets and in health food stores.

Look for seeds that are intact, and inspect them when you get home. Discard those that are cracked or otherwise damaged.

If you buy seeds from a bin, make sure they are

Pumpkin seed may help prevent and/or treat:

Anemia (iron deficiency)	Heart disease
Arthritis, rheumatoid	Triglycerides, high
Benign prostatic hypertrophy (BPH)	Urinary incontinence
Cholesterol problems (high total cholesterol, high "bad" LDL cholesterol, low "good" HDL cholesterol)	

Pumpkin seed pairs well with these spices:

Black cumin seed	Coriander	Oregano
Cardamom	Cumin	Sesame seed
Chile	Garlic	Sun-dried tomato
Cocoa	Onion	Thyme

and complements recipes featuring:

Cakes	Muffins	Sauce
Chicken	Pork	Soups
Cookies	Salads	

plump, free of moisture, with no insect damage. Smell them to make sure they're not musty or rancid.

Pumpkin seeds can be kept in the refrigerator in an airtight container for about two months.

You can purchase pumpkin seed oil in specialty markets or online. Read the label carefully to make sure you're getting 100 percent oil. (The oil is expensive and is sometimes diluted with sunflower seed oil to reduce the price.)

Pumpkin seed oil is a deep, rich green, and may have a red tinge when you look at it through the bottle in bright light. Some of the best oils come from Austria. Keep the oil in a cool, dark place.

Green Pumpkin Seed Sauce

This is an easy version of the famous Oaxaca Mole Verde de Pepitas. *Serve it on top of grilled, sautéed, or baked chicken.*

1 cup pumpkin seeds, hulled
6 red chiles
1 cup chopped onions
2 cloves garlic, diced
2 romaine lettuce leaves
½ cup cilantro, chopped
1 teaspoon ground cumin
1 teaspoon dried oregano, preferably Mexican
¼ teaspoon dried thyme
½ teaspoon salt
2 cups chicken broth
2 tablespoons olive oil
½ cup light cream

1. Dry roast the pumpkin seeds in a heavy skillet over high heat until they start to pop. Start to shake the skillet and continue to roast until they turn golden, about three to five minutes. Transfer to a plate to cool. Place in a spice mill and grind to a fine powder.

2. Put the chiles, onions, garlic, lettuce, cilantro, cumin, oregano, thyme, salt, and the ground pumpkin seeds in a food processor and process until smooth. Add 1½ cups of the chicken broth through the feed tube and process until smooth.

3. Heat the oil in a skillet and add the sauce and cream. Cook over medium heat for five minutes, stirring constantly until the sauce thickens. Reduce the heat and add the remaining broth, if needed, and simmer partially covered for 10 minutes. The sauce can be made ahead of time and kept in a sealed container until ready to use. When ready to use, bring to a simmer in a saucepan and run it through the food processor again, if necessary, to get a smooth consistency.

Makes about 3 cups.

In the Kitchen with Pumpkin Seed

You can dry your own pumpkin seeds from your Halloween jack-o'-lantern. Here's how:

Scoop out the seeds with a strong metal spoon and wipe off the pulp with a paper towel. Lay the seeds out on a clean kitchen towel in one layer and let them air dry overnight. A pumpkin can contain as many as 600 seeds.

To roast pumpkin seeds: Put the seeds in a single layer on a pastry sheet, sprinkle with oil and salt, and bake them in a 300°F oven for 20 to 30 minutes, or until golden.

You can use pumpkin seeds whole or ground, in both sweet and savory dishes.

Here are a few ways to add more pumpkin seeds to your diet:

- Toss them with any of the dry spice mixes described in this book, sprinkle with a little Worcestershire sauce, and roast them as instructed above. Add them to chicken and tuna fish salads or toss them over salad greens.
- Grind the seeds and add them to vinaigrette or creamy salad dressings.
- Mix whole or ground seeds into oatmeal and other hot cereals.
- Use pumpkin seeds instead of nuts when making brittle.
- Grind the seeds and use them as a thickener in sauces.
- Add ground seeds to muffin and cake recipes.
- Add whole seeds to yeast and quick breads.
- Add whole seeds to homemade granola recipes.

ROSEMARY *Cancer Guard for the Grill*

Rosemary is at home at a backyard barbecue. Its robust aroma accents the powerful flavor of red meats. Grill jockeys sprinkle it on roasts, add it to marinades, and throw rosemary sprigs on hot coals to infuse steaks and chops with a smoky rendition of its pine-like aroma.

But rosemary also does another important (though little known and rarely acknowledged) job at a barbecue. It guards your health by keeping away unwanted intruders known as HCAs—a gang of carcinogens that are out to ruin your fun.

The Real Hamburger Helper

Nothing spoils a good cookout like hearing that the juicy hamburger you're enjoying is loaded with *carcinogens*. But scientists were spoilsports about 30 years ago, when they let the public know that grilling, frying, broiling, or smoking (but not baking) at high temperatures causes molecules in certain foods to break down and produce toxic chemicals called *heterocyclic amines*, or HCAs. When consumed, HCAs are readily absorbed, and traces of them have been found in human colon, breast, and prostate cells. They've also been found to induce DNA damage in test animals. Population studies over the years link a high intake of grilled meat with an increased risk of various cancers, including colon, breast, prostate, and pancreas.

Studies conducted during the last three decades consistently have found that HCAs start to build up on *all* flesh foods—meat, poultry, and even fish (but not vegetables and fruit)—four minutes after the temperature reaches 352°F. The longer the cooking time and the higher the temperature, the greater the toxic build-up. In one study, for example, food fried at 435°F contained six times as many HCAs than the same type of food fried at 352°F.

High temperature defines what grilling, frying, broiling, and smoking are all about. The

standard household oven broiler is set at 500°F, and high-end steakhouses cook meats at 600°F and higher.

Saying you shouldn't enjoy a grilled hamburger or Porterhouse steak would almost be un-American. In fact, there's been lots of debate over the years as to how carcinogenic, or even harmful, HCAs really are. However, the US Department of Health and Human Services categorizes them as "reasonably anticipated to be a human carcinogen" that can increase the risk of certain types of cancers.

What to do?

Well, the backyard barbecue has *not* been declared hazardous to your health and probably never will be, but the International Agency on Cancer Research says you can minimize this potential risk by cutting back on high-temperature styles of cooking and avoid eating charred food.

Or you can take *rosemary* to all your cookouts. Studies show that this spice is a potent antioxidant that can wipe out HCAs.

When researchers in Austria fried hamburgers at a relatively moderate temperature of 356°F for 20 minutes, they found HCAs continued to rise as the meat was being cooked. When they sprinkled rosemary on another set of burgers before putting them on the grill, however, and fried them at the same temperature for the same amount of time, 61 percent fewer HCAs were detected.

Researchers at Kansas State University have been experimenting with HCAs and rosemary extract for the last few years. They consistently found putting a little edible rosemary extract on hamburgers significantly decreased levels of HCAs. In some instances HCAs could not be detected at all.

"Lower temperatures can affect taste adversely," noted Kansas State researcher and food science professor J. Scott Smith. "The better way may be to use rosemary extracts so temperatures can still be kept high."

A Super-Sized Antioxidant

Rosemary's carcinogen-killing talent comes from a special blend of antioxidants—*rosmarinic acid*, *carnosic acid*, and *carnosol*. Together they make rosemary one of the most powerful antioxidants on earth. Studies show that rosemary possesses more antioxidant strength than BHA and BHT, manmade antioxidants strong enough to keep fats such as butter and lard from going bad.

Rosemary can even do better than that; it can help keep the immune system from going bad. One study found that just *breathing* rosemary essential oil reduced levels of the stress hormone cortisol in a group of volunteers. This is significant, because high levels of cortisol are associated with an increase in oxidative stress, a kind of internal rust that ages and damages cells. In fact, oxidative stress plays a role in *all* chronic diseases, including heart disease, cancer, and Alzheimer's—and in aging itself.

Rosemary is such a potent antioxidant that it can reduce the misery of radiation sickness (a mega-oxidizer) and prolong the lives of experimental animals exposed to a massive dose of gamma rays, according to a study in the *Journal of Environmental Pathology, Toxicology, and Oncology*. In another animal experiment, Korean researchers found rosemary prevented neurological damage (caused mostly by oxidation) from the toxic pesticide dieldrin (which is now banned in the US, though not in other parts of the world).

It appears rosemary may even be powerful enough to protect your skin from one of the most powerful and penetrating oxidizers on earth—the sun.

A Natural Skin Saver

Laboratory and animal studies suggest that rosemary might act like a protective shield against the sun's ultraviolet (UV) radiation, which causes premature aging (photoaging) and increases the

Rosemary may help prevent and/or treat:

Anxiety	Liver disease
Arthritis, osteo- and rheumatoid	Memory loss (age-related, mild cognitive decline)
Blood clots	
Cancer	Stress
Depression	Stroke
Dermatitis	Ulcer
Diabetes, type 2	Urinary tract infection
Gout	Wrinkles
Heart disease	

risk of skin cancer. In a study in the *European Journal of Dermatology*, rosemary extract protected human skin cells from damage when they were exposed to simulated UV radiation. The experiment, reported the French researchers, "supports this extract as a promising agent for the prevention of skin photo-damage."

In another study showing rosemary can literally save your skin, researchers at Rutgers University in New Jersey injected two groups of test animals with carcinogens that cause skin cancer. One group was treated with carnosol before each injection. After four months, the mice treated with carnosol developed 61 percent fewer tumors.

In another animal experiment, researchers in Italy found rosemary extract significantly reduced the growth of two different types of melanoma.

A Spice with Many Talents

Traditional healers have long believed rosemary contained special curative powers. They used it to treat diabetes, respiratory illnesses, arthritis, and dizziness. People inhaled rosemary boiled in wine to sharpen the mind. A medical text from the 17th century praised it as "a remedy for weakness and coldness of the brain." Rosemary oil was put in hair rinses to promote vigor and growth.

Many of these uses are proving to be scientifically valid. We know, for example, that rosemary possesses nutrients that can help fight inflammation, bacteria, and viruses. It can also stimulate the central nervous system. The cosmetics industry has enough faith in rosemary's traditional use to put it in formulas to treat wrinkles and oily skin.

To date, more than 500 studies have looked at rosemary and its constituents in the search to help cure and prevent a myriad of conditions. Among them are:

Dermatitis. A cream containing rosemary extract significantly decreased the oozing and swelling in 21 patients with severe dermatitis. The patients reported improvement in dryness, itchiness, and other symptoms. The study was reported in my book *Molecular Targets and Therapeutic Uses of Spices.*

Memory. Several studies show that the smell of rosemary can enhance thinking and total recall. One study of 144 people, reported in the *International Journal of Neuroscience*, found that smelling rosemary essential oil while performing mental tasks improved memory. Another found that sniffing the essential oil decreased anxiety before a test.

Cancer. More than 50 animal and test tube studies show that carsanol, carnosic acid, and other components of rosemary can suppress and kill cancer cells. For example, researchers in Israel, reporting in the journal *Oncology*, found that rosemary increased survival time in mice with leukemia. And researchers at the University of Illinois, in a study in *Cancer Letters*, found rosemary extract could "significantly inhibit the initiation and promotion" of breast cancer in animals exposed to carcinogens.

Cirrhosis. Rosemary protected animals exposed to the liver toxin carbon tetrachloride from the damage typical of cirrhosis of the liver, according to Mexican researchers, reporting their results in *Phytotherapy Research*.

Researchers in Mexico also found that daily doses of rosemary improved the structural integrity of liver cells in mice and protected them from liver damage, despite repeated exposure to toxic substances; their findings were in the *Journal of Ethnopharmacology*.

Blood clots and stroke. Two studies by researchers in Japan found that adding rosemary to the daily diet of test animals fed a high-fat diet improved blood flow through the carotid artery (in the neck) into the brain. It also "significantly inhibited" blood platelets from clumping, reducing the risk of a blood clot. A high-fat diet contributes to the build up of plaque in arteries that can lead to a heart attack or stroke.

Arthritis. US researchers found that a supplement containing rosemary extract reduced pain by up to 50 percent in people with arthritis. They reported their results in *Phytotherapy Research*.

Studies in Mexico found that adding rosemary to the diets of test animals helped alleviate the pain and inflammation from chemically induced arthritis. "This study reinforces the folk medicinal use of the plant in pain and anti-inflammatory disorders such as arthritis and gout," the researchers concluded in the *Journal of Ethnopharmacology*.

Repeated treatment with rosemary extract "dramatically reduced" pain and inflammation and helped restore "nearly normal" joint health in test animals with experimentally induced rheumatoid arthritis, according to a study in the *Journal of Rheumatology*. "This effect could be beneficial in clinical [human] settings," the researchers concluded.

Diabetes. Treatment with rosemary extract helped lower blood sugar levels in both normal and diabetic rabbits, according to a study in the *Journal of Ethnopharmacology*. The spice was just as effective as the diabetes drug glibenclamide (Glynase).

Ulcer. Rosemary "might have a therapeutic potential in the treatment of diseases such as peptic ulcer," concluded scientists from the

University of Illinois after evaluating the gastrointestinal healing potential of 25 spices and plants, according to a study in *Phytotherapy Research*.

Urinary tract infection. Researchers in Morocco found that rosemary increases urine flow similar to diuretic medication, according to a study in the *Journal of Ethnopharmacology*. They concluded that the research supports the Moroccan common practice of using rosemary to treat urinary tract infections.

Depression. Treatment with rosemary extract worked as effectively as fluoxetine (Prozac) in treating depression-like symptoms in animals, according to Brazilian researchers, in a study in *Progress in Neuro-Psychopharmacology & Biological Psychiatry*.

Getting to Know Rosemary

Rosemary is a legendary—and holy—spice. In a story told in the Christian tradition, the Virgin Mary threw her blue robe over a bush with white flowers when she stopped to rest while fleeing to Egypt with the baby Jesus. When she retrieved her robe, the flowers had turned the color of her robe, the same blue color found on the flowers of the rosemary bush today. "Robe of Mary" eventually became "rosemary."

In ancient Greece and Rome, rosemary had traditional uses at both weddings and funerals. Brides put rosemary sprigs in their bouquets as a sign of fidelity and newlyweds planted rosemary on their wedding day. Rosemary branches were placed in the hands of the dead and, according to legend, grew to cover the entire corpse. Rosemary sprigs were placed on the graves of loved ones as a symbol of remembrance.

In premodern Europe, the French burned rosemary and juniper berries in hospitals to purify the air and prevent disease, and rosemary leaves were burned as incense in English courtrooms to protect officials from contracting contagious diseases from prisoners.

Today, rosemary is especially popular in the Mediterranean region, where it thrives in dry,

Rosemary pairs well with these spices:

Ajowan	Coriander	Paprika
Basil	Garlic	Sage
Bay leaf	Marjoram	Sun-dried
Cinnamon	Nutmeg	tomato
Clove	Oregano	Thyme

and complements recipes featuring:

Chicken	Pizza
Game	Pork
Grilled vegetables	Rabbit
Lamb	Tomato sauces

Other recipes containing rosemary:

Basic Barbecue Rub (p. 272)	Pizza Spice Blend (p. 272)
Hungarian Goulash (p. 61)	Roast Chicken with 40 Cloves of Garlic (p. 134)
Mediterranean Vinaigrette (p. 160)	Rosemary Barbecue Rub (p. 272)
Penne and Sausage with Fennel Tomato Sauce (p. 117)	Spaghettini with Basil-Tomato Sauce (p. 42)
	Spice de Provence (p. 271)

sunny, sandy scrublands near the sea, and grows on retaining walls in backyard gardens. However, nowhere is it more enthusiastically used than in the cuisines of Italy and the Provence region of France, where it is a popular ingredient in both sweet and savory dishes.

Italian butchers often dress meat with rosemary or give rosemary sprigs to customers. Italians combine rosemary with honey, garlic, chiles, and wine, and use it to baste grilled lamb, goat, beef, fish, shellfish, and rabbit. Rosemary bread is a specialty in almost every region of Italy. Perhaps the most famous is *pan di ram-*

erino, a Florentine bread flavored with rosemary and raisins that is a tradition at Easter time. Rosemary is used in Italian pizza topping mixes, and some Italian pizzas are flavored with nothing but rosemary.

Rosemary grows wild and is cultivated in backyard gardens all over Provence. Just about every restaurant table in Provence features a bottle of olive oil seasoned with a sprig of rosemary, chiles, and other spices. Rosemary and garlic are featured spices in the Provencal vegetable dish ratatouille and it is hard to find a lamb dish that doesn't make use of rosemary. Rosemary is used to spice French liver pâté and is used to flavor grilled whole fish.

How to Buy Rosemary

Rosemary's stiff woody stalks with thin, dark green, pine-like leaves make it one of the most recognizable of culinary plants. On top, the leaves are glossy, with a vertical crease down the middle; the underside is pale gray-green.

There are actually two kinds of rosemary that produce the edible spice: a five-foot stiff bush that is often used as a hedge around homes and a low-growing variety that inhabits rocks and retaining walls. Upright rosemary is the more pungent variety. The only difference in appear-

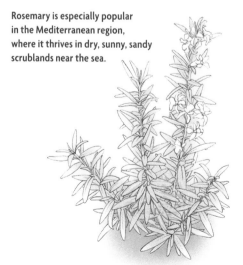

Rosemary is especially popular in the Mediterranean region, where it thrives in dry, sunny, sandy scrublands near the sea.

ance between the two varieties, other than size, is that the leaves on the upward-growing rosemary are about an inch long, while those of the low-growing rosemary are about one-half inch.

You can purchase rosemary fresh or dried (whole, chopped, crushed, or ground). There is not much of a difference between fresh and dried; they're both equally strong. (And unlike most other spices, rosemary retains its flavor and volatile oils when ground.) Both are available year round in well-stocked supermarkets.

Fresh rosemary is easy to grow in backyards or container gardens in warm weather. Newly snipped or freshly purchased rosemary keeps for a week or more immersed in clean fresh water. You can also wrap it in foil, put it in a plastic bag, and freeze.

Rosemary's leathery leaves and tough stems make it perfect for drying. It must be dried immediately after harvesting to preserve volatile oils. Hang fresh-cut branches upside down in a dark, well-aired warm place for a few days. When dried, the edges roll into tight scrolls and lose their flat appearance.

Once dried, the leaves are easy to strip from the stem. Hold them upside down and pull each leaf from the stem. This prevents ripping a piece of stem with the leaf. Snip them into quarter-inch pieces to make them easier to use.

Most of the rosemary imported to the US comes from Spain.

In the Kitchen with Rosemary

Rosemary has a pine-like aroma with a minty almost pepper-like balsamic taste. Its flavor is strong and can easily overpower a dish. If used carelessly or in excess, it will dominate all other spices and flavorings.

Rosemary does not lose its flavor in long, slow cooking. Because it contains a lot of oil, it dissolves quickly in fatty liquids. Again, it will take over a dish if the liquid is not degreased. The subtlest way to use rosemary is to throw a handful of sprigs on the coals near the end of grilling and let the smoke lightly scent the food.

Grilled Rack of Lamb with Rosemary Rub

This entree can also be roasted. Place the lamb racks on top of two rosemary sprigs on a rack in a roasting pan. Roast at 400°F for 20 minutes.

2 racks of lamb, trimmed and the bones frenched, about 2 pounds each
2 tablespoons Rosemary Barbecue Rub (p. 272)
3 sprigs fresh rosemary

1. If using a charcoal grill, set the grill for indirect cooking and place a dripping pan in the center. Preheat the grill to medium.
2. Rub the lamb racks generously with the rosemary barbecue rub and let sit at room temperature for at

least 30 minutes. When ready to grill, coat the grill with oil and set the rack, fat side up, on the grill over medium heat until medium rare, or until it reaches the desired doneness, about 20 minutes. The lamb is medium rare when an instant-read thermometer measures 140°F. Throw the sprigs of rosemary on the coals five minutes before the rack is finished. Let the rack sit for 15 minutes before carving.

Makes 6 servings.

Being a hardy spice, it is best used with full-bodied foods such as roast lamb, chicken, pot roasts, and stews. It also goes well with starchy foods, such as scones, bread, and dumplings. It complements vinegars nicely.

When using fresh rosemary, strip the leaves from the stalk and crumble at the last minute to release their oil. The leaves of dried rosemary should be used in the same way.

Here are some ways to add more rosemary to your diet:

- Put whole sprigs under roast lamb or place a sprig in the cavity of a whole chicken or fish. Whole sprigs used this way should be removed and discarded.

- Finely chop the leaves and add to tomato-based soups.
- Finely chop and add to biscuit and bread mixes.
- Add rosemary sprigs to sugar syrup for poached pears and peaches.
- Infuse a rosemary stalk in vinegar and sprinkle on bread you're going to grill.
- Use rosemary to flavor strong vegetables, such as brussels sprouts, cabbage, and eggplant.
- Combine a big sprig of rosemary, 2 or 3 crushed red chiles, a few fresh sprigs of thyme, a bay leaf, 1 tablespoon of oregano, 1 teaspoon of fennel seeds, and add to a bottle of extra-virgin olive oil.

SAFFRON *Lifting Your Spirit*

Saffron is the world's most expensive—and exquisite—spice. Its golden-red threads—as brilliant as a summer sunset—are worth their weight in gold. Well, almost. A pound of dried saffron goes for about $5,000, about 25 percent of the price of a pound of gold. Thank goodness saffron is sold by the gram!

The *stigma* is the pollen-gathering part of the flower—and saffron is the dried stigma of the blue saffron crocus. It's easy to see why saffron is the most expensive spice in the world when you consider that it takes 80,000 crocus flowers and a quarter million dried stigmas to produce one pound of saffron!

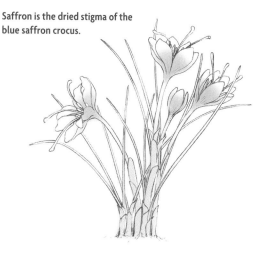

Saffron is the dried stigma of the blue saffron crocus.

The stigmas are picked by hand as the fall-blooming flower begins to open, a task that takes on ceremonial proportions during the two to three weeks of harvest in Iran, in the Kashmiri region of India, and around La Mancha in Spain, where a lot of the world's saffron is grown. Saffron is commonly grown on a family farm in these regions—and every family member lends a hand, working round the clock to pick, pluck, and dry the stigmas, and ready them for market. The hard work is often followed by a happy celebration—the euphoria coming, perhaps, from such a large infusion of mood-boosting saffron!

Mother Nature's Prozac

"In Persian traditional medicine, saffron is used for depression," wrote a team of psychiatrists from the Tehran University Medical Center in the *Journal of Ethnopharmacology.*

And that's why the psychiatrists decided to test the spice to see if it might work to beat depression. And also because they figured it might work a lot better than antidepressant drugs.

"Although a variety of pharmaceutical agents are available for the treatment of depression, psychiatrists find that many patients cannot tolerate the side effects, do not respond adequately, or finally lose their response," said the researchers.

It turned out that saffron brightened a lot of blue days.

As good as fluoxetine (Prozac). The researchers studied 40 people with mild to moderate depression, dividing them into two groups—one took fluoxetine; the other took saffron (15 milligrams, twice a day). After two months, saffron was as effective as fluoxetine, relieving depression in 25 percent of the study participants.

An effective treatment. In a second study from Iran, psychiatrists again studied 40 people with mild to moderate depression, dividing them into two groups—one took 30 mg of saffron a day and the other took a placebo. After six weeks, those taking the saffron had much lower scores on the standard test for depression (Hamilton Depression Rating Scale). The findings were in *Phytomedicine.*

Another team of Iranian researchers—studying 40 people for six weeks who took either saffron or a placebo—saw an even stronger effect for the spice. Their results were reported in *Phytotherapy Research.*

As effective as imipramine (Tofranil). In another study from Iran, researchers compared saffron to the antidepressant imipramine (Tofranil), which is a *tricylic antidepressant.* Thirty people with mild-to-moderate depression were divided into two groups, with one taking the spice and one taking the drug. Saffron was just as effective as the drug. The results were in *BMC Complementary and Alternative Medicine.*

The active ingredient. The spice may work in exactly the same way that many antidepressants do, say Iranian researchers: two compounds in saffron (*crocin* and *safranal*) protect levels of several brain chemicals (*serotonin, dopamine,* and *norepinephrine*) that boost and stabilize mood.

Chinese researchers investigated the antidepressant mechanism of saffron, in animal research. They concluded that crocin was the active ingredient in the spice, and that this saffron compound "should be considered as a new plant material for curing depression." Their findings were in the *Journal of Natural Medicine.*

Saffron, On and On

There are many other ways that saffron may help you stay healthy or feel better.

Atherosclerosis. Twenty people—10 healthy, 10 with heart disease—took 100 mg a day of saffron. After six weeks, the oxidization of cholesterol (the key process in forming artery-clogging plaque) was decreased by 43 percent in the healthy individuals and 36 percent in those with heart disease.

Alzheimer's disease. Researchers studied 54 people with mild to moderate Alzheimer's disease, dividing them into two groups—one received 30 mg a day of saffron and one received donepezil (Aricept), a drug often prescribed to slow the disease. After five months, saffron was as effective as donepezil at slowing mental decline, but without the side effects. The study was reported in the journal *Psychopharmacology*.

Menstrual cramps. Researchers studied 180 women, aged 18 to 27, who suffered from menstrual cramps, dividing them into three groups. For three menstrual periods (from Day 1 to Day 3), one group received a daily herbal remedy containing 500 mg of saffron; another group received daily mefenamic acid (Ponstel), a non-steroidal anti-inflammatory drug similar to ibuprofen; a third group received a placebo. Both those taking saffron and Ponstel had a "significant reduction" in the intensity and duration of pain during the periods—with the greatest reduction seen in those taking saffron. The study was reported in the *Journal of Midwifery and Women's Health*.

Premenstrual syndrome (PMS). An estimated 70 to 90 percent of women experience PMS, with 10 to 40 percent saying the symptoms—mental, emotional, and physical discomforts of all kinds, starting mid-cycle and continuing until menses—interfere with daily life. Researchers studied women with PMS, aged 20 to 45, dividing them into two groups—for two menstrual cycles, one received 30 mg a day of saffron and one didn't. "Saffron was found to be effective in relieving the symptoms of PMS," wrote the researchers in

BJOG: An International Journal of Obstetrics and Gynecology.

Infertility (male). Fifty-two infertile men were put on a daily dose of 50 mg of saffron. After three months, their percentage of normally shaped sperm (morphology) rose by 21 percent, and the number of sperm with normal movement (motility) doubled. The findings were in *Urology Journal*. It's probably crocin, the powerful antioxidant in saffron, that protected and regenerated the sperm, producing these "promising results," said the researchers in *Urology Journal*.

Erectile dysfunction. Researchers studied 20 men with erectile dysfunction (ED), giving them 200 mg of saffron a day. After 10 days, they had a 44 percent improvement in their scores on the International Index of Erectile Function, a standard questionnaire to determine the severity of ED. The findings were in *Phytomedicine*.

Cancer. Saffron has stymied many types of cancer in test tube and animal studies, including lung, colon, breast, liver, pancreatic, bladder, and cervical cancer, and leukemia. Saffron "may have potential to prevent and/or to treat certain forms of cancer," concluded a team of researchers, after reviewing more than 30 studies on saffron and cancer, in the journal *Acta Horticulturae*.

Anxiety and insomnia. "Saffron is used for insomnia and anxiety in traditional medicine," noted a team of scientists in *Phytotherapy Research*. In an animal experiment, they found saffron extracts reduced anxiety-like activity and increased total sleep time.

Memory loss. Researchers in Greece found that compounds in saffron improved memory in experimental animals. The findings were in *Behavioral Brain Research*.

Age-related macular degeneration. This gradual destruction of the macula—the center of the retina—is the leading cause of blindness in the US. Doctors at Texas A&M University College of Medicine found that crocin-derived compounds could "significantly increase the blood flow in the retina" and "could be used to treat . . .

age-related macular degeneration." They reported their results in the *Journal of Ocular Pharmacology and Therapeutics*.

Parkinson's disease. In this neurodegenerative disease, there's a gradual and progressive destruction of the area of the brain that produces dopamine, leading to a range of symptoms, such as tremors, muscular rigidity, apathy, and dementia. In an animal experiment, researchers in India found the crocetin in saffron protected dopamine-generating brain cells, and stabilized dopamine levels. Crocetin, wrote the researchers, "is helpful in preventing Parkinsonism and has therapeutic potential in combating this devastating neurological disorder." The results were reported in *Pharmacology Biochemistry and Behavior*.

Multiple sclerosis. Researchers in Pakistan used saffron to reduce the symptoms in animals with experimentally induced multiple sclerosis, an autoimmune disease that destroys the sheath around nerve cells, causing a wide range of neuromuscular symptoms, such as difficulty walking. Saffron "may be potentially useful for the treatment of multiple sclerosis," concluded the researchers.

Getting to Know Saffron

There are nearly 100 varieties of crocus flowers but there is only one that contains the stigmas that become the spice saffron—the leafless blue crocus. The orange-red stigmas are attached to a membrane in the base of the flower called a style. And when the flowers open in the fall, the fragile stigmas must be quickly removed from the styles by hand. Care is taken not to remove bits of style along with the stigmas. (Getting a little style in a batch of saffron is okay, but too much ruins the quality and reduces the price.) Once dried, the stigmas become a matted mass of curly, thread-thin strands so light a small breeze can sweep them away.

Because the styles must be picked as soon as the flowers open, an entire harvest is usually completed in a few around-the-clock days. The

---

Saffron may help prevent and/or treat:

Alzheimer's disease	Macular degeneration, age-related
Anxiety	
Atherosclerosis	Memory loss (age-related, mild cognitive decline)
Cancer	
Depression	
Erectile dysfunction	Menstrual cramps
Fatigue	Multiple sclerosis
High blood pressure (hypertension)	Parkinson's disease
	Premenstrual syndrome (PMS)
Infertility, male	
Insomnia	

Saffron pairs well with these spices:

Almond	Cumin
Cinnamon	Mint
Clove	Nutmeg
Coriander	

and complements recipes featuring:

Chicken	Lamb	Rice
Couscous	Nuts	Shellfish
Curries	Polenta	Soups
Flan	Puddings	

---

blue crocus is native to Iran, but crocus farms are now found in many countries (Iran, India, Spain, Greece, and England are among the most productive) and are mostly family owned.

Saffron is as old as civilization. The ancient Greeks used the spice to scent and purify their temples. The ancient Romans bathed in saffron water. Cleopatra used it as a facial mask. (Or so the legends say. I sometimes wonder if there are any spices Cleopatra *didn't* use in her facial masks.)

Throughout medieval times, saffron had great

commercial importance in Europe, especially as a culinary spice, saffron is most popular in the regions where it's harvested. Spain and Portugal make great use of saffron, and you'll find its telltale hue in their myriad fish and seafood broths. Spain's national dish *paella*, a large collection of meats and seafood, gets its signature brilliant golden color from saffron.

Provencal cooking features saffron as an essential ingredient in bouillabaisse and in *rouille*, a garlic mayonnaise spiked with saffron and red chile.

But saffron colors rice dishes everywhere, including Indian *biryanis*, and the Indian rice pudding *kheer*, and Iranian pilafs and the Iranian rice pudding *shola*. Saffron is also the key spice in classic Italian risotto Milanese.

Saffron is used in India's grand Moghul cuisine. Lamb is marinated for three days to make the elaborate *Shahi raan*, royal roast leg of lamb with saffron raisin sauce.

Arabs use saffron with cardamom to flavor coffees.

Scandinavians celebrate the feast of the patron saint Santa Lucia on December 13 by baking saffron bread called *Lussekatter* (Lucy's kitten), which is traditionally served by a daughter in the household wearing a long white robe, carrying a candle, and wearing a crown of lingonberries.

The Pennsylvania Dutch—German immigrants who settled in eastern Pennsylvania—use saffron to color and flavor their famous potpie, which isn't a pie at all but a chicken stew buried under large, square noodles. The original settlers brought crocus and saffron with them from Germany and grow the spice from their own backyards.

How to Buy Saffron

Because it is so expensive, saffron is also the most adulterated (and fabricated) spice. In 16th-century Germany, camouflaging safflower, turmeric, and other inexpensive substances to look like saffron was a big business—and a crime. In fact, the Germans took the offense so seriously that they formed a group of inquisitors called the Safranschau, who pursued, tried, and punished "adulterers."

Though saffron is grown in many regions throughout the world (220 tons are produced a year), Spanish saffron from La Mancha is considered the best, with Kashmiri Indian a close second. Australia's Tasmanian saffron is a new contender for high-quality saffron, and is possibly the most expensive. However, 90 percent of the world's saffron is produced in Iran.

Saffron comes in two standard grades: pure stigmas, which have no style, and filaments, with a piece of pale style attached. Words like *coupé* (Spanish), *morga* (Indian), *poshal* (Iranian), and *stigmata* (Greek) all denote pure stigmas. These are also subgraded according to the amount of crocin in the saffron. Higher crocin means better quality. The darker the color, the more crocin in the saffron. Saffron can range in color from yellowish orange to deep burgundy. Greek saffron from the town of Krokos is strictly controlled and its producers claim it has the highest crocin content. The least expensive saffron comes from Mexico.

Filaments are easy to spot, as an end of the stigma will be pale or yellow in color. Within this grade are also subgrades, based on the amount of other floral waste in the product. Typically, filaments are about 20 percent cheaper than stigmas. Iranian *sargoal* (a filament) can sell for ⅔ the cost of stigmas.

Generally, saffron is sold as 1/20 of an ounce—about a tablespoon—in a glass vial or small plastic case. Most of the saffron sold in the US is filament from La Mancha.

Saffron is also sold ground, but unless you are absolutely certain that it is the real thing, you are better off buying the threads.

A typical vial of saffron runs from $10 to $20 or more. If you see saffron any cheaper it's likely an imposter. Turmeric powder, which is inex-

Shellfish in Saffron Broth

This is a classic shellfish stew from Catalonia. It is best made ahead of time so the flavors gel and richen.

2 dozen clams or mussels, or a mixture of the two
½ cup white wine
½ cup chopped onions
½ red bell pepper, chopped
2 garlic cloves, minced
1 carrot, julienned
1 celery stalk, julienned
1 red-skinned potato, peeled and cut into small cubes
2 tablespoons butter or olive oil
2 cups chicken broth
⅛ teaspoon saffron, crumbled and dissolved in ¼ cup hot water
8 large shrimp
8 large scallops, sliced
4 ounces salmon, cut into small pieces
1 teaspoon dried basil
1 teaspoon dried mint
1 teaspoon dried parsley
1 tablespoon diced scallions

1. Bring the white wine to a low boil in a deep skillet. Add the clams and mussels and steam, shaking the pan occasionally, until they open. Reserve the clams and the liquid.

2. Sauté the onions, red pepper, garlic, carrots, celery, and potatoes in a medium dutch oven in the butter or oil over medium heat until tender, about 10 minutes.

3. Add the chicken broth and saffron mixture and bring to a simmer. Stir in the shrimp, scallops, and salmon. Cover and cook until the shrimp and salmon turn pink, about 3 minutes. Add the clams in their shells, cover and simmer for 5 minutes. Add the basil, mint, and parsley and cook 1 minute more. Ladle in bowls and sprinkle with the scallions.

Makes 4 servings.

pensive, is often passed off as saffron, especially to tourists shopping in foreign spice markets. Safflower is so frequently made to resemble saffron threads it got the nickname "bastard saffron." It has no taste.

There is only one sure way to tell if your saffron is the real thing. Saffron is soluble in water and starts to bleed its color almost instantly when put in a bowl of warm water.

Saffron will keep in a dry, dark place for three years or longer. It should not be stored in the refrigerator and does not take to freezing.

In the Kitchen with Saffron

The taste of saffron varies depending on where it was grown and the amount of crocin it contains. The aroma is often likened to oaky wine, and the taste honey-like, with a bitter, lingering aftertaste. Once it meets water, its flavor intensifies,

so only a pinch is needed in any dish serving four people.

Saffron only works in liquids and must always be infused in warm water or milk before it is added to a recipe. It will bleed most of its color within the first 10 minutes, though infusing it for longer (even hours) is okay. Never infuse saffron in oil, as it will trap the volatile oils in the threads and they will not bleed.

Break or grind the threads in a mortar and pestle before adding them to liquid. The threads are easier to grind if you give them a quick, light toasting in a dry pan first.

Classic ways to use saffron include shellfish stews, soups, curries, rice dishes, and creamy sauces. There is no reason to go overboard using saffron. Increasing the quantity will not increase the flavor.

SAGE *Improving Memory and Mood*

Want some sage medical advice? Make sage a staple of your spice cabinet.

Starting thousands of years ago, traditional healers—practitioners of traditional Chinese medicine, Ayurvedic physicians, healers in ancient Greece and Rome, Native-American medicine men—have been advising people to use sage. The tradition is so notable that even its botanical name, *Salvis officinalis*, comes from the Latin *salvare*, meaning *to save* or *to cure*. As a proverb from a medieval Italian manuscript states, *Why should he die who has sage in his garden?*

Well, if 21st-century scientists wrote proverbs, one might say, *Why should he or she have memory loss when sage is available?*

Clearer Mind, Better Mood

A supplement of sage might not make you "profoundly wise," the dictionary definition of a sage. But it might make you profoundly grateful—as it brightens your mood, refreshes your concentration, and sharpens your memory. That's exactly what several scientific studies show sage *can* do—confirming centuries of traditional use of the spice to improve memory and prevent age-related mental decline.

Better, faster recall. In a study by UK psychologists, researchers asked 24 healthy men and women (average age, 23) to take a series of 11 challenging memory tests—for example, seeing a different word flashed every two seconds for 30 seconds, and then having one minute to remember and write down as many of those words as possible. They repeated the tests several times a day on three separate days—and on some days they took a supplement containing sage extract before the tests, and on some days they didn't. On the days they took sage, they could recall more, and they could recall it faster.

More calm and contentment. But the students didn't only remember better when they took sage—they *felt* better, too. Calmer, more content,

and more alert—for up to six hours after taking the spice. "The improvements in mood are possibly the most striking findings," wrote the researchers in the journal *Physiology & Behavior*. (In a follow-up study several years later, the researchers again found that sage improved mood—and also reduced anxiety.)

The researchers theorize the spice improves memory and mood in several ways. Sage may block the action of *cholinesterase*, an enzyme that destroys acetylcholine, a brain chemical (neurotransmitter) that plays a role in memory, attention, and alertness. Sage might improve the functioning of the *cholinergic receptors* on brain cells that receive acetylcholine, like a dock receives a ship. Sage might boost levels of hormones that refresh the brain. Sage might dampen neuron-harming inflammation. Sage might do all that—and more. The power of sage, said the researchers, is probably caused by "a number of different mechanisms."

Preventing age-related memory loss. In another study, the researchers used the same series of tests to discover if sage could improve the memory-power of older adults—20 people with an average age of 72. Once again, a supplemental dose of sage extract improved the ability to process and remember information.

A "particularly important" finding, said the researchers in the journal *Psychopharmacology*, was a test that showed sage could reduce by half the ability of cholinesterase to destroy acetylcholine. That loss of acetylcholine in the brain is the main factor behind the advancing stages of memory loss in older people—starting with age-related memory loss, progressing to mild cognitive decline, and disastrously developing into dementia (60 to 80 percent of which is Alzheimer's disease).

"The benefits in the present study thus reflect a substantial reversal of the deterioration in memory which typically occurs over approximately five decades of normal aging," concluded the researchers. "Sage therefore has potential as an agent not only for general enhancement of cognition in older people, but also in Alzheimer's disease, either alone or as an adjunct to more conventional therapies."

Treating Alzheimer's. And one study *has* tested sage in people with Alzheimer's, with promising results. Doctors in Iran gave sage extract for four months to people diagnosed with mild to moderate Alzheimer's disease. Sage "produced a significantly better outcome on cognitive functions" compared to another group with Alzheimer's who didn't take the spice, reported the researchers in the *Journal of Clinical Pharmacy and Therapeutics.*

"The results of this study indicate the efficacy of sage in the management of mild to moderate Alzheimer's disease," concluded the researchers. They also noted that sage may "reduce agitation," a common problem in people with Alzheimer's.

Sage from Head to Toe

But sage is good for more than the brain. It might help the rest of your body, too.

Sore throat. In a German study involving nearly 300 people, a spray containing sage extract was "significantly superior" to a placebo in quickly easing the pain and inflammation of a sore throat. The spray provides "a convenient and safe treatment," concluded the researchers in the *European Journal of Medical Research.* In another study of 154 people with sore throats, a sage/echinacea spray was more effective in reducing symptoms than a spray combining the antiseptic chlorhexidine and the anesthetic lidocaine.

Heart disease. The root of a variety of sage (*Salvia miltiorrhiza*) called "Chinese sage," "red sage," and "danshen" is used in traditional Chinese medicine to treat cardiovascular disease. In a study by Chinese doctors in the journal *Phytotherapy Research*, stroke patients treated with danshen were less likely to have a second stroke. In another study, in the *Journal of Alternative and Complementary Medicine*, danshen slowed the buildup of arterial plaque in people with heart disease.

Psoriasis, eczema, and contact dermatitis. German researchers found that a topical lotion containing sage extract worked as effectively as over-the-counter hydrocortisone cream in clearing up irritant-induced skin rashes. Sage extract "might be useful in the topical treatment of inflammatory skin diseases," concluded the researchers.

Cancer. Research shows sage has the power to prevent skin cancer in experimental animals and kill colon cancer cells in the test tube.

Diabetes. In animal research, sage stabilized blood sugar in chemically induced diabetes.

Herpes. In laboratory research, German scientists found sage extract killed the virus that causes cold sores and genital herpes.

Ulcers. In animal experiments, Brazilian researchers found sage protected against the development of stomach ulcers.

Getting to Know Sage

Sage was used as a medicine for millennia before it became a culinary curiosity among Europeans, sometime during the 16th century. Over time,

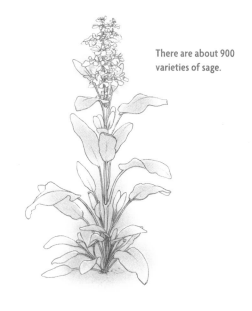

There are about 900 varieties of sage.

cooks came to appreciate sage for its grease-cutting action on game and sausage.

Sage is a prominent feature of Italian cuisine. It puts the flavor in the rolled veal and prosciutto dish *saltimbocca alla Romana*, and no ravioli worth its filling is laced with anything but browned butter sage sauce. *Pasta fagioli* is a meatless pasta and bean dish flavored with sage. *Fegato alla salvia*—liver with sage—is a popular dish in Venice. Sage is one of the secrets of authentic Italian pizza.

The Germans use sage in pork, lamb, and mutton dishes. A popular German dish is *aal in salbei*, skinned eel braised in onions, butter, and sage. The French put sage in cured meats and other *charcuterie*.

The English started the custom of smothering sage in onions and adding it to bread and sausage as a stuffing for holiday game birds. They also use it in mince pies. The English drank sage tea long before black tea became the afternoon tradition. They also made sage ale. But the best known use of sage in England is adding it as a flavoring to cheese. The green marbling in Sage Derby cheese comes from the liquid squeezed from sage and spinach leaves. Sage Lancashire contains chopped sage leaves.

In the US, many artisanal cheese makers in Vermont make their own version of sage cheese. Sage is also popular in the US as a spice in chowders, stuffings, sausage dishes, baked fish, baked pork chops, meatloaf, and melted cheese dishes. It is synonymous with the flavor of Thanksgiving turkey.

In the Middle East, fresh sage leaves are added whole to salads.

Sage is native to the Mediterranean. The perennial plant is easy to grow in most temperate climates, and makes a highly aromatic and attractive plant in the backyard garden, where its delightful violet-pink flowers attract bees.

How to Buy Sage

There are about 900 varieties of sage, but only a few are used for culinary purposes. Common

---

Sage may help prevent and/or treat:

Alzheimer's disease	Genital herpes
Anxiety	Heart disease
Cancer	Memory loss
Cold sores	(age-related, mild
Dermatitis, contact	cognitive decline)
Diabetes, type 2	Psoriasis
Eczema	Sore throat
Fatigue	Stroke
	Ulcer

Sage pairs well with these spices:

Almond	Marjoram	Parsley
Basil	Mint	Rosemary
Bay leaf	Onion	Sun-dried
Clove	Oregano	tomato
Garlic	Nutmeg	Thyme

and complements recipes featuring:

Butter	Gravies	Scones
Calf's liver	Meatloaf	Turkey
Fatty fish	Pizza	
Goose	Polenta	

Other recipes containing sage:

Basic Barbecue Rub (p. 272)	Roast Chicken with 40 Cloves of Garlic (p. 134)
Pizza Spice Blend (p. 272)	

---

sage (the variety Americans are most familiar with, and considered the most flavorful) has slender gray-green leaves with a downy texture on the top and a shiny, deep-veined underside.

Sage has a piney balsamic taste that is pungent and warm, like the taste of fall (just as mint is fresh and cool, like the taste of spring).

Sage Sausage and Apricot Stuffing

This recipe is just enough to stuff an 18-pound turkey. Cut it in half for a smaller bird or to stuff a goose. Cut to a third and it will stuff 4 Cornish hens. If you want to serve it as a dressing rather than a stuffing, put it in a baking dish coated with non-stick spray and lightly cover with tin foil. Bake in a 350°F oven for 30 minutes, or until heated through.

24 dried apricots	1. Soak the apricots in enough hot water to cover for 45 minutes. Remove, dice, and set aside.
3 tablespoons canola oil	
3 cups diced onion	2. Heat the oil in a large skillet over medium-high heat. Add onions and celery and cook until soft, turning continually until soft but not browned. Add the baharat and stir continually until the spices become fragrant, about five minutes. Stir in the sage. Set aside to cool.
3 cups diced celery	
1 tablespoon *baharat* (p. 268)	
2 teaspoons dried sage	
1 pound veal sausage	
8 cups cubed day-old bread	
1 cup chopped almonds	3. Remove sausage from casing and put in a large bowl. Add the bread, almonds, and cooked onion mixture. Add the chicken broth and wine and combine. Add the parsley and season to taste.
1 cup chicken broth	
¼ cup red wine	
1 cup chopped fresh parsley	
Salt and freshly ground black pepper to taste	4. Loosely stuff in the cavity of the bird just before roasting.

Makes about 4 cups.

Common sage is grown in greenhouses and is usually available year round. Other varieties of sage are also becoming available. Pineapple sage, from Mexico, has an unmistakable fruity accent. Clary sage is sweet and milder than common sage. Greek sage is stronger and has more camphor-like notes.

Buy fresh sage with bright full leaves that stand straight. Leaves that look dry and wilted are past their prime. Fresh sage will stay fresh for a week standing in a glass of clean water. The leaves will start to discolor in a few days if left in the refrigerator.

Dried sage is made from Dalmatian sage (native to Croatia, on the eastern coast of the Adriatic sea) and is sold whole, minced, chopped, crushed, rubbed (coarsely ground), or finely ground.

Rubbed sage is gray and woolly with a greenish tinge. It has a high oil content, which gives it a dusty finger feel. Because it is minimally ground, rubbed sage holds its aroma longer than finely ground sage.

Here's how to dry your own sage: Trim the leaves from the stem and lay them on a cutting board close to a sunny window, turning the leaves each day until they are dry. This will take several days.

Dried sage will retain its flavor for up to a year if kept in an airtight container in a dark, dry place.

In the Kitchen with Sage

Because of its robust flavor, sage is best in hearty dishes. This makes it especially well-suited for the slow, long-cooking foods of fall and winter. Because it has an affinity for fatty food, it is an important spice to complement duck, goose, pot roast, sausages, meatloaf, stuffings, and organ meats such as liver. It also goes well with fall vegetables, such as squash, sweet potatoes, and apples.

Dried sage is stronger than fresh but both will dominate a dish, so use it sparingly. Mate it with other spices in order to deflect its dominance.

Here are some ways to add more sage to your diet:

- Deep fried sage leaves make a fashionable garnish. Dredge the leaves in flour, dip in whipped egg white, and fry in a layer of hot oil. Fried sage leaves take on a flavor reminiscent of artichoke. Throw them over pasta or fish.
- To make sage butter, melt a stick of butter in a pan, add a teaspoon of dried sage, and stir until the butter is lightly browned. Pour over pasta or pumpkin ravioli and sprinkle with toasted pumpkin seeds.
- Sprinkle rubbed sage on cheese pizza.
- Add rubbed sage to macaroni and cheese.
- Add sage to meatloaf recipes.
- Add sage to eggplant and tomato recipes.
- Sprinkle sage on onions sautéed in preparation for long-cooking stews.
- Use diced fresh sage instead of dill on smoked salmon.
- Sprinkle a little sage on a fresh apple eaten out of hand.

SESAME SEED *Oiling Your Circulation*

"Open Sesame!"

Those well-known words—the password to a cave filled with riches, overheard by the fictional Ali Baba in "Ali Baba and the Forty Thieves"— are probably based on the fact that the pod of the sesame plant bursts open at maturity, scattering its seeds.

The wild sesame plant, native to West Africa, was also domesticated in India, where sesame seeds are a symbol of immortality in the Hindu religion, and sesame oil plays a key role in the ancient Ayurvedic system of health and natural healing. Charaka—the Hippocrates of Ayurvedic medicine—called it the "best of all oils," and Ayurveda recommends it for *abhyanga*, a daily, whole-body self-massage for purification and vitality. In his book *Ayurveda: The Science of Self-Healing*, noted Ayurvedic physician Dr. Vasant Lad recommends a daily sesame oil massage of the gums, and rubbing the soles of the feet with sesame oil before bedtime to produce calm, quiet sleep.

Sesame seeds are so oily that they even *feel* oily when you rub them between your fingers. Forty to 60 percent of the seed *is* oil—including lots of heart-healthy monounsaturated fat (the same type as in olive oil). Sesame is also loaded with vitamin E, an antioxidant that supports the heart. It's rich in *phytosterols*, cholesterol-like plant compounds that block the absorption of dietary cholesterol. And it's loaded with *lignans* such as *sesamin* and *sesamolin*, a type of *phytoestrogen* (a weak estrogen found in plants) also linked to heart health. So it's no surprise that scientific research shows the tiny seed can play a big role in the health of your circulatory system, possibly reducing the risk of heart attack and stroke.

Open Arteries!

High blood pressure is a major risk factor for heart attack and stroke. Blood pressure medications can control the problem. Blood pressure medications *and* sesame seed oil might cure it.

Curing high blood pressure. Researchers in India studied nearly 398 people with very high blood pressure, all of whom were taking the drug nifedipine (Procardia), a calcium channel blocker, to control the problem. For two months, 356 of the study participants were asked to use sesame oil

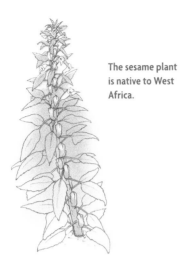

The sesame plant is native to West Africa.

as their only dietary oil. Two months later, the researchers could hardly believe the results.

"The consumption of sesame oil remarkably reduced the blood pressure," said the researchers. Systolic pressure (the upper reading) fell from an average of 166 to 134, while diastolic (the lower reading) fell from 101 to 85. Looked at another way, the average blood pressure fell from what medical experts say is the "very high" level of stage 2 hypertension, to the "caution" level of prehypertension—in other words, the participants no longer had high blood pressure, as it is medically defined!

And that's not all. They had lower blood levels of sodium and higher levels of potassium, a sign of effective blood pressure management. They had a big drop in the oxidation of blood fats, the process that creates artery-clogging plaque. And they had large increases in blood levels of several artery-protecting antioxidants, such as *superoxide dismutase*.

"These results suggest that dietary substitution of sesame oil, in nifedipine-taking hypertensive patients, has an additive effect in the reduction of blood pressure," conclude the researchers in the *Journal of Dietary Supplements*.

In another study by the same team of researchers, 32 hypertensives on one of two pressure-lowering medications—either diuretics

or a beta-blocker—were asked to use nothing but sesame oil as their dietary oil for 45 days. Once again, their blood pressure normalized! Then the participants *stopped* using sesame seed oil for 45 days—and their blood pressure zoomed back up! The findings were in the *Yale Journal of Biological Medicine*.

Lowering cholesterol in postmenopausal women. The drop in artery-protecting estrogen at menopause means a rise in the incidence of heart disease. Taiwanese researchers studied 24 postmenopausal women, dividing them into two groups. One group included 50 grams (about 1½ ounces) of sesame powder in their diet for two weeks, and one group didn't. Compared to those who didn't use sesame, those who did had bigger drops in total cholesterol and "bad" LDL cholesterol, and a more heart-healthy ratio of LDL to "good" HDL cholesterol. They also had less oxidation of LDL. And they had higher blood levels of biomarkers of estrogen. "Sesame ingestion benefits postmenopausal women," concluded the researchers in the *Journal of Nutrition*.

Boosting the protective power of vitamin E. "The tocopherols"—the components of vitamin E—"are believed to play a role in the prevention of age-related diseases such as cancer and heart disease," wrote a team of researchers from the University of Hawaii Cancer Research Center in the journal *Nutrition and Cancer*. But, they noted, little is known about which foods *really* increase blood levels of vitamin E and the cell-protecting "functional activity" of the nutrient. Animal research, they explained, points to the necessity of raising levels of *gamma-tocopherol* for vitamin E to function. (The more familiar *alpha-tocopherol* is found in most vitamin E supplements.) And sesame seeds are rich in gamma-tocopherol.

In their study, the researchers fed nine people muffins baked with either sesame seeds (rich in gamma-tocopherol), walnuts, or soy oil (other good sources of gamma-tocopherol). After three days, *only* the sesame seed muffins "significantly elevated" blood levels of gamma-tocopherol.

Little Seed, Big Results

Animal and test tube research reveals promising possibilities for sesame's power to prevent and treat various diseases.

Alzheimer's disease. Researchers in Korea found that sesamol, a compound in sesame, could stop the formation of amyloid beta, the protein found in the plaque that riddles the brain of a person with Alzheimer's disease. Sesame "may hold promise in the treatment of Alzheimer's disease," concluded the researchers in *Biological and Pharmaceutical Bulletin.*

Cancer. Many studies show that sesame and its components may have anti-cancer potential. In the laboratory, Japanese researchers found sesamin stopped the growth of breast cancer cells, and also reduced the activity of genes linked to lung, bone, kidney, and skin cancer. Another team in Japan found sesamol killed leukemia cells. US researchers found that both sesamol and sesame oil reduced the number of tumors in animals with chemically induced skin cancer.

Huntington's disease. This genetic disease of the central nervous system typically appears in middle age, eventually causing near-paralysis and dementia. Researchers in India used a chemically induced animal model of Huntington's disease to test the protective power of sesamol, an antioxidant in sesame. They found it helped prevent loss of muscle control and mental decline. "Sesamol could be used as an effective agent in the management of Huntington's disease," wrote the researchers in *Basic Clinical and Pharmacological Toxicology.*

Wound healing. Indian researchers found that a compound prepared from sesame seeds and sesame seed oil sped up wound healing in animals.

Getting to Know Sesame Seed

People have been enjoying sesame seeds for a while now—a depiction of bakers sprinkling bread with sesame seeds is carved into a 4,000-year-old Egyptian tomb. And to this day, sesame seeds are used as a topping for breads, biscuits, buns, and bagels. (A third of all the sesame seeds grown in Mexico are purchased by McDonald's for its sesame seed buns.)

Most of the world's sesame seeds, however, are used as a source of dietary oil rather than as a spice. Cold-pressed sesame seeds produce a highly stable oil that doesn't turn rancid in heat and humidity. That's why sesame oil has become such an integral ingredient in Asian stir-fries and other dishes. (Sesame oil is also called "gingelly oil.")

Seeds fresh from the plant come in a range of colors—yellow, brown, black, and red—but once hulled they are a creamy white. This is the seed used throughout the US and Europe. Unhulled black sesame seeds are used in addition to white in the Middle East, India, and Asia.

The Middle East has many sesame specialties. *Halva* is the popular confection—dense and sweet—made from compressed ground sesame seeds and sweet syrups. Tahini, a paste made from ground sesame seed, is used as a dip and spread, and accompanies the deep-fried chickpea patty called a *falafel*, and the seasoned eggplant dish called *baba ghanoush*. Hummus—a food found in just about every US supermarket—is mashed chickpeas made with tahini, olive oil, and spices. *Simsmiyeh* is a chewy sesame candy popular in Lebanon. Sesame is a key ingredient in the nutty Egyptian spice blend *dukkah*.

In India, black and white sesame seeds, called *gingili*, have many roles in cooking. They are sprinkled on breads, pastries, and biscuits, and in rice pilafs, sauces, and stuffings. The India region of Gaya is famous for its *tilkut*, a sweet savory confection made from sesame seeds.

One of the most innovative uses of sesame seeds is found in Japan's *shoujin ryori* cuisine, a vegan style of eating created by monks. The cuisine offers one of the few dishes starring sesame seeds: *goma dofu*, sesame seeds ground to a paste and into a block (just as tofu, another Japanese dish, is specially processed soybeans in a block). Japanese cuisine also uses white seeds to flavor teriyaki and black and white seeds in sushi.

Sesame seed may help prevent and/or treat:

Alzheimer's disease

Cancer

Cholesterol problems (high total cholesterol, high "bad" LDL cholesterol)

Heart disease

High blood pressure (hypertension)

Huntington's disease

Wounds

Sesame seed pairs well with these spices:

Allspice	Garlic	Pumpkin seed
Cardamom	Ginger	Thyme
Chile	Mint	Vanilla
Cinnamon	Mustard seed	Wasabi
Clove	Nutmeg	
Coriander	Onion	

and complements recipes featuring:

Breads and biscuits	Salad greens
Chicken	Salmon
Chickpeas	Stir-fries
Noodles	Tuna
Pork	

Other recipes containing sesame seed:

Dukkah (p. 268)	Wasabi Orange Chicken with Toasted Almonds (p. 260)
Grilled Lamb Patty Pockets with Cucumber Mint Sauce (p. 165)	

Shichimi is a popular sesame-based spice blend and a common Japanese table condiment. The Japanese also mix sesame seeds with MSG and salt and use it just as Americans use regular table salt. In both Japan and China, sesame seeds are ground into a paste and served over noodles.

In Mexico, sesame seeds are used frequently in mole recipes, complex sauces that are the hallmark of many regional cuisines.

Sesame seeds didn't appear in the US until the 17th century, brought here from West Africa with the slave trade. In most of the South, sesame seeds are still referred to as benni (*benni* is the West African name for sesame seed), and benniseed cookies are a Southern specialty.

How to Buy Sesame Seed

Sesame seeds are pearly white, flat, tear shaped, and tiny. They are readily available in well-stocked markets. Look for seeds that have an even creamy color.

The oily seeds don't have a long shelf life. If they've been in your spice cabinet for more than a few months, smell them before using. If they smell rancid, throw them out. For the longest shelf life, keep sesame seeds in an airtight container in a cool, dark place.

You can find hulled black sesame seeds in Indian and Asian markets. There isn't much of a difference in taste or texture between black and white seeds. (Cooks often choose one or the other based on how the garnish affects the appearance of the dish.)

Most of the world's sesame seeds come from China and India, but they're also cultivated in Guatemala, Mexico, and the southern US. Most of the sesame seeds used in the US are from Mexico.

In the Kitchen with Sesame Seed

Raw sesame seeds taste stale and bland. You need to toast them to bring out their appealing nutty essence. But toast with care, as they can burn easily. The easiest way to toast them is in a dry iron pan. Heat the pan on medium-high for just a few minutes until they turn golden. Continually stir, so they do not burn. If they start to hop around, it's a clue that they're done.

Sesame oil is strong—a little goes a long way. Use only a quarter to a third of sesame oil compared to other oils you use. The oil adds a

Sesame Seared Tuna with Pickled Ginger and Vanilla Slaw

You can find wasabi powder and pickled ginger at any market that sells take-out sushi or at an Asian market.

For the slaw:
1 cup sour cream
¾ cup rice vinegar
¼ cup sugar
1 teaspoon vanilla extract
¼ teaspoon salt
Freshly ground white pepper
2 cups shredded napa cabbage
2 cups julienned carrots
⅔ cup chopped scallions
½ cup chopped roasted peanuts
1 green pepper, cored, seeded, and coarsely chopped
1 red pepper, cored, seeded, and coarsely chopped
1 jalapeño, cored and seeded
For the tuna:
⅓ cup white sesame seeds
⅓ cup black sesame seeds
4 teaspoons wasabi powder
2 tablespoons sesame oil
4 six-ounce sushi-grade tuna steaks, 3" x 3" each
½ cup pickled ginger

1. *To make the slaw:* Put the sour cream in a small bowl and slowly whisk in the rice vinegar. Add the sugar, vanilla, salt, and pepper and stir. Set aside for 30 minutes.
2. Combine the cabbage, carrots, scallions, peanuts, green and red peppers, and jalapeño in a large bowl. Pour the dressing over the slaw and refrigerate while you make the tuna.
3. *To make the tuna:* Combine the sesame seeds and wasabi powder on a plate. Rub the tuna steaks with the sesame oil and dip the steaks in the sesame mixture to coat them.
4. Lightly coat a large heavy-bottomed frying pan with non-stick spray and put over high heat. When the pan is hot, sear the tuna on all sides until the seeds are golden, about one minute on all sides. Divide slaw among four plates and top with tuna. Divide the ginger and place on top of the tuna.

Makes 4 servings.

pleasing nutty taste to Asian stir-fries, especially poultry and vegetables.

The sky's the limit as to what you can do with toasted sesame seeds. You can use black and white seeds interchangeably; if you don't have black seeds, substitute white. (The only thing you'll lose is a little drama in the presentation.)

Here are a few ways to get more sesame seeds into your diet:

- Put toasted seeds in green salads or fruit salads.
- Add toasted seeds and fried garlic to steamed spinach.
- Use sesame seeds instead of breadcrumbs on pan-fried chicken.

- Sprinkle toasted seeds on top of or into lentil soups.
- Sprinkle toasted seeds on ice cream.
- Sprinkle black and white toasted seeds on deviled eggs.
- Add toasted white seeds to your recipe for hot wings.
- Sprinkle toasted white seeds on baby back ribs during the last few minutes of grilling, after you smear them with spicy barbecue sauce.
- Make a seasoning for grilled meats by combining 2 tablespoons of black and white seeds, 2 tablespoons of coarse salt, 1 teaspoon of hot pepper flakes, and lots of cracked black peppercorns.

STAR ANISE *Beautiful and Healthful*

In the beauty pageant of spices, star anise wears the tiara, with auburn skin, a firm body, curves in the right places, and a scent that beckons. Its literally stellar looks—a eight-pointed star of slender pods, each pod cradling a seed—makes it the most admired spice in the world. And its beauty is far more than skin deep.

The Official Flu Fighter

For thousands of years, practitioners of traditional Chinese medicine (TCM) have used the licorice-tasting spice for: clearing mucous from the respiratory tract (the spice is a classic *expectorant*, thinning and liquefying mucous so it can be expectorated, or coughed up), for arthritis, as a digestive aid to relieve gas and bloating, and to spark appetite.

Today, a compound in star anise is used as the "starter ingredient" for oseltamivir (Tamiflu), the most commonly prescribed drug for treating the flu—a fact that caused the price of the already-expensive spice to spike during the swine flu pandemic. The compound is *shikimic acid*, which is naturally abundant in the spice. It takes more than 30 pounds of star anise to get one pound of shikimic acid.

But shikimic acid is only one among many compounds that scientists have found (and are continuing to find) in star anise. Like shikimic acid, these compounds can play a role in fighting infection—viral, bacterial, or fungal—and the inflammation that infection leaves in its wake. Chief among them is *anethole*, the volatile oil (and proven antioxidant) that gives the spice its sweet, licorice-like flavor. (Anethole is the same compound that flavors aniseed, though the two spices are not botanically related.)

A few of the ways the spice has been shown to fight microbes in the laboratory:

Epstein-Barr virus. Japanese researchers found that star anise can inhibit the growth of the virus that causes mononucleosis.

Septic shock. In an animal experiment, researchers in Korea found that compounds in star anise could reduce the deadliness of septic shock, an often-fatal, system-wide bacterial infection.

E. corrodens. This bacteria in the mouth and respiratory system is responsible for causing infections from bites, and it can also run amok in people with head and neck cancer. Italian researchers found compounds in star anise stopped its growth.

Herpes simplex 1. When German researchers investigated the virus that causes cold sores they found that a compound in star anise could limit "viral infectivity" by 99 percent.

HIV. Researchers in China and Germany found that compounds in star anise were active against the virus that causes HIV/AIDS.

Hepatitis B. Chinese researchers found compounds in star anise could defeat the virus that causes this liver infection.

Streptococcus mutans. Another team of Chinese researchers found new compounds in star anise which showed "significant activities" against the oral bacteria that cause cavities.

The Fallen Star

A few years ago, star anise was pulled from the shelves in several countries after health officials in the US, Italy, Spain, and the Netherlands got frantic calls from parents about children and babies falling ill when star anise tea was used as a home remedy to ease respiratory illness and quell colic. Seventy cases were reported; symptoms were serious, including seizures, but they always cleared up within two or three days, and there were no reports of long-term illness.

An international investigation pointed to an imposter. Japanese star anise—a poisonous look-alike—had tainted a supply of star anise tea. The real spice was cleared of all suspicions, with the FDA reaffirming that it is safe for human consumption.

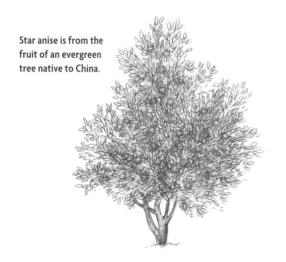

Star anise is from the fruit of an evergreen tree native to China.

Star anise may help prevent and/or treat:

Cancer	Hepatitis B
Cold sores	HIV/AIDS
Dementia, non-Alzheimer's	Mononucleosis
	Septic shock
Flu	Tooth decay

Star anise pairs well with these spices:

Allspice	Cinnamon	Fennel seed
Black pepper	Cumin	Mint
Cardamom	Curry leaf	Nutmeg
Chile	Ginger	Vanilla

and complements recipes featuring:

Chicken	Mango
Custards	Pork
Duck	Soups
Fish casseroles	Stir-fries
Fruit desserts	Syrups

Caution: The FDA considers star anise safe, but advises against giving star anise tea to small children and babies for colic. The FDA also cautions breastfeeding mothers against drinking star anise tea to prevent colic in their infants. If buying star anise tea, make certain it is not adulterated with Japanese star anise. The best strategy: buy the tea from a retailer you trust.

Other recipes containing star anise:

Caribbean Curry Paste (p. 287)	Chinese Five-Spice Powder (p. 268)

In other laboratory research, compounds in star anise have been found to kill cancer cells and reduce damage to brain cells.

Getting to Know Star Anise

Star anise is the spice from the fruit of an evergreen tree native to China—and it's not an exaggeration to say that the spice is one of the (if not the) most important ingredients in Chinese cuisine—the signature flavoring in nearly every Chinese regional cuisine. It is, for example, what gives Peking duck and Chinese spare ribs the distinctive taste that American cooks find so hard to duplicate in their kitchens.

A traditional Chinese cook wraps star anise in a muslin sack and puts it in "master stock"—a stock that continually cooks and melds as it is used and new ingredients are added. In fact, a master stock can stay in use for months or even years. (A traditional name for a master stock: Thousand-Year Sauce.) Many Chinese households have a master stock recipe and keep the ingredients a family secret.

Star anise (along with cinnamon) is also a key ingredient in the famous Shanghai braising method called red cooking. And it is the key ingredient in the well-known Chinese five-spice powder and other Asian spice mixes.

The spice is almost as frequently used in Vietnamese and Malaysian cuisines, where it appears in soups, marinades, and stews, and is ground and rubbed along with other spices into barbecued roasts and meats. It is a key ingre-

Pears Poached in Port and Star Anise

This recipe produces delicious thick syrup. Keep any leftover syrup to spoon warm or at room temperature over ice cream or frozen yogurt.

4 ripe Bosc pears
2 cups ruby port wine
⅔ cup sugar
½ cup water
4 whole star anise
Pinch of cinnamon

1. Peel the pears, leaving the stems intact. Combine the port, sugar, water, star anise, and cinnamon in a saucepan large enough to hold the pears. Bring to a simmer, cover, and cook for 10 minutes.

2. Add the pears to the liquid using a slotted spoon and simmer, uncovered, for 20 minutes. Turn the pears occasionally so they turn an even deep red color. The liquid should turn to a thin syrup-like consistency. Cool the pears in the syrup.

3. Divide the syrup among individual dessert dishes and add the pears whole with a scoop of vanilla or cinnamon ice cream. Or slice the pears, fan style, on a plate and drizzle with the syrup.

Makes 4 servings.

---

dient in the Vietnamese beef soup called *pho*. Malaysians use it to add sweetness to curries.

In Thailand, star anise is mixed with other spices to make tea.

It is also popular in India, where it is used in Kashmiri cooking.

It took until the 17th century for star anise to find its way to Europe, where nowadays it's most popular as a flavoring in confections, jams, syrups, and cordials.

How to Buy Star Anise

Star anise's unusual looks make it easy to identify—eight seed-holding pods (or carpals) in the form of a star. You can purchase it whole, in broken pieces, or ground.

Look for stars that are intact. (This is more for aesthetics than taste or freshness. Broken pieces are not necessarily a sign of age; more likely, they're a sign of aggressive handling during shipping or packaging.)

To test for freshness, break off one of the pods and squeeze it between your fingers until the seeds pop out. You should be able to detect its aroma immediately. No aroma means it is past its time.

Up until a few years ago, star anise was consid-ered a gourmet spice and was difficult to find in a typical supermarket. These days, most markets carry it. You can also find it in Asian and Indian markets. A four-ounce jar can cost anywhere from $4 to $10, depending on where you shop.

Whole star anise has a long storage life and will keep for five years in a glass jar with an airtight lid. Ground star anise will keep for a year under the same conditions.

Japanese star anise, which the Chinese call "mad herb," is not sold on the open market—because it's poisonous! However, supplies of true star anise have been known to get adulterated with the Japanese variety. (For more information, see the box on page 221.) Make sure you purchase this spice from a retailer you trust. However, it is also easy to recognize the difference between the two. True star anise always has eight carpals, but Japanese star anise has 10 or more. And rather than smelling like licorice, Japanese star anise smells like turpentine or denatured alcohol.

In the Kitchen with Star Anise

Star anise is sweet, due to its large quantity of anethole, which is 13 times sweeter than sugar. Its flavor is strong—licorice with a slight taste of cinnamon and clove—so a little goes a long way.

One whole star anise, or a pinch of ground, is enough to aromatize a vegetable stir-fry. Using too much will make a dish bitter.

One of the secrets to Chinese cooking is the way cooks use star anise when working with meat, simmering it in onions and soy sauce, which produces sulfur and phenolic aromatics that intensify the flavor.

The star itself is not edible (except in powdered form), but many cooks will use the star from the pot and put it on a platter or plate as a garnish. The seeds, however, are edible and have an interesting nuttiness. When grinding, use the pod and seed.

Here are a few ways to put more star anise in your diet:

- Use it in soups, stews, and casseroles that require long cooking.
- Put it in the pan when making roast chicken and duck.
- Add it to braising liquid for meats and fish.
- Add star anise to stewed apples or plums.
- Add it to the liquid when poaching chicken or fish.
- Make a rub for poultry or game by combining 2 ground star anise with 1 tablespoon of sugar, 1 teaspoon black mustard seeds, 10 black peppercorns, and 1 teaspoon of salt. It makes about ¼ cup, enough for a whole bird.

SUN-DRIED TOMATO *Guardian of Men's Health*

The tomato has baffled botanists since they started categorizing the plants in Mother Nature's garden: is it a fruit or a vegetable? Even in the 21st century, the confusion continues—botanists define it as a fruit, while consumers call it a vegetable. Well, sometimes the tomato is *neither*—when it's sun-dried. Then it's a *spice*.

Tomatoes are officially "sun-dried" when all the moisture is taken out. At the same time, all the nutrients are left in—delivering a super-concentrated dose of the healthful vitamins, minerals, and phytochemicals for which the tomato is justifiably praised. The most notable of these is *lycopene*, the pigment that colors tomatoes red. Lycopene is also the strongest member of the formidable family of antioxidants known as *carotenoids*. Antioxidants play a key role in human health because they help protect your body from the ravages of *reactive oxygen species* (ROS), cell-damaging, disease-causing molecules created in excess by many features of modern life, such as air pollution, a sugary or fatty diet, and second-hand smoke.

Unlike some other nutrients, lycopene isn't manufactured by the body. Food is our only source—and 85 percent of the lycopene in the diet comes from tomatoes and tomato products. And while it's hard to beat the juicy taste of a red-ripe tomato plucked right from the summer vine, ounce for ounce you'll get more disease-fighting lycopene from sun-dried tomatoes. When researchers tested a wide range of tomato products to find out which was tops in lycopene, sun-dried was the winner by a big margin. No surprise, considering it takes 10 tomatoes to produce one *ounce* of sun-dried tomato.

Prostate Cancer Protection

Lycopene first caught the attention of researchers nearly three decades ago when studies showed that death rates for all forms of cancers were lowest in older Americans who had the highest intake of tomatoes. But the nutrient really gained notoriety when studies started to show that it might help protect men against prostate cancer.

To date, dozens of studies have been conducted on tomato, lycopene, and prostate cancer. Results aren't consistent, but many show that regular consumption of tomato-based foods can help prevent and treat the disease. For example:

In a report in *Cancer Epidemiology, Biomarkers and Prevention*, researchers analyzed 21 studies on tomato intake and prostate cancer. Men who had eaten the most cooked tomatoes had a 19 percent lower risk of prostate cancer, compared to men who had eaten the least.

In another study, men newly diagnosed with prostate cancer were put on a diet that included pasta dishes made with tomato sauce. After three weeks, their blood levels of PSA (prostate-specific antigen), a biomarker for prostate cancer activity, declined by 20 percent.

In India, scientists studied a group of men with life-threatening metastatic prostate cancer, in which the disease has spread outside the organ. Since testosterone fuels the growth of prostate cells, all the men had opted for medical treatment to reduce the hormone, but half also took lycopene supplements. Two years later, PSA levels were lowest in those taking lycopene.

More Anti-Cancer Power

Lycopene shows promise in reducing the risk of several other cancers.

Breast cancer. Cellular and animal studies show that lycopene helps kill breast cancer cells, even the types most resistant to cancer drugs.

Colon cancer. Researchers measured blood levels of lycopene in people with and without colorectal adenoma, an intestinal growth that can turn into cancer. Those with polyps had 35 percent less lycopene.

Brain cancer. A study in animals found that lycopene treatments inhibited the growth of malignant brain cancer (glioma) cells. Growth slowed even more when the animals were given lycopene before being injected with the cancer cells.

Pancreatic cancer. A study in the *Journal of Nutrition* found that those with the highest intake of lycopene had a 31 percent lower risk of pancreatic cancer.

Studies also have reported encouraging results

Tomato may help prevent and/or treat:

Blood clots	Heart attack
Cancer	Heart disease
Cholesterol problems (high total cholesterol, high "bad" LDL cholesterol)	High blood pressure (hypertension)
	Infertility, male
	Osteoporosis
Dementia, non-Alzheimer's	Parkinson's disease

for lycopene in battling cancers of the bladder, cervix, liver, lung, stomach, and blood.

Red Alert: Tomatoes Are Good for Your Heart

Tomato plants thrive in warm sandy soil, and some of the world's best tomatoes are grown and dried in the exquisitely sun-drenched coastal regions along the Mediterranean Sea—where people eating the healthy foods (and sipping the red wine) of the Mediterranean diet enjoy a lower incidence of heart disease than people in the United States and many other countries. There's a lot of debate over which foods or combination of foods in the Mediterranean diet are the cause of healthier hearts. But a new study in the *British Medical Journal* shows that high vegetable consumption is right up there—including the lycopene-rich tomato.

In one study on lycopene and heart disease, researchers looked at the dietary intakes of 1,400 people, half of whom had suffered a heart attack. Focusing on three powerful antioxidants—vitamin E, beta carotene, and lycopene—they found that only lycopene was linked to a lower rate of heart attacks. Lycopene may play a role in the protective effect of vegetable consumption on heart attack risk, concluded the researchers in the *American Journal of Epidemiology*.

In another study, Harvard researchers tracked the tomato consumption of nearly 40,000 middle

The Poisonous Tomato

They say it was a brave man who first tasted an oyster, but perhaps that distinction should go to the first person to bite into a tomato. Tomato plants were around for a century or so before tomatoes found their way into European kitchens—people resisted the tempting red ball of flavor because they feared it was *poisonous*.

When tomato seeds first landed in Europe via Spain in the mid-16th century, people were shocked to find that it was kin to a plant with a deadly reputation: *belladonna*, the most notorious member of the nightshade family of plants. According to food historians, there is no evidence the tomato was eaten or used in cooking for over 100 years after its arrival in Europe. The first mention of tomatoes in a recipe did not appear in any continental cookbooks until the mid-1700s, and it took another 50 years until it became common.

How the tomato eventually overcame this misconception is unclear, but it might have had something to do with its fabled reputation for being an aphrodisiac. Perhaps like Adam, a curious person couldn't resist it. Hence, its 18th-century moniker: love apple.

By the way, early fear-mongers were not totally wrong. The *leaves* of the tomato plant do contain a poisonous alkaloid. In small doses, it's not strong enough to harm people, but could sicken a dog or cat. In fact, some cooks add a tomato leaf or two at the end of making a tomato sauce to restore some of the fresh taste lost in cooking.

---

age and older women with no known heart disease. After seven years, those who had eaten only 1½ or fewer servings a week of lycopene-rich tomato products had a 29 percent higher risk of developing cardiovascular disease than those eating 7 to 10 weekly servings.

Studies show that lycopene helps keep the heart strong and arteries flexible in three ways: by blocking the formation of "bad" LDL cholesterol, by thinning blood, and by lowering high blood pressure.

In a study reported in *The British Journal of Nutrition*, 21 healthy people spent three weeks eating a diet loaded with lycopene, with a daily intake of two cups of tomato juice and one ounce of ketchup. After three weeks, their LDL had dropped by 13 percent and their total cholesterol by 6 percent. The researchers also found that the tomato-rich diet cut the oxidation of LDL, reducing its ability to turn into artery-clogging plaque.

Researchers from Scotland found that a tomato extract (a pill equal to six whole tomatoes) reduced the ability of blood to clot—a risk factor for a heart attack—by 72 percent.

As for high blood pressure, researchers in Israel asked 54 people with high blood pressure that wasn't controlled by medication (an ACE inhibitor, calcium channel blocker, or diuretic) to also take either a tomato extract or a placebo. After six weeks, those taking the tomato extract had a "clinically significant" drop in blood pressure—systolic blood pressure fell from an average of 146 to 132, and diastolic blood pressure from 82 to 78. At the same time, their blood levels of lycopene tripled. In those taking the placebo, there was no change in lycopene levels or blood pressure.

Bone Up on Lycopene

More than 10 million Americans have the bone-weakening disease osteoporosis—approximately 15 percent of women and 4 percent of men over the age of 50. Another 10 million or so have osteopenia—bone density that is below normal and may lead to osteoporosis. And every year, two million people with osteoporosis have a so-called "osteoporotic fracture," usually of the hip, spine, or wrist.

You might want to throw some tomatoes at poorly performing bones. Cellular studies from researchers in the Department of Nutritional Sciences at the University of Toronto showed that lycopene might play a role in bone-building—stimulating osteoblasts (the cells that add to bone) and blocking osteoclasts (the cells that destroy bone). "Our research suggests that prevention and treatment of osteoporosis through the consumption of tomatoes and tomato products rich in lycopene may offer a viable alternative to medication for osteoporosis," said Leticia Rao, PhD, one of the researchers.

Those same researchers also say that ROS might spur the development of osteoporosis, just as they do heart disease. In a study on postmenopausal women (the main victims of osteoporosis), the Canadian researchers found the women with a lycopene-rich diet had much lower levels of a biomarker linked to high levels of ROS and bone destruction. "These results suggest that the dietary antioxidant lycopene reduces oxidative stress and the levels of bone turnover markers in postmenopausal women, and may be beneficial in reducing the risk of osteoporosis," wrote the researchers in *Osteoporosis International*.

The Brain-Lycopene Connection

Several studies show that lycopene may play a role in dementia, Parkinson's disease, and other

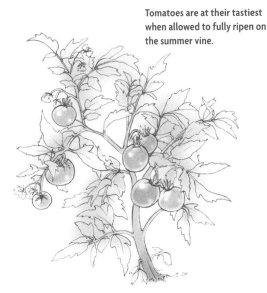

Tomatoes are at their tastiest when allowed to fully ripen on the summer vine.

forms of age-related decline. For example:

Low blood levels of lycopene levels were found in people with vascular dementia (the second most common kind, after Alzheimer's) and with Parkinson's disease. And in a study of 88 elderly nuns in a nursing home, researchers linked higher blood levels of lycopene with an improved ability to perform self-care tasks.

Researchers speculate that lycopene might protect the brain by reducing damage from ROS.

Male Fertility Pill

An estimated 7 to 10 percent of men in their prime reproductive years (age 20 to 50) are infertile. In one out of four of those men, doctors can't find a cause. It could be ROS—studies show that 25 percent of men with unexplained infertility have significant levels of ROS in their semen, whereas fertile men have no detectable levels. Could lycopene help?

Researchers in India studied 50 infertile men between the ages of 21 and 50, treating them with eight milligrams (mg) of lycopene a day for one year. On average, the men had significant improvements in sperm quality—and 36 percent of their partners went on to have successful pregnancies.

Is It Tomatoes or Lycopene?

Lycopene may be the tomato's crown jewel, but the fruit contains other nutritional gems. Tomatoes are also rich in vitamin C. And they're loaded with plant compounds (phytochemicals) such as coumaric acid, chlorogenic acid, and tomatine, all of which have anti-disease activity.

Many lycopene studies used tomato products as the source of the nutrient. This means lycopene may not act alone. Rather, it may derive its disease-fighting strength from working *with* other nutrients.

So even though lycopene is available as a dietary supplement, I don't recommend it. In my view, your best bet is to *eat* more tomatoes and tomato-containing foods such as tomato sauces, soups, juices, and ketchup—and always have a jar of sun-dried tomatoes in your refrigerator. In fact, it's a good idea to eat sun-dried tomatoes and other tomato products *daily*. When you stop eating tomatoes, lycopene levels plummet.

The Whole World Loves Tomatoes

The tomato is used in virtually every cuisine in the world to flavor just about every food. The total number of dishes in which tomato is the main ingredient numbers in the thousands.

Needless to say, Italian cuisine would be a lot less appealing if it weren't for the tomato. The tomato is also a staple in the Indian diet—it's frequently used as the liquid that balances the spices in curries and is a common ingredient in chutneys. Tomato is the ingredient that adds a sweet acidic flavor to many dishes in Southeast Asia, and the Chinese use tomato in sweet-and-sour sauces. It's the main ingredient in vegetable-spice mixes such as Latin American and Mexican salsas, Indonesian sambals, and Spanish sofritos.

Currywurst—a sausage topped with a tomato sauce spiked with curry powder and paprika—is a national dish in Germany. (It's sold on street corners in Berlin just like hot dogs are sold on the streets of Manhattan.) The French slow roast tomato into a *confit* as a rich full-bodied flavor enhancer. In Spanish Catalonia, people rub tomato into grilled bread for a snack called scrubbed toast. The tomato has even generated its share of geographical controversy: New Englanders were up in arms when New Yorkers replaced the cream in their famed clam chowder with tomato and renamed it Manhattan clam chowder.

Tomatoes are grown fresh in numerous colors and sizes—there are green, yellow, orange, red, and purple tomatoes, and varieties ranging from the size of a grape to a baseball.

Tomatoes are at their tastiest—and most health-giving—when allowed to fully ripen on the summer vine. Lycopene gives tomatoes their rich, red hue, and the pigment saturates the tomato only when it's vine-ripened.

As for taste: while tomatoes contain gel-like substances that makes them juicy, the flavor comes from the wall, the flesh just inside the skin. That flavor intensifies as sugar and acids build up during ripening. So it's no wonder that supermarket tomatoes are derided as "flavorless produce"—they're picked and shipped when

---

TOMATOES CAN BE DRIED
IN AN HOUR OR TWO WITH
A FOOD DEHYDRATOR.

---

they're still green and then exposed to ethylene gas, which triggers ripening in mature fruit.

My recommendation: unless you grow your own tomatoes, or can buy local tomatoes at a farmer's market, use canned or jarred tomatoes. They're actually healthier. Studies show that lycopene is much better absorbed from cooked tomatoes. One study showed *triple* the absorption after a tomato product was heated. In another, the lycopene in tomato paste was nearly four times better absorbed than that from fresh tomatoes.

The variety of tomato products is almost endless. There are an infinite number of soups, juices, sauces, pastes, and stews. Cooked tomatoes come whole, diced, crushed, stewed, pureed—and, of course, as a sun-dried spice.

Getting to Know Sun-Dried Tomato

Sun-dried tomatoes have probably been around since, well, since tomatoes. They're a staple of Mediterranean and Italian diets—traditionally, Italian families put some of their tomato crop on the rooftop to dry, so they'd have enough tomatoes to last through winter and into the next growing season. Recently, they've become popular in the US—some estimates say that more are consumed here than in Italy!

Sun-dried tomatoes are so named because they're left to bask in the sun day after day until they shrivel up and dry. This can take anywhere from 4 to 14 days. The process isn't difficult, but it requires just the right environment. The tomatoes need good ventilation, protection from critters, and have to be brought in at night. If you're planning to dry tomatoes yourself, it requires a lot of patience. Remember, too, that it takes a *lot* of fresh tomato to make a little sun-dried. A baseball-size tomato will shrink to the size of a pinky ring.

Their intense flavor, and the painstaking process of producing them, classifies them as gourmet items—with a price to match. A small eight-ounce jar—available at most supermarkets and gourmet stores—can cost six dollars or more. Compare that to the 60 cents you pay for the same sized can of tomato sauce.

There is, however, a relatively easy way to dry a tomato, without ever exposing it to the sun: slow roasting. You can use any type of ripe tomato, though the Roma is considered best because it has fewer seeds than other varieties. Here's how to do it:

1. Cut the stem end out of each tomato and slice the tomatoes in half lengthwise. Line the tomato halves up on a pastry sheet, making sure that they do not touch, and sprinkle them with salt and your favorite spices.

2. Put them in a pre-heated 200°F oven and leave them there for the next 8 to 10 hours. Check them every hour or so. They are done when they are dry with no sign of moisture. They may not all bake uniformly—and if the tomato isn't fully dried, the remaining moisture can collect bacteria. So, if necessary, remove them from the oven one by one, as they finish.

Another way to dry them is with a food dehydrator. A drawback is the initial expense of the

Oven-Roasted Tomatoes

Long before there were sun-dried tomatoes, the French were capturing the concentrated goodness of the fruit by making a *confit*.

The method for making *tomato confit* is similar to sun-dried tomatoes, except the tomatoes are taken out of the oven when they are still soft. They are then jarred, to use in salads, on pasta, or in anything that would be enhanced by a rich, pure tomato flavor.

To make tomato confit, quarter whole tomatoes and put them on a baking sheet lined with tinfoil. Sprinkle them with salt, pepper, dried thyme, and a little confectioner's sugar. Place a garlic sliver in the middle of each tomato and bake in a 200°F oven for an hour. Turn, baste, and bake for another hour.

dehydrator, which can cost $150 or more. But the advantage is that the tomatoes dry in an hour or two. Look for a device with a temperature gauge (maintaining the right temperature while drying keeps bacteria at bay) and follow the manufacturer's directions.

You can keep dehydrated tomatoes in plastic freezer bags. They'll keep in a cool, dry place for about two months or in the freezer for six to nine months. Before storing, make sure all the air is squeezed out.

As for oven-dried tomatoes: once properly dried (meaning *totally* dried), you can pack them in an airtight container and keep them in the pantry indefinitely. (You will have to reconstitute them before using.) Or you can also pack them in a jar with olive oil, where they will keep refrigerated for about two weeks.

To reconstitute sun-dried tomatoes, put them in warm water for about 30 minutes. If you reconstitute sun-dried tomatoes but don't use them right away, you must refrigerate them.

Here are some ways to enjoy sun-dried tomatoes:

- Eat them as a luscious snack.
- Stir them into soups, stews, and sauces

just before serving, to give the dishes a rich color.
- Use them in place of fresh tomatoes in sandwiches.
- Chop and add to tuna, chicken, or green salads.
- Slice and serve them in pasta dishes.

In the Kitchen with Tomato

Tomatoes originated in South America and fresh tomatoes don't take kindly to cold. Keep them out of the refrigerator, which chills the taste right out of them. Instead, keep them in a *cool* place—their ideal temperature is 55°F. And keep them out of the sun.

If for some reason you refrigerate fresh tomatoes, let them sit at room temperature for at least a half hour before eating. You'll get back most (but not all) of the flavor.

Tomatoes yield to slight pressure when ripe. If you buy tomatoes that aren't quite ripe, you can hasten the ripening process by putting them in a brown paper bag with a banana, which releases ethylene gas.

Here are some other ways to optimize the flavor and nutrition of tomatoes:

Go for gazpacho. This raw, tomato-based soup is good for you. Researchers at Tufts University asked a group of volunteers to eat gazpacho twice a day for a week. Their blood levels of vitamin C went up an average of 25 percent and their levels of three biomarkers for inflammation (a risk factor for heart disease) went down.

Whole is better. Whether fresh or canned, favor whole tomatoes. Studies show they're nutritionally superior to skinned-and-seeded varieties. (Don't remove the seeds and juice from fresh tomatoes unless the recipe calls for it—doing so changes the flavor balance in favor of sweetness.)

Strike oil. Tomatoes and olive oil are the mainstays of the Mediterranean diet—and they team up to beat disease, because olive oil increases the body's ability to absorb lycopene. When Harvard researchers analyzed the

Tomato pairs well with virtually *all* spices, but particularly well with:

Basil	Garlic	Parsley
Chile	Onion	Rosemary
Fennel seed	Oregano	Thyme

and complements recipes featuring:

Beef	Green beans
Chicken	Pasta
Cheese (feta, Parmesan, ricotta, Romano)	Poultry
	Sandwiches
Corn pie	Shrimp
Eggs	Soups
	Stews

Other recipes containing tomato:

All-American Chili con Carne (p. 110)	Mussels with Thai Red Curry Sauce (p. 156)
Bloody Mary Soup with Jumbo Lump Crabmeat (p. 70)	Onion and Tomato Chutney (p. 113)
Boeuf Bourguignon (p. 240)	Penne and Sausage with Fennel Tomato Sauce (p. 117)
Brussels Sprouts Kulambu (p. 123)	Potato Cauliflower Curry (p. 252)
By-the-Bay Fisherman's Chowder (p. 46)	Prawns with Almond Hot Pepper Sauce (p. 26)
Hungarian Goulash (p. 61)	Spaghettini with Basil-Tomato Sauce (p. 42)
Madras Beef Curry (p. 106)	

diets of 40,000 women, they found the highest lycopene levels in women who ate foods with tomatoes *and* olive oil (that includes pizza!). Those women had a 34 percent reduced risk of heart disease, compared to 29 percent for tomato-lovers who didn't routinely add oil to

Roasted Tomato Soup with Fennel and Mint

The tomatoes in this soup are slow roasted to produce concentrated flavor in the same way you make sun-dried tomatoes. You just take them out of the oven a lot sooner. The soup can be served warm or chilled. It makes a nice dinner starter or a light lunch with a salad. You can also stir in cooked crab. To dress it up, place a butterflied shrimp in the center of the soup and top with a dollop of sour cream or guacamole.

2 pounds tomatoes
Sea salt
2 teaspoons dried mint
2 teaspoons dried oregano
2 teaspoons dried parsley
2 teaspoons dried thyme
1 teaspoon fennel seeds
3 cups chicken stock
Fresh mint sprigs, for garnish

1. Cut the stem end out of the tomatoes. Slice the tomatoes in half and place them on a pastry sheet lined with tin foil. Sprinkle with sea salt.
2. Combine the mint, oregano, parsley, and thyme in a dish. Separate out 1 teaspoon of the mixed herbs and set aside. Sprinkle the larger portion of the spices on top of the tomatoes. Put in a preheated 275°F oven for 3 hours or until the tomatoes give off all their juices. Remove from the oven and cool.
3. Meanwhile, dry roast the fennel seeds. Heat a small heavy skillet and add the seeds, shaking the pan so they do not burn until they emit an aroma and darken. Set aside to cool.
4. Put the chicken stock in a medium saucepan and heat to a simmer. Remove from the stove. Put the roasted tomatoes in the bowl of a food processor. Add the fennel seeds, the rest of the spice mixture, and the chicken broth and process until smooth. Return to the saucepan and heat. Serve garnished with mint sprigs.

Serves 6 as a starter and 4 as a main course.

their tomato-based meals. So don't be shy—pour on the olive oil.

Team up tomato with broccoli. As a member of the cruciferous family of vegetables, broccoli is a well-known cancer fighter. In animal research at the University of Illinois, scientists found that broccoli and tomato together more effectively reduced the risk of prostate cancer than either one alone.

Here are some other tips for working with tomatoes in the kitchen:

- Take advantage of tomatoes in season (and get more lycopene!) by buying in bulk and making large batches of sauces. Freeze the sauce in small containers for ease of use.
- Perk up commercial pasta sauce by adding a cup or two of canned chopped tomatoes while it is cooking.
- Enhance the taste and healing power of tomato dishes by sprinkling them with *baharat*, a popular Middle Eastern spice mix. You'll find a recipe for the mix on page 268.
- When making a puree from scratch, you'll get a smoother sauce by starting with fresh tomatoes or canned crushed rather than whole canned tomatoes. This is because canners frequently add calcium salts to whole canned tomatoes to help keep the cell walls intact. This interferes with the disintegration during cooking. If you want to make a fine-textured dish using canned tomatoes, check the labels and look for a brand that doesn't list calcium among the ingredients.
- Adding a little sugar to tomato sauce as it's cooking intensifies the flavor.

- Make a fast and tasty barbecue sauce by combining 1 cup of ketchup with a few cloves of diced garlic, 2 tablespoons of diced ginger, 2 tablespoons of rum, and ¼ cup each of brown sugar, soy sauce, and distilled white vinegar.
- Pan roast tomatoes by cutting them in half and putting them in a pan of hot olive oil. Puncture the sides of the tomatoes with a sharp knife, so the liquid seeps out. Cook

for 10 minutes, turn, sprinkle with salt and spices and cook another 10 minutes.
- Here's how to make scrubbed toast, a classic favorite in the Catalonian region of Spain. Grill or broil thick crusty bread. While it's still hot, rub the bread with a crushed garlic clove. Cut a large tomato in half and scrub it into the bread until it absorbs the juices and the seeds coat the bread.

TAMARIND   *A Beloved Folk Remedy*

Never heard of tamarind? Well, it's likely you've *tasted* it. Tamarind is the key spice that gives Worcestershire sauce its defining flavor—and long shelf life.

In many African countries, the pod and seeds of the tamarind tree aren't famous as a food but as a folk remedy, used to fight respiratory infections, fevers, digestive upset, and constipation, help speed wound healing, and prevent sunstroke. (A recent review in the *Journal of Ethnopharmacology* of tamarind's use as a traditional medicine in West and East Africa cited more than 60 scientific references.) Around the world, tamarind is used for many other health problems, including as a gargle for sore throats and a liniment to ease aching joints. The spice is so potently curative that in animal experiments Indian researchers found it could neutralize venom from one of the world's deadliest snakes, the Russell's viper.

Tamarind's healing action comes from its powerful antioxidants, including *tartaric acid* (also found in bananas and grapes), which are concentrated in the seedpods. Tartaric acid is also what gives tamarind its characteristic sour taste. Additionally, tamarind pulp is a good source of calcium, and the B vitamins riboflavin, niacin, and thiamine. Together, these and other phytonutrients make tamarind a healing spice with a diverse set of talents.

Eyeing the Healing Power of Tamarind
Preliminary research shows that tamarind may help protect and heal the eye.

Dry eye syndrome. Dry eyes are the number one reason for visits to the eye doctor, with 30 percent of Americans suffering from dry eye disorder—the stinging, burning, and grittiness that comes from a tear film that's not functioning at its best. Italian researchers treated 30 people with dry eye syndrome, using either eye drops made from hyaluronic acid (a common treatment) or tamarind. After three months, the patients using tamarind reported significantly better levels of relief from several symptoms—burning, trouble blinking, and the sensation of having something in the eye. The researchers theorize that tamarind extract works so well to stay on and soothe dry eyes because its molecular structure is similar to the *mucins* (the proteins in mucous) that are found on the cornea and in the tear duct.

The research is preliminary, and as of this writing eye drops with tamarind seed extract, or *tamarind seed polysaccharides* (TSP), are not yet available.

Bacterial keratitis. In animal research TSP drops used with an antibiotic helped speed the healing of a corneal infection called *bacterial keratitis*.

Pink eye. Similarly, TSP drops helped speed the

healing of conjunctivitis (pink eye) in experimental animals.

Cataracts and age-related macular degeneration. Exposure to cell-damaging UVB radiation from the sun isn't only a risk factor for skin cancer—it also raises the risk of cataracts and age-related macular degeneration, two common eye problems in older people. In a test tube study, Italian researchers found tamarind drops helped protect corneal cells from UVB damage.

The Many Talents of Tamarind

Scientists are finding several other ways tamarind may prevent and heal disease.

High cholesterol. Researchers in Pakistan asked 30 healthy people to take either tamarind extract or a placebo for one month. Those taking tamarind had a 13 point drop in total cholesterol and a 20 point drop in "bad" LDL cholesterol. They also had a small drop in diastolic blood pressure (the lower reading).

In animal research, scientists in Brazil found tamarind decreases total cholesterol, lowers "bad" LDL, increases "good" HDL, and lowers triglycerides, another blood fat. "Together these results indicate the potential of tamarind extracts in diminishing the risk of atherosclerosis development in humans," the researchers concluded in *Food and Chemical Toxicology*.

In a test tube study, the same team of researchers found that tamarind affected human immune cells (neutrophils) in a way that could reduce the inflammation that underlies the development of cardiovascular disease.

Kidney stones. Tamarind is eaten daily in the tropical south of India, where the cuisine is hot and mostly vegetarian, both of which take well to an infusion of the sour spice. Kidney stones are rare in the people of South India compared to people who live in the North, where tamarind isn't as popular. Could there be a connection between eating tamarind and the low rate of kidney stones in South India? To find out, researchers at the National Institute of Nutrition in Hyderabad asked four men to eat a diet rich in

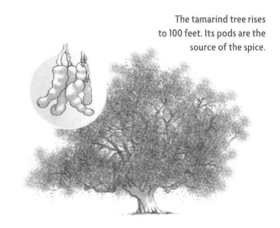

The tamarind tree rises to 100 feet. Its pods are the source of the spice.

foods likely to form the calcium oxalate crystals that comprise most kidney stones. After one week on the diet, the men added tamarind extract. The researchers tested the men's urine before and after adding tamarind—and the addition of the extract lowered levels of several parameters that increase the risk of forming stones. "Consumption of tamarind offers some protection against the recurrence of calcium oxalate stones in men," concluded the researchers in the journal *Nutrition Research*.

Cancer. Indian researchers found that tamarind extract slowed the growth of colon cancer in experimental animals.

Diabetes, type 1. Tamarind is a traditional treatment for diabetes in India. In animal experiments, Indian researchers lowered blood sugar in animals with drug-induced type 1 diabetes (the autoimmune disease that destroys the cells of the insulin-generating pancreas). Tamarind "may have beneficial effects in Type-1 diabetes mellitus," the researchers concluded in the *Journal of Ethnopharmacology*.

Getting to Know Tamarind

Native to tropical Africa, the majestic tamarind tree—which rises to 100 feet and spans 30 feet—is appreciated for the shade it supplies in the countries of the "tropical belt" that circles the world. Tamarind trees are practically indestructible. The deep root system and big burly

The "Secret" of Worcestershire Sauce

Worcestershire sauce is an English invention that came about by accident during the mid-1840s. According to culinary legend, the owners of a chemist's shop in Worcester (bordering the scenic Cotswolds in the English countryside) made a barrel of spiced vinegar according to an old Indian recipe for a customer who never showed up to claim it.

The concoction sat and fermented in the shop's cellar for years. The owners, John Wheeley Lea and William Henry Perrin, figured it had spoiled and told a clerk to throw it out. The clerk, however, got a whiff of the concoction and decided to taste it. The barrel was not spoiled and had, in fact, undergone an intriguingly tasty change.

The owners bottled the sauce and sold it as Lea and Perrin's Worcestershire Sauce. The rest, as they say, is history. The sauce, now distributed and well-known worldwide, is used to flavor grilled meats and is a popular ingredient in the Bloody Mary cocktail. The American ketchup-making company H. J. Heinz purchased Lea and Perrin's in 2005 and still sells the condiment under the original label.

The recipe is said to be secret, though it is known to contain tamarind, cloves, anchovies, onions, and garlic. There are many imitation brands of Worcestershire, but connoisseurs say none come close to matching Lea and Perrin's secret recipe.

---

trunk help the tree survive high winds, and it is highly resistant to drought. Mysteriously, no other vegetation grows beneath its widespread canopy of pale-green flowering leaflets that sag like a weeping willow, making the shady circle of a tamarind tree the perfect spot for an afternoon picnic (or nap). The leaflets are stunning as they bend from the weight of the elongated pods and then close up at night. As the pods brown in the sun, they produce the spice's hallmark prune-like sourness.

Unlike many tropical spices that must be hand-picked and tenderly handled, all that's required to harvest tamarind is a person brave enough to climb the tree and shake the pods.

When harvested, the shells and seeds are removed and the pulp compressed into acidifying cakes. As the pulp is exposed to air it begins to oxidize and turn dark, almost black. It takes on a sharp, tingly, and intensely acidic taste, making it a perfect souring agent.

Tamarind is to the East what lemon is to the West. It is the most popular souring agent in most tropical countries, and is a key ingredient in the cuisines of India, Thailand, Indonesia, and Malaysia. It is used as a paste, syrup, and juice. Only the paste is strong enough for the cuisine

of South India, where it is used to flavor fiery fish curries, vindaloos, and vegetarian dishes. It also goes in chowder-like vegetarian stews called *sambars* and soups called *rasams*. A tamarind dip is made for deep-fried snacks called *samosas*. In North India, batter-fried dumplings called *dahi vada* float in a sauce made from tamarind and yogurt.

Tamarind, which is called *assam* in Asia, is used in the marinade to made Malaysia's famed satays, and is in the dipping sauces that accompany them. It is also used in the hot and sour soups of China, Thailand, and Singapore. Tamarind paste gives a tang to Asian stir-fries. In Thailand, the pulp is dusted with sugar and eaten as a sweetmeat. In the West Indies, the seeds are sugared and compressed into patties. In the Philippines, sweet potatoes are added to the patties to make a sweet treat called *champoy*.

In Jamaica, tamarind is used in jams, syrups, and in Jamaican pickapeppa sauce, a condiment popular in the US.

Tamarind has a cool, refreshing taste, which makes it popular as a beverage in tropical lands. In India, the drink is infused with rosewater and lemon juice and sipped after dinner on hot evenings. Tamarind is diluted and sugar is added to

Tamarind may help prevent and/or treat:

Cancer	Dry eye syndrome
Cataracts	Eye infection, bacterial keratitis
Cholesterol problems (high total cholesterol, high "bad" LDL cholesterol, low "good" HDL cholesterol)	Heart disease
	High blood pressure (hypertension)
	Kidney stones
Conjunctivitis (pink eye)	Macular degeneration, age-related
Diabetes, type 1	Triglycerides (high)

Tamarind pairs well with these spices:

Ajowan	Clove	Sun-dried tomato
Amchur	Galangal	
Chile	Garlic	Turmeric
	Ginger	

and complements recipes featuring:

Asian soups	Peanuts
Chutneys	Pickled foods
Curry pastes	Stir-fries

Other recipes containing tamarind:

Brussels Sprouts Kulambu (p. 123)	Onion and Tomato Chutney (p. 113)

make a soft drink in Jamaica and Latin American countries.

Throughout the Caribbean, Mexico, and Latin America, tamarind makes a popular sweet and sour candy. Sweetened balls of tamarind are rolled in sugar and sometimes spiced with chile, which is called *pulparindo* (as well as other names).

In addition to Worcestershire sauce, tamarind is also an ingredient in another popular American cocktail condiment—Angostura bitters.

How to Buy Tamarind

Most Indian and Asian grocers sell tamarind in plastic-wrapped blocks—a sticky fibrous mass of oxidized dark brown-to-black pulp. You extract the flavor by soaking the paste in hot water and squeezing it out. Tamarind blocks are imported from India and Thailand. The two are quite different in texture and taste, though both deliver the desired sourness. Indian tamarind is fairly dry, with a paper-like texture. The Thai variety is cleaner-looking, but very sticky. Thai is more appealing aesthetically but the Indian tamarind is easier to handle.

Tamarind is also sold as a concentrate, and as a dried and ground powder. They, too, must be diluted. The concentrate is easiest to work with; many Indians living in the US buy and use the concentrate for its convenience. You can find it in large jar containers in any Indian grocery store, where it looks a lot like apple butter. If you're not familiar with tamarind, you might want to consider buying a concentrate for your first try. Tamarind powder, called cream of tamarind or assam powder, is harder to find.

Due to its high acid content, tamarind is very stable and requires no special storage conditions. Blocks should be kept in airtight packages to prevent them from drying out.

In the Kitchen with Tamarind

Tamarind tastes like lemon or lime with an edge. It is nose-puckering sour, so keep this in mind when cooking with it. A little goes a long way. Tamarind delivers a tang and adds an appetizing rich dark color to gravies, stir-fries, soups, stews, curries, chutneys, and sauces that you cannot get from a lemon or lime.

You'll come across the pulp as an ingredient most often in Indian recipes, which are heavy on spices. Usually, however, the recipe calls for tamarind water or tamarind juice. The terms "tamarind water" and "tamarind juice" are used interchangeably and refer to the same thing. The water/juice can be made out of tamarind in all its forms.

Tamarind Sauce

This savory-sweet sauce from the Caribbean is superb over baked, grilled, and fried fish. It also makes a great dipping sauce for Asian dumplings and a topping for baked brie.

⅓ cup tamarind water
5 tablespoons brown sugar
½ cup diced onions
1 clove garlic, diced
2 dried red chiles, seeded and chopped
3 tablespoons soy sauce
3 tablespoons pineapple juice
¼ cup chopped cilantro
Freshly ground black pepper

1. Combine the tamarind water (see the instructions for making tamarind water below) and brown sugar in a medium saucepan over low heat and stir until the sugar dissolves. Add the onions, garlic, and chiles and stir for three minutes. Add the soy sauce and pineapple juice and stir. Cover and simmer for 10 minutes. Stir in cilantro and black pepper.

Makes about 1 cup.

To make tamarind water from a block, break off a piece about one inch in diameter and soak it in ½ cup of hot water for about 15 minutes. Stir and press it. Strain it, squeezing out as much water as possible and discard the dried pulp.

To make tamarind water from a concentrate, soak ¼ cup of tamarind in 1 cup of boiling water for about 15 minutes and strain. It doesn't have a lot of staying power to stay fresh in the refrigerator for more than a few days, but you can make it in large batches and freeze it in ice cube trays. When you want to make a sweet and sour dish, or you need a souring agent to perk up a recipe, just plop in a cube of tamarind water.

Tamarind *pulp* and tamarind water *cannot* be used interchangeably.

THYME *Anti-Microbial, Pro-Health*

Once upon a time—maybe about 5,000 years ago, before the Romans distributed the plant throughout their empire—there was probably just one thyme. Now there are many. There's the French thyme that most of us cook with. There are also the varieties of thyme that a canny plant-lover might spot in a walk around a typical suburban neighborhood, peeking into backyard gardens, such as lemon thyme, orange thyme, anise thyme, and silver thyme. Worldwide, there are more than *one hundred* varieties of thyme, each with a subtly different flavor. But all those varieties have one factor in common: the volatile oil *thymol.*

Thymol is one of Mother Nature's most powerful *antiseptics*—when applied to your skin or the mucous membranes inside your mouth, it kills germs. (Thymol is a primary antiseptic in the mouthwash Listerine, famous for the slogan, "Kills Germs on Contact.") And while there's lots of preliminary research in test tubes and experimental animals on the power on thymol (and other powerful compounds in thyme) to defeat a variety of diseases, the gold-standard human research is all about germs—particularly the viruses and bacteria that cause *acute bronchitis.*

Calming Coughs
Acute bronchitis is a viral or bacterial infection of the bronchial tract that often develops three or four days after you've gotten over a cold or flu.

In response to the infection, the bronchi pump out mucous—and intense "coughing fits" to clear the mucous are the condition's most prominent symptom, sometimes accompanied by a flu-like sore throat, fever, and chills. Thyme can calm the coughing down.

Researchers in Germany studied 361 adults with acute bronchitis, dividing them into two groups. One took a natural formula containing thyme and primrose root; the other took a placebo. For the next 11 days, the researchers counted the number of daily coughing fits experienced by the participants. Those taking the thyme/primrose mixture had 16 percent fewer coughing fits than those taking the placebo, and their other symptoms improved more rapidly.

In another study from Germany, researchers gave a syrup containing thyme and ivy (Bronchipret) to more than 1,200 children and adolescents with acute bronchitis. After four days of treatment, the severity of symptoms had decreased by 46 percent; after 10 days, by 86 percent. The number of coughing fits decreased by 81 percent after 10 days. Nearly 9 out of 10 children found relief from the formula. "Acute bronchitis . . . can be treated safely and effectively with thyme and ivy syrup," concluded the researchers.

In a study on adults, the thyme/ivy combination decreased coughing fits by 21 percent more than a placebo, and led to a much faster resolution of other symptoms.

And when researchers from Switzerland tested the thyme/ivy product on cough not only from bronchitis, but also from the common cold and *any* respiratory infection with excess mucous, they found it "good or very good" in clearing up cough in 90 percent of cases.

Protecting Teeth from Decay

Thymol can brighten your breath *and* your teeth. More than a dozen studies have been conducted on a tooth "varnish" that combines thymol and the antiseptic chlorhexidine (Cervitec and CervitecPlus). It works in:

Thyme may help prevent and/or treat:

Aging	bowel disease)
Alcohol abuse	Cough
Blood clots	Flu
Bronchitis, acute	Heart attack
Cancer	Infection, bacterial
Cold sores	Stroke
Colds	Tooth decay
Colitis (inflammatory	Ulcer

The elderly. In a study in the *Journal of Dentistry*, researchers in Spain found that the thymol-containing varnish helped prevent cavities in older people in an assisted-care residential home.

Teens with braces. Researchers in Sweden found the varnish helped lower levels of cavity-causing bacteria on the molars of adolescents with braces. Their findings were in the *Journal of Clinical Dentistry*.

Children. Another team of Spanish researchers found using the varnish in six- and seven-year-olds with their first permanent teeth helped prevent cavities. A study by Brazilian dentists, published in *Caries Research*, showed the same results.

Thyme Is Anti-Disease

Thymol is in a class of phytonutrients (plant compounds) called *monoterpenes*, that includes the volatile oils carvacrol and geraniol. They're all powerful antioxidants and powerfully anti-inflammatory, taming the twin processes that underlie and worsen most chronic diseases. And they're all being investigated by scientists for their potential to protect and heal.

Anti-aging. In two animal studies, Scottish researchers tested thyme's ability to slow the sands of time. In the first study, animals fed thyme oil had less age-related reductions in the antioxidants superoxide dismutase and glutathione peroxidase than animals who didn't receive it. In the second study, the researchers found that supplementing with thyme oil protected neurons in the brains of aging rats.

Anti-cancer. There are scores of studies investigating monoterpenes as possible cancer-fighters, showing they protect DNA (DNA damage is the genesis of cancer), and have activity against liver, skin, and uterine cancer, and leukemia.

Anti-clot. In animal studies from Japan, adding thyme to a high-fat diet reduced the formation of blood clots, a risk factor for heart attacks and strokes.

Anti-herpes. In a laboratory study, German researchers found that thymol stopped the herpes simplex-1 virus (the cause of cold sores) from replicating.

Anti-infection. Researchers in Germany found that thyme oil (as well as other essential oils) is effective against bacteria that are becoming resistant to antibiotics—particularly the "flesh-eating" bacteria, *Staphylococcus aureus* (MRSA).

Anti-colitis. Researchers in Croatia found that a combination of thyme and oregano oils (both rich in thymol) lessened the severity of colitis (inflammatory bowel disease) in experimental animals.

Anti-ulcer. Researchers in Iran found that several components of thyme oil—thymol, carvacrol, b/neol, and others—effectively killed the *Helicobacter pylori*, the bacteria that causes stomach ulcers.

Anti-alcoholism. Egyptian researchers found adding thyme to the diet of experimental animals fed excessive alcohol helped protect their livers and brains from alcohol-related damage. "Thyme," concluded the researchers in *Food and Chemical Toxicology*, "may play a part in protecting the body against the hazardous effects caused by alcohol abuse."

Getting to Know Thyme

The ancient Egyptians used thyme in mummification. The ancient Greeks used it as an incense in their temples, to freshen and cleanse the air.

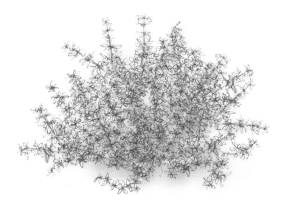

There are more than 100 varieties of thyme.

(The Greek word *thymon* means "to fumigate.") The ancient Romans believed thyme promoted vigor, and used it in their baths.

Garden-variety thyme—the kind that shows up on the supermarket spice shelf—is the most potent source of thymol among all the thymes. The stiff and bushy perennial shrub with small green furry leaves is native to the Mediterranean and is among the ingredients credited with making the Mediterranean diet one of the healthiest on the planet. Thyme is also one of the planet's most pleasantly aromatic spices, which is why it is popular worldwide.

Thyme plays a major role in giving French food its notable flair. The smoky scent and intense taste of thyme enriches rich cream sauces, soups, and stews. Thyme is the key spice in Julia Child's famous *boeuf bourguignon* (and is one of the few spices used repeatedly throughout her classic bestseller, *Mastering the Art of French Cooking*). A sprig of thyme is found in the traditional French *bouquet garni*. It is also rumored to be among the 27 plants and spices used to make bénédictine, the French liqueur (the recipe is a closely guarded secret).

Thyme grows wild in the Provence region of France—the scent fills the air on a warm breezy day, and in the hot sun of a Provencal summer you can find thyme nearly dried right on the vine. Sprigs of thyme are added to the pot of

Provencal *bouillabaisse* and *bourrides*, the area's signature fish stews.

Thyme is also popular in the Middle East and North Africa. The thyme cultivated in the Middle East is particularly pungent and is called *za'atar*, the same term used to describe a spice mix that includes thyme, toasted sesame seeds, sumac, and salt. Morocco cultivates a variety with a distinct scent of pine called *z'itra*.

Thyme is one of the most common spices in the American spice cabinet. It is used in stuffings, vegetable soups, stews, and casseroles. It was the only spice used in the original recipe for New England and Manhattan clam chowders (though many modern-day versions don't include any spice except salt and pepper). It is also one of the spices in the rubs used in Cajun cooking to make blackened foods.

How to Buy Thyme
When thinking thyme, think *dried* thyme. It's preferred for cooking because it's more pungent and holds up better in the pot. It's also cheaper. A bunch of fresh thyme that lasts a week costs more than a jar of dried thyme that lasts a year.

The generic dried thyme that you find in the supermarket is "French thyme" from the Mediterranean (though most French thyme actually comes from Spain). Top chefs consider it the best. Dried thyme leaves are gray-green in color. Make sure the bottle is free of debris, which is sometimes found in brands with inferior packaging.

Lemon thyme has become popular in the US in recent years; you can find it dried in most supermarkets. Lemon thyme is a cross between French thyme and the large, wild thyme that grows as ground cover. It is less pungent in flavor and has (no surprise) a lemony tang, which comes from its higher concentration of geraniol.

You can find fresh thyme year round in many supermarkets, and in the summer at many farmer's markets. Store fresh thyme in the refrigerator, wrapped in a slightly damp towel. It stays fresh for up to a week.

Thyme pairs well with these spices:

Ajowan	Nutmeg
Basil	Onion
Bay leaf	Oregano
Coriander	Pumpkin seed
Garlic	Rosemary
Marjoram	Sage
Mint	Sun-dried Tomato

and complements recipes featuring:

Beef	Potato salad
Casseroles	Ripe olives
Chicken	Sauces
Fish	Soup
Lobster	Stuffings
Meat loaf	Tomatoes
Pâtés	

Other recipes containing thyme:

Basic Barbecue Rub (p. 272)	Jamaican Jerk Marinade (p. 269)
Boeuf Bourguignon (p. 240)	Pizza Spice Blend (p. 272)
Bouquet Garni (p. 271)	Roast Chicken with 40 Cloves of Garlic (p. 134)
By-the-Bay Fisherman's Chowder (p. 46)	Roasted Tomato Soup with Fennel and Mint (p. 231)
Dukkah (p. 268)	
Green Pumpkin Seed Sauce (p. 200)	Spice de Provence (p. 271)
Hungarian Goulash (p. 61)	

Dried thyme is hardier than most spices and keeps well in an airtight container out of direct sunlight for about 18 months.

Boeuf Bourguignon

This is an adaptation of the original boeuf bourguignon from Julia Child's Mastering the Art of French Cooking *that was featured in the 2009 hit film* Julie and Julia. *(Just don't leave it in the oven too long, as Julie did!) The dish improves with age, so make it a day ahead, if possible, and reheat it on the stove top. Serve it with noodles or rice and a green salad.*

4 bacon slices
3 pounds lean beef cubes
1 cup sliced carrots
1 cup sliced onions
1 teaspoon salt
¼ teaspoon fresh ground black pepper
2 tablespoons flour
3 cups full-bodied red wine
3 cups beef stock
1 tablespoon tomato paste
2 garlic cloves, mashed
½ teaspoon thyme
1 bay leaf
4 tablespoons butter
24 small white onions
Bouquet garni (p. 271)
1 pound button mushrooms, cleaned and
    quartered
6 sprigs fresh parsley

1. Fry the bacon over medium-high heat in a heavy large Dutch oven until crisp. Transfer the bacon with a slotted spoon to a plate and set aside.
2. Dry the beef with paper towels and sauté it a few pieces at a time until it is browned on all sides. Set aside with the bacon. If you need more fat, add vegetable oil to the pan.
3. Brown the sliced carrots and onion in the same fat. Put the beef and the bacon back in the pan with the vegetables. Sprinkle with the salt, pepper, and flour and toss the beef around to coat it with the flour. Set the beef, uncovered, in a preheated 450°F oven for 4 minutes. Toss the meat and bake it for 4

minutes more. Remove the casserole from the oven and lower the oven temperature to 325°F.

4. Put the casserole on the stove top over low heat and add the wine, 2 cups of stock, tomato paste, garlic, thyme, and bay leaf. Stir to blend. Bring to a simmer. Cover the casserole and set it in the lower third of a preheated oven for 3–4 hours. The meat is done when you can pierce it easily with a fork.
5. Meanwhile, melt 2 tablespoons butter in a small saucepan. Add ½ cup of stock and bring to a simmer. Add the onions and bouquet garni. Cover and simmer for 20 minutes or until the onions are tendered when pierced with a fork. Set aside.
6. Melt the remaining butter in a medium-size skillet and sauté the mushrooms until they lose their moisture and reabsorb the moisture in the pan. Sprinkle mushrooms with salt and pepper and set aside.
7. When the meat is tender, pour the contents of the casserole into a sieve over a saucepan. Wipe out the casserole with a paper towel and return the beef and bacon to it. Add the onions and mushrooms to the beef.
8. Skim fat off the sauce and simmer for about 5 minutes, skimming fat off as it rises. Raise the heat and boil down rapidly until you have about 2½ cups and the sauce thickens enough to coat a wooden spoon. Pour the sauce over the meat and vegetables. Cover the casserole and simmer for five minutes. Serve with the parsley sprigs.

Makes 6 to 8 servings.

In the Kitchen with Thyme

Thyme is one of the most subtle and versatile spices, and its agreeable aroma, both fresh and dried, gives depth to just about any savory dish.

Thyme can enliven gravies and sauces, especially rich, cream-based sauces. If you want the flavor of thyme to meld into a gravy or sauce, use it in the early steps of the recipe. If you want the gravy or sauce to have a perfume of thyme, use it toward the end.

Thyme adds nice flavor rubbed into the skin of a chicken before grilling or baking. It also goes with beef, especially ground meat. It works particularly well in tomato sauces and dishes and in casseroles featuring potatoes.

Thyme also helps cut the mouth feel of fatty food, so sprinkle it on the flesh of goose and duck while they are roasting.

Be careful when using fresh thyme: it turns black in an acidic environment, such as dishes containing tomato or lemon. It also quickly loses its volatile oils when exposed to heat.

Here are some ways to add more thyme to your diet:

- Add dried thyme and lemon or lemon thyme to melted butter for boiled lobster or shrimp.
- Sprinkle fresh or dried thyme with chives or by itself on baked potatoes.
- Sauté dried thyme, garlic, and reconstituted sun-dried tomato with mushrooms to go along with grilled steak.
- Sprinkle dried thyme over root vegetables.
- Put fresh thyme branches in with pot roasts or roast an eye roast sitting on the branches.
- Infuse a thyme branch in olive oil or in a bottle of vinaigrette dressing.
- Make the Middle East spice blend *za'atar* by combining 1 tablespoon of dried thyme with 2 tablespoons of toasted sesame seeds, 2 teaspoons of sumac, and salt.
- Sprinkle dried thyme over a salad made of tomatoes, cucumbers, ripe olives, and feta cheese.
- Sprinkle dried thyme into extra-virgin olive oil and use it for dipping bread.
- Add dried thyme to scrambled eggs.

TURMERIC *Leading Crusader against Disease*

Once disparagingly called poor man's saffron because of its brilliant deep yellow hue, turmeric is now considered Indian gold. The reason for turmeric's status as a spice superstar: the good health of the people who eat it daily, and its emerging scientific reputation as one of nature's most powerful healers.

Turmeric is a kitchen staple in India, found in just about every dish that crosses the table—a fact that has not been lost on researchers, who observed 30 years ago that the incidence of chronic illnesses among people in India is significantly lower than in most Western countries, especially the United States.

Turmeric owes its preventive and curative skills to its active ingredient: *curcumin*, a compound so diverse and powerfully rich in antioxidant and anti-inflammatory actions that it has been shown to protect and improve the health of virtually every organ in the body. To date, thousands of animal and human studies from around the world have found that curcumin can combat more than 70 maladies, including some of the biggest health threats, such as cancer, heart disease, type 2 diabetes, and Alzheimer's disease. And the list just keeps on growing.

In fact, international research shows that turmeric, taken as supplemental curcumin,

Marco Polo's Faux Pas

Talk about rumors that are hard to kill!

When Marco Polo "discovered" turmeric in China in 1280, he likened it to expensive saffron, the spice that turns a brilliant yellow when added to liquid. He couldn't have been more wrong. Saffron and turmeric share nothing in common but their color. This mistake is the reason why, some 700 years later, turmeric is *still* considered to be an inexpensive substitute for saffron.

Like saffron, turmeric gives a dish a yellow hue—but it's not a substitute for saffron, any more than saffron is a substitute for turmeric. As culinary spices, their flavor and aroma is completely different.

is *as* effective and, in some cases, even *more* effective than pharmaceutical drugs—without their side effects. Recently, my colleagues and I at the University of Texas M.D. Anderson Cancer Center compared curcumin to anti-inflammatory and pain-killing medications, and to cancer drugs, testing those agents for their effectiveness in reducing inflammation and stopping the proliferation of cancer cells. Curcumin proved to be *more* effective at reducing inflammation than over-the-counter aspirin and ibuprofen, and *as* effective as the more powerful prescription drug, celecoxib (Celebrex). It also proved as effective in thwarting breast cancer cells as tamoxifen, a drug widely used to stop the spread or recurrence of breast cancer. These results are nothing less than astounding.

"If I had only one single herb to depend upon for all possible health and dietary needs, I would choose the Indian spice turmeric," said Dr. David Frawley, founder and director of the American Institute for Vedic Studies in Santa Fe, New Mexico. It is a spice, he said, that everyone "should get to know and live with."

I heartily agree: currently, there is no spice under more scientific scrutiny in the US and around the world—and no spice offering more promise for better health—than turmeric.

How Turmeric and Curcumin Work

Turmeric has more than 50 healing actions, from relieving pain to improving circulation—which is why healers in India (and China) have been using it for more than 2,000 years to treat a range of ills.

For example, traditional healers have used turmeric as:

- an antacid to sooth digestive problems.
- a powder to speed wound healing and prevent infection (bandages in India often contain turmeric).
- an analgesic to relieve headache (curcumin is an ingredient in Tylenol).
- a stimulant to improve blood flow.
- a topical paste to clear skin problems.
- a decongestant to clear nasal passages (some nasal sprays contain curcumin).

As a folk remedy, it has been used to treat some 60 maladies—from measles, chicken pox, and colic to colds, gum disease, flatulence, indigestion, and stress.

But its ranking as the superstar of spices comes from the fact that it is an *antioxidant* with powerful *anti-inflammatory* abilities. Why is that so important?

Oxidation is a kind of internal rust caused by what scientists call *reactive oxygen species* (ROS)—molecules that are missing an electron from their outer ring, or shell, and steal an electron from other molecules, creating *oxidative damage*, or *oxidative stress*. ROS are created by numerous factors, such as sunlight, pollution, a high-fat diet, and even aging itself. The oxidative stress they cause in turn leads to chronic low-grade inflammation, an insidious version of the same type of immune-triggered redness, heat, and swelling that accompanies a wound. And chronic inflammation has been shown to trigger or advance many of the diseases of modern life. That includes cardiovascular disease (CVD), which causes heart attack and stroke; type 2 diabetes, which quadruples the risk of CVD, and can also cause kidney failure, blindness, and amputation; Alzheimer's and Parkinson's disease; asthma; and autoimmune diseases such as rheumatoid arthritis and psoriasis. In experiments with cell cultures, animals, and humans, antioxidant and anti-inflammatory curcumin has been found effective against all of those conditions.

But turmeric's strength as an antioxidant has gotten the attention of mainstream medicine in the United States and around the world mostly because of its scientifically shown ability to fight *cancer*.

The Anti-Cancer Spice

Even the toughest skeptic would have a hard time questioning more than 1,000 research studies with the same result: curcumin is anti-cancer. Research demonstrates that the curcumin found in turmeric can fight cancer on many levels. It can:

- inhibit the activation of genes that trigger cancer.
- inhibit the spread (proliferation) of tumor cells.
- inhibit the transformation of a normal cell into a cancer cell.
- kill cells that mutate into cancer.
- shrink tumor cells.
- prevent tumors from spreading to other organs.
- prevent the development of the blood supply necessary for cancer cells to form and spread.
- enhance the cancer-destroying effects of chemotherapy and radiation.

Curcumin has exhibited some or all of these actions against 22 different types of cancer, including the biggest killers—breast, colon, lung, and prostate. It also slowed the progression of some of the toughest-to-beat cancers, such as brain, bone, blood, esophagus, liver, pancreas, stomach, uterine, and melanoma (the deadliest form of skin cancer). There is no other natural

Turmeric may help prevent and/or treat:

Acne	Flatulence
Allergies	Gallbladder disease
Alzheimer's disease	Gout
Arthritis, osteo- and rheumatoid	Gum disease
	Heart disease
Asthma	High blood pressure (hypertension)
Blemishes	
Cancer	Itching
Cholesterol problems (high "bad" LDL cholesterol, low "good" HDL cholesterol)	Liver disease
	Macular degeneration, age-related
	Overweight
Colitis (inflammatory bowel disease)	Pain
Cystic fibrosis	Parkinson's disease
Depression	Pollution side-effects
	Psoriasis
Dermatitis, contact	Rash
Diabetes, type 2	
Eczema (atopic dermititis)	Scleroderma
	Stroke
	Wounds
Eye infection, uveitis	

substance that has been found to possess this degree of anti-cancer power. Here are reports on some of the studies on curcumin and cancer.

Breast cancer. Some of curcumin's most remarkable results have been against breast cancer, and it is showing promise against even the most drug-resistant forms of the disease. In one study, when researchers added curcumin to paclitaxel (Taxol), a common chemotherapy drug for breast cancer, it not only enhanced the effects of the drug, but also decreased the drug's side effects, making the chemotherapy regime more tolerable for patients. In another study, reported in the journal *Menopause*, researchers found that curcumin lowered the risk of breast cancer in women who took combined estrogen and progestin hormone replacement therapy (HRT), a proven risk factor for the disease.

Colon cancer. Numerous animal studies have found that curcumin can help prevent and delay the onset of colon cancer, and human studies are beginning to show the same results. In one study, researchers at UCLA found that curcumin prevented the formation of polyps (fleshy growths on the lining of the large intestine) in people with familial adenomatous polyposis (FAP), an inherited condition that can lead to colon cancer. In another study, people with FAP who took 480 milligrams (mg) of curcumin plus 20 mg of quercetin (the active phytochemical in onions) had fewer and smaller polyps.

Cervical cancer. Curcumin has been found to kill human papillomavirus, the leading cause of cervical cancer. It has also been found to fight the precancerous cellular changes that often precede the disease.

Lung cancer. Several animal studies have found that curcumin may protect against tobacco-induced lung cancer. In one study, 16 smokers took 1500 mg of curcumin a day. After 30 days, urine samples showed they had excreted significantly more tobacco-related toxins than six other smokers who didn't take curcumin.

Pancreatic cancer. Both human and animal studies have found curcumin holds promise in fighting pancreatic cancer, a particularly lethal form of the disease that doesn't respond well to chemotherapy drugs. In our labs at M.D. Anderson, we found that curcumin taken in combination with the chemotherapy drug gemcitabine (Gemzar) enhanced the action of the drug in animals.

In another study, 34 patients with advanced pancreatic cancer—normally lethal within one year—were given high daily doses of curcumin. In 64 percent of the patients, the spice slowed the expected progression of the disease.

Prostate cancer. In a study reported in the journal *Cancer Research*, researchers gave mice prostate cancer, then divided them into four groups, each with a different treatment. One group

of mice received curcumin, a second received a chemotherapy drug, the third radiation, and the fourth no treatment. Among the four treatments, curcumin worked best at controlling the progression of the disease. In another study, researchers at Rutgers University found that a combined regimen of curcumin and isothiocyanate (an anti-cancer compound found in cruciferous vegetables such as cauliflower, cabbage, and kale) reversed the growth of prostate tumors in mice.

Skin cancer. In our labs at M.D. Anderson Cancer Center, we injected mice with substances that produce melanoma. We treated half the mice by putting curcumin in their chow and the other half by applying curcumin as a paste to the cancerous lesions. In both cases, curcumin halted the progression of the disease in a majority of mice. In another experiment, we tested curcumin in lab-grown melanoma cells to see if the spice could stop the cells from surviving and reproducing. The more curcumin we added to the melanoma, the more cells died.

In addition, studies have found that cancer rates are the lowest in countries with the highest dietary intake of turmeric. I believe it is no coincidence that the rates of the most common cancers—lung, breast, colon, and prostate—are 10 times lower in turmeric-loving India than in the United States.

Protection against Cancer-Causing Pollution

The incidence of childhood leukemia has risen 50 percent since 1950, and many researchers suspect that one factor is prenatal and postnatal exposure to pollutants such as benzene, a carcinogen found in industrial waste. Turmeric to the rescue . . .

At a recent conference on childhood leukemia, researchers from Loyola University Medical Center in Chicago reported evidence that eating foods spiced with turmeric could reduce the risk of childhood leukemia. The researchers, who have been studying turmeric for 20 years, believe the spice works by pro-

Reduce Wrinkles with Turmeric

Indian women use turmeric as a beauty aid to keep the face smooth, radiant, and free of wrinkles and blemishes. Mrs. Aggarwal offers this formula for a facial mask, which you can use as often as you like. Many Indian women use it daily.

To make the mask, Indian women use sesame oil made in India, but any odorless oil, such as vegetable or canola, will do. To use sesame, you must get the sesame oil found in Indian markets, as the sesame oil generally found in supermarkets has a strong smell and is expensive.

This formula, which should last for several uses, feels as fresh and clean as a spa facial—at a fraction of the cost!

½ cup garbanzo (chickpea) flour
1½ tablespoons turmeric
Odorless cooking oil
Water

Mix the flour and turmeric in a container with a tight fitting lid. Keep it in a dry place in or near the bathroom.

To make the mask, mix about 1 tablespoon of the flour mixture in a small dish with about 5 drops of oil. Add enough water to make a paste. It should be the consistency of cake batter.

Pull your hair back or cover it with a towel. Using your fingertips, spread the mixture on your face and neck, making sure to stay clear of the eyes. Let the mixture stay on your face until it dries, about 15 minutes. Wash it off in the shower.

tecting children against harmful environmental chemicals.

Researchers have also found that curcumin has the strength to:

- inhibit the toxicity of polycyclic aromatic hydrocarbons (PAHs), cancer-causing chemicals in the environment. PAHs also form on meat, poultry, and fish when they are grilled or fried at temperatures exceeding 352°F.
- inhibit damage caused by ionizing radiation, such as radiation from the sun, x-rays, and other medical tests.
- prevent the formation of suspected cancer-causing compounds found in processed and cured foods.

Here's a tasty health hint. To make turmeric even more potent against cancer-causing environmental hazards, sprinkle turmeric *and* black pepper together in your food. Studies show that both curcumin in turmeric and pepperine in black pepper fight environmental insults. Plus, pepperine enhances the absorption of curcumin.

Promise for Alzheimer's Disease

During the last 25 years, the rate of the memory-robbing brain disease Alzheimer's has doubled in the United States. In fact, it is increasing almost everywhere in the world—except in India, where it affects less than one percent of the population. The reason might be turmeric and curcumin.

Alzheimer's is caused by an accumulation of plaque between brain cells (neurons), which thwarts communication between those cells. Scientists don't know *why* these plaques form, but they do know *how* they develop. The trigger is a protein called amyloid-A. In healthy brains, this protein is broken down and eliminated. In Alzheimer's, the protein clumps together and hardens. Animal studies show that curcumin binds to amyloid-A, stopping it from clumping together and blocking neural activity.

Current medications for Alzheimer's slightly reduce the symptoms and slow the disease, but no drug is considered highly effective. Curcumin might be the drug of the future. Not only can it disarm amyloid-A, studies show it can also: slow oxidative damage to neurons; reduce damage to neural synapses, the pathways of communication between brain cells; and reduce levels of toxic metals in the brain that might contribute to Alzheimer's.

Regular intake of turmeric is also proving to be a natural safeguard against the decline in memory and brain function that can accompany age. Asian scientists conducted a study of turmeric consumption and mental acuity among older people who didn't have Alzheimer's and found that those who consumed the most turmeric-rich foods scored higher on standardized mental tests than those who rarely or never eat turmeric.

Help for Parkinson's Disease

Parkinson's disease is a degenerative condition caused by the death of brain cells that manufacture *dopamine*, a brain chemical (neurotransmitter) that controls many functions, including the connection between the central nervous system and muscles. Both oxidative damage and inflammation have been implicated in the disease, which led researchers at Johns Hopkins University School of Medicine to wonder if curcumin could help protect cells from dying.

To test the theory, the researchers created a laboratory model of Parkinson's disease, in which nerve-like cells produced a protein that eventually killed 50 percent of the cells. Adding curcumin to the cellular model reduced the rate of cell death to 19 percent—and also dramatically reduced the rate of oxidative damage in the cells. "These results suggest that curcumin is a potential candidate for inhibiting the oxidative damage that leads to Parkinson's disease," said Wanli Smith, PhD, an assistant professor of psychiatry and behavioral science at Johns Hopkins. "This common spice could be a weapon to protect the brain."

Easing Arthritis

Inflammation is a hallmark of the most common forms of arthritis—osteoarthritis (the destruction of the cartilage that covers and cushions the end of bones), rheumatoid arthritis (an autoimmune disease that attacks joints), and gout (an excess of sharp-edged uric acid crystals, which destroy joints).

To combat inflammation, many people with arthritis take a non-steroidal anti-inflammatory drug (NSAID) such as aspirin, naproxen (Aleve, Naprosyn), or ibuprofen (Motrin). While they help reduce inflammation, NSAIDs can also irritate the lining of the gastrointestinal (GI) tract—nearly one in three of the 13 million people taking NSAIDs suffers from GI problems, which hospitalize 103,000 people yearly and kill more than 16,000, with sudden and massive bleeding from an ulcer. The new class of NSAIDs called Cox-2 inhibitors, such as celecoxib (Celebrex), were supposed to spare the GI tract—but ended up dramatically increasing the incidence of heart disease and stroke!

No wonder people with arthritis are looking for a *safe* and effective anti-inflammatory agent. Curcumin just might be it.

Recently, researchers in Thailand proved curcumin's anti-inflammatory power when they tested the spice against ibuprofen in an experiment involving 107 older people with severe chronic osteoarthritis of the knee. Half took 800 milligrams (mg) of ibuprofen, while the other half took 2,000 mg (2 grams) of an extract containing the active compound in curcumin. Every two weeks for six weeks, the researchers measured their pain levels, their knee flexibility, their ability to walk up and down stairs, and the time it took to walk 328 feet (a little longer than a football field).

The researchers found that curcumin "might be just as effective as ibuprofen in alleviating knee pain and improving knee function."

In a study of 18 people with rheumatoid arthritis, researchers found that 1,200 mg of curcumin taken for two weeks was just as effective in reducing arthritis symptoms as phenylbutazone (Butazolidine), a powerful NSAID. People who took the curcumin reported a reduction in morning swelling and stiffness, and an increase in the ability to perform everyday tasks.

A study in animals shows *how* curcumin works. In the experiment, researchers from the University of Arizona induced arthritis

Turmeric Versus Curry Powder

Don't confuse turmeric with curry, a "spice" that can be found everywhere—except India and most parts of Asia.

Curry powder is *not* one spice. Rather, it's a combination of spices the English invented in the 18th century as a shortcut to the seemingly arduous task of creating a variety of spice combinations to enhance different curries. Well, they may have saved some time, but they also homogenized the flavor. So, if all your curries taste the same, you can blame curry powder.

The spices in curry powder typically include coriander, cumin, fenugreek, black pepper, and, always, turmeric, the spice that gives curry powder its yellow hue.

Since it was first introduced, curry powder has become popular all over the world. Some countries, such as France and Denmark, even invented their own versions. But the "one type fits all" curry powder never caught on in India or other regions where creating curries is an art—and using a standard blend of spices is seen as anything but creative. In Asian cuisine, different curries call for different spice combinations that impart a special flavor to *that* particular dish. (You'll find out for yourself, when you make the spice and curry blends in Part III.)

Two more curious facts about curry powder:

It's often erroneously reported as being a rich source of curcumin. But it's only as rich as the amount of turmeric in the powder, and turmeric levels vary.

Curry powder has nothing to do with *true spice curry*. That spice is derived from the curry leaf, which (in spite of its similar name) is from a different botanical family. There is no curcumin in the true spice curry.

in laboratory animals—and then found that giving turmeric to the laboratory animals *before* arthritis was induced prevented joint inflammation. "Turmeric . . . demonstrated a profound inhibition of induced arthritis that is rarely seen," said Janet L. Funk, MD, the study leader. In animals with arthritis, turmeric cut cartilage destruction by 66 percent and bone destruction by 57 percent, compared to animals not receiving the spice.

When the researchers investigated the *mechanism* of turmeric, they found it derailed the genetic and molecular mechanisms of arthritis. Specifically, the spice influenced the action of *nuclear factor-kappa B*, a so-called "transcription factor" that switches genes on and off—in this case, turmeric helped the factor switch off key inflammatory genes that result in the destruction of cartilage and bone.

Fights Heart Disease and Stroke

ROS do some of their greatest damage against healthy arteries, so it's no surprise that researchers in France recently reported that curcumin has the ability to help prevent clogged arteries, a key risk factor for heart attacks and stroke. In their study, the researchers fed two groups of mice the same artery-clogging diet, giving one group a curcumin supplement along with the diet. After 16 weeks, the mice fed the curcumin had 26 percent fewer fatty deposits in their arteries. The researchers also confirmed what previous studies have found: curcumin has the ability to alter the genetic signaling involved in plaque build-up.

But curcumin's artery-protecting prowess doesn't stop there. In another animal study at the Medical College of Georgia, curcumin was found to reduce the size of blood clots involved in hemorrhagic stroke, the type caused by a ruptured blood vessel in the brain. In the experiment, researchers induced stroke in animals, then gave them injections of curcumin every hour for three hours. The curcumin "significantly reduced" the size of the clots, reported the researchers.

In another animal study, the same researchers found that turmeric reduced the risk of cerebral vasospasm, a life-threatening narrowing of an artery sometimes triggered by a stroke or traumatic brain injury (TBI). As a result of the study, the researchers recommended turmeric as a possible additional therapy to "both prevent the development of cerebral vasospasm and to reduce oxidative brain injury" in people who've had a stroke or TBI.

Curcumin also fights artery-clogging cholesterol. In one study, Indian researchers asked 10 healthy men to take a 500-milligram curcumin supplement every morning. After just one week, "bad" LDL cholesterol dropped an average of 33 percent and "good" HDL cholesterol increased 29 percent.

One reason curcumin is a stellar cholesterol fighter: it works in the liver, where it increases the production of proteins that attach to LDL particles and escort them out of the body. Curcumin also stimulates the liver to produce more bile, which helps break down and eliminate excess cholesterol.

In addition, animal studies have found that curcumin has the ability to help:

- lower triglycerides, another artery-clogging blood fat.
- block the production of homocysteine, an amino acid linked to higher rates of heart disease and stroke.
- regulate blood pressure.
- reduce damage from a heart attack.

Guardian of the Liver

Virtually everything that goes in the body, both good and bad, makes a stop in the liver. When functioning at its peak, the liver can filter almost two quarts of blood per minute and easily dismantle toxins. The liver, however, takes a lot of abuse. Alcohol, pollution, second-hand smoke, allergens, poor diet, and even stress can take their toll on the liver, making it sluggish. Curcumin, however, can help keep the liver healthy, and it does so in two ways: by promoting the production of enzymes that detoxify the liver and by promoting flow of bile that cleanses the liver and rejuvenates its cells.

Not only does turmeric help keep the liver in peak condition—animal studies in the United States, Finland, and China suggest that turmeric has the strength to prevent alcohol-induced cirrhosis of the liver and liver cancer.

Help for Problem Skin

According to Indian folklore, turmeric is the secret to smooth and radiant skin. It is a tradition in India for brides and grooms to apply turmeric mixed in milk to their skin before the marriage ceremony to enhance their skin's vibrancy. Indian women use a paste made with turmeric as a daily mask to prevent blemishes and wrinkles. And in India and many other parts of the world, turmeric is a common ingredient in cosmetics.

Modern science has confirmed what Ayurvedic doctors in India have known for centuries: turmeric is an effective remedy for all kinds of skin ailments. That includes: acne, blemishes, itching, and rashes; stubborn conditions such as contact dermatitis, an allergic reaction; and serious chronic conditions such as psoriasis and scleroderma.

And in an experiment with laboratory animals, wounds healed faster, with less scarring, among animals treated with topical curcumin.

A Spice Fat-Buster

Research at Tufts University showed that turmeric may play a role in preventing overweight.

In their experiment, the researchers put two groups of mice on a high-fat diet intended to promote weight gain, but one group was also given a daily curcumin supplement. After 12 weeks, the mice receiving curcumin gained less weight and accumulated fewer fat cells. (Their cholesterol was lower, too.)

"Weight gain is the result of the growth and expansion of fat tissue, which cannot happen unless new blood vessels form, a process known as angiogenesis," explained Mohsen Meydani, PhD, a study researcher. "Based on our data, curcumin appears to suppress angiogenic activity in the fat tissue of mice fed high-fat diets." And the

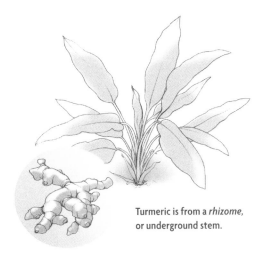

Turmeric is from a *rhizome*, or underground stem.

researchers concluded that turmeric and curcumin hold promise as a way for us humans to prevent weight gain, too.

A Cornucopia of Healing

There are many other conditions that turmeric and curcumin may help fight. They include:

Inflammatory bowel disease (Crohn's disease and colitis). Several animal and preliminary human studies indicate that curcumin is effective against Crohn's disease and can help maintain remission in people with ulcerative colitis. In one study, curcumin produced significant improvement in the symptoms of 207 people with inflammatory bowel disease.

Cystic fibrosis. This fatal disease strikes children and young adults, causing the lungs to fill with thick mucus. In animal research, Yale scientists found that curcumin corrected a defect that produces the excess mucus. A protective dose would be well tolerated in humans, they said.

Depression. Animal studies found that curcumin reduced depression-like behavior in mice and increased levels of the serotonin and dopamine, two brain chemicals often depleted in depression.

Type 2 diabetes. Animal and human studies show that curcumin helps control blood sugar levels and also reduces the risk of complications associated with the disease, such as diabetic retinopathy, a destruction of blood vessels in the eye that can lead to blindness. Curcumin also can strengthen the pancreas, which produces insulin, the hormone that regulates blood sugar levels.

Eye diseases. Uveitis is a serious eye infection that can lead to blindness. In a study of 32 people, curcumin was as effective as corticosteroids in treating the infection. And in a study reported in *Phytotherapy Research*, an eye drop containing turmeric extract (Ophthacare) was effective in treating a number of eye problems, including pink eye (conjunctivitis), dry eye, and problems in postoperative cataract care.

Gallbladder disease. A study in people with gallbladder disease found that 20 mg a day of supplemental curcumin reduced the formation of gallstones and improved the health of the gallbladder.

Age-related macular degeneration (AMD). This disease gradually destroys the macula, the central area of the retina that is responsible for focus and sharp vision. It afflicts 20 percent of Americans ages 65 to 74, and 35 percent over 75, and is the *number one* cause of blindness. Animal research at the University of Oklahoma Health Sciences Center shows that curcumin may offer natural protection against AMD by protecting the retina from damage caused by light and oxidative stress. Animal studies have found that curcumin may protect against cataracts in the same way.

Pain. Numerous studies show that turmeric reduces pain and inflammation. In one, 45 surgical patients were given three daily doses of either 400 mg of curcumin, 100 mg of phenylbutazone, an anti-inflammatory drug, or a placebo. The curcumin provided significant relief, without the side effects of the drug.

How Much Do You Need?

Eating a lot of turmeric-rich food is a great way to promote good health. In India, the average person ingests about a teaspoon of turmeric daily, spread out over three meals—enough

Turmeric pairs well with these spices:

Allspice	Fennel seed
Black pepper	Galangal
Caraway	Garlic
Cardamom	Ginger
Cinnamon	Mustard seed
Coconut	Onion
Coriander	Sun-dried tomato
Cumin	

and complements recipes featuring:

Curries	Tomato sauces
Lentils	Vegetables of all
Rice	varieties, especially
Soups	cauliflower and onions

for Indians to enjoy a remarkably low incidence of Alzheimer's disease, cancer, and type 2 diabetes.

I also recommend taking a daily 500 mg curcumin supplement for general health. (Recommended dosages for specific health conditions can be found in Part IV, "Index of Healing Prescriptions.")

Rest assured that supplemental curcumin is safe to take: there have been no serious side effects and no toxicity reported from taking up to 16 grams of curcumin a day. In culinary terms, that would be like eating a daily cup of turmeric!

A curcumin supplement is best taken on an empty stomach about an hour before eating. You can improve the absorption of a curcumin supplement by taking it with: grapefruit juice, pineapple juice, milk, or pepperine (the supplemental form of black pepper), or with a meal containing oil (such as olive oil) or dairy (such as yogurt).

Getting to Know Turmeric

You only *think* turmeric is foreign to American taste buds. Turmeric is a flavoring in some of America's all-time favorites. It's what puts the bright yellow color in American cheese and in the mustard on ballpark franks. It's also used to color butter, margarine, canned chicken broth, bread-and-butter pickles, yellow cake, and popcorn.

When it comes to cuisine, turmeric is best known as a key ingredient in *curry*, the variety of spicy dishes that accompany every meal in India. In fact, turmeric is so well-loved in India, it is used in just about *everything*. And it is a common ingredient in many spice blends, known as *masalas*.

Moroccans combine turmeric and saffron to make *harira*, a soup traditionally eaten at the end of Ramadan, and it is also a key ingredient in the Moroccan spice mixture *ras-el-hanout*. The Lebanese use it to make a yellow cake called *sfouf*. Throughout the Middle East, it is a key ingredient in *chermoula*, a marinade used to flavor fish and other foods.

The Japanese are also fond of turmeric. They put it in tea, bottle it in vinegars, add it to noodles, and even put it in dog food. They also put it in soaps, lotions, and creams.

In England you can find turmeric in dairy products, cough drops, and even veterinary medicine. It is also the main ingredient in the British favorite *piccalillo*, a pickled chutney-like vegetable dish that is served with meats, especially at Christmas time.

Turmeric is the star ingredient in *kapitan* chicken, a mild curry popular in Malaysia.

In Thailand, cooks often use *zedoary*, a spice also known as white turmeric. Though it comes from the same family, it bears little resemblances to turmeric—it is used as a thickener in place of arrowroot and contains very little curcumin.

And turmeric is used to flavor *momas*, Nepal's version of a dumpling.

How to Buy Turmeric

Most of the world's turmeric comes from two places in India: Alleppey and Madras. I recommend buying turmeric from Alleppey, if possible, as research has shown it contains nearly two times more curcumin than turmeric from Madras. It is also a deeper color (bright yellow) and has a mellower flavor.

M OST OF THE WORLD'S
TURMERIC COMES FROM INDIA,
AND MOST INDIAN TURMERIC
COMES FROM EITHER
ALLEPPEY OR MADRAS.

Turmeric (sometimes spelled tumeric) can also be found in the spice section of most supermarkets. If you are buying at a spice market, you might notice a difference in the color from bag to bag. Don't worry—it's not a sign of deterioration.

Turmeric comes from the rhizome (an underground stem of a bushy perennial plant), and it's very hard to grind. For this reason, it is almost always sold already ground. The fresh rhizome is sometimes found in Asian and Indian markets.

If possible, buy turmeric in a quantity that you will use up in a few months, as it tends to lose its aromatic flavor over time.

In the Kitchen with Turmeric

Turmeric is the only readily available edible source of curcumin, so you want to make sure to get it in your diet as much as possible. When cooked, it has a mild fragrance, somewhat reminiscent of ginger and orange, with a slight peppery taste.

Turmeric is still relatively new to Western dishes and taste buds—and it's a rare cook who will use up a bottle before its expiration. That should change, however, once you get the true culinary sense of what turmeric is all about. Even Indians agree that raw turmeric is rather harsh, which is why they always *cook* it. The spice will mellow as it is cooked. Just heat a little oil in a pan and sprinkle it with turmeric, stirring it with a wooden spoon so it doesn't burn. Within seconds, your senses will enjoy its deliciously aromatic perfume—and you will discover why Indians are so fond of the spice! If you can't smell its perfume, your turmeric is past its prime.

Here are some tips for putting more turmeric in your dishes:

- Heat oil in a pan and add turmeric as just described, and add vegetables to make a stir-fry.
- Try the same thing using sliced apples.
- Add turmeric to your standard meat,

Other recipes containing turmeric:

Ajowan Parathas (p. 17)

All-American Chili con Carne (p. 110)

Brussels Sprouts Kulambu (p. 123)

Caribbean Curry Paste (p. 287)

Coconut Meatballs with Peanut Sauce (p. 101)

Colombo Powder (p. 270)

Ginger Carrot and Squash Soup (p. 140)

Hot Curry Powder (p. 284)

La Kama (p. 266)

Malaysian Curry Paste (p. 287)

Ras-el-hanout (p. 266)

Sambaar Masala (p. 265)

Spiced Vegetable Fritters (p. 36)

Vindaloo Curry Paste (p. 286)

Potato Cauliflower Curry

Called aloo gobi *in India, this popular dish originated in the north of the country and is served in every Indian home. The combination of turmeric, onion, pepper, garlic, ginger, and cruciferous vegetables make it a potent cancer fighter.*

2 tablespoons vegetable oil
2 teaspoons turmeric
1 teaspoon cumin seed
1 medium onion, thinly sliced
3 cloves garlic, chopped
1 twenty-eight-ounce can diced tomatoes
1 medium head cauliflower, cut into florets
1½ pounds russet potatoes, peeled and cut into large chunks
½ teaspoon diced fresh ginger
½ teaspoon chili powder
¼ teaspoon freshly ground black pepper
1 tablespoon *garam masala* (p. 264)
Salt, to taste
¼ cup chopped cilantro (optional)

1. Heat the oil in a large pot over medium heat. Add the turmeric and cumin seeds until the spices render their aroma, about 30 seconds. Add the sliced onions and garlic and sauté, stirring frequently, until the onions are soft, about eight minutes.
2. Stir in the diced tomatoes, cauliflower, potatoes, ginger, chili powder, and ground pepper. Reduce the heat, cover partially, and cook for 40 minutes, stirring frequently. If the curry appears too dry and the vegetables start to stick to the pan, add some water.
3. Add the garam masala, simmer five minutes. Turn off the heat and keep covered until ready to serve. Sprinkle with cilantro, if using, and serve.

Makes 6 servings.

poultry, and fish recipes that call for sautéing or searing in a pan.
- Add a teaspoon or two to meat and vegetables stews in recipes serving two to four. Add more for larger portions.
- Add turmeric to fried onions. (One study, reported on page 244, found that onions and turmeric together work synergistically to protect against cancer.)
- Use turmeric in dishes featuring cruciferous vegetables for extra protection against breast, prostate, and other types of cancer. Cruciferous vegetables are good for more than prostate cancer; in fact, intake is associated with lower levels of all kinds of diseases. This includes cabbage, cauliflower, broccoli, brussels sprouts, kale, and watercress.
- Eat more yellow mustard.
- Add turmeric to scrambled eggs and other egg dishes. Not only does it add flavor, it also gives eggs an intensely yellow appearance.

- Use it as they do in India, as the spice in dishes featuring lentils.
- Add it to dips and salad dressings.
- Blend it in melted butter and drizzle it over cooked vegetables.
- Add a tablespoon of turmeric to a large pot of chicken noodle soup.
- Heat turmeric in a little oil before adding the liquid to make basmati rice.
- Add 1 teaspoon of turmeric to homemade chili.
- Use it as a flavoring for seafood stews and dishes using coconut milk.

Turmeric is not recommended for dishes calling for dairy, which masks the spice's delicate flavor.

Caution: During ancient times, turmeric had a secondary use as a fabric dye to make colorful clothing for the rich. So be careful about spills—it can be difficult to get out of fabric and can even leave a stain on your kitchen counter.

VANILLA *Health in Your Dessert*

New York cheesecake, Boston cream pie, crème brûlée. Sit down to enjoy any sweet dessert, and you'll most likely find vanilla in it.

Vanilla is among the most used—and most enticing—flavors in the world. Some 10,000 tons a year are produced of this expensive spice, with demand far exceeding supply. (That's why there's so much imitation vanilla extract on store shelves.)

The Orchid Spice

Perhaps it's not surprising that vanilla is so alluring when you consider its botanical pedigree. It's the only edible member of the Orchid family, considered by many to be the loveliest of flowers. And perhaps vanilla's association with the sensuous orchid is why this spice also has an aphrodisiacal reputation for enhancing romance. An *ancient* reputation.

Vanilla is native to Mexico, and its first domesticators—the Totonac culture of Mesoamerica, rivals of the Aztecs—told this lusty legend of its origin: the tropical vanilla orchid sprouted from the blood of the goddess Princess Xanat, beheaded by her father after she disobeyed him and ran away with her mortal lover. In the 18th century, husbands in Europe were told to drink a vanilla-rich tonic to increase their virility and fertility. And beginning with its introduction into Europe, vanilla has been an inspiring ingredient in perfumes.

But the traditional use of vanilla as a tonic went beyond the bedroom, according to Jenna Deanne Bythrow of Georgetown University, in an article on the spice in *Seminars in Integrative Medicine*. The Aztecs wore it as a "medicinal charm." Spanish friars used it to treat patients who were "coughing and spitting up blood." In the New World and the Old, it was an oft-used remedy for "woman's troubles," such as hysteria and depression. In European herbals of the 18th and 19th centuries, it was touted as a "nerve stimulant." And a 19th-century American medical text praises its powers to "exhilarate the brain, prevent sleep, increase muscular energy, and stimulate the sexual energies." Let's all have another serving of Boston cream pie!

Investigating Vanillin

More than 200 phytonutrients—bioactive plant compounds—have been discovered in vanilla, and in the last two decades scientists have begun to investigate their healing potential. The compound receiving the most scrutiny is the spice's main constituent: *vanillin*. Studies show it may play a promising role in two conditions:

Cancer. In the worldwide search for natural compounds to beat cancer, scientists have taken a close look at vanillin, in the test tube and in experimental animals.

In Malaysia, scientists found vanillin could kill human cancer cells, leading them to declare "it could be a useful colorectal cancer preventive agent."

In Thailand, researchers found vanillin could limit *metastasis*—the movement of cancer cells from their original site to the rest of the body. It worked by turning off cancer-promoting enzymes

Make Your Own Extract

An ounce of pure vanilla extract and a vanilla bean cost about the same—around $2.50. You can save money without losing flavor by making your own extract. It's easy. Here's how:

Take two vanilla beans, split them in half, and place them in a clean jar with an airtight lid. A used mayonnaise jar will work.

Pour in a half cup of vodka—any kind will do—and tightly seal. Put it in a cool place out of sunlight. Turn the jar every day for six weeks. That's it.

You can remove the beans or keep them in the jar, adding more vodka as you start using the extract.

(proteins that spark biochemical action) and by inhibiting *angiogenesis*, the creation of a new blood supply for the tumor. Japanese researchers found the same effects, concluding that vanillin "may be of value in the development of anti-metastatic drugs for cancer treatment."

In China, researchers found that bromovanin—a vanillin derivative—stopped the advance of a "broad spectrum" of human cancers, and suggested the compound was "very appealing for the development" of a new anti-cancer drug.

And researchers at the New York University School of Medicine found that vanillin is *anti-mutagenic*. In human cells, it reduced by up to 73 percent the ability of toxins to "mutate" DNA, the genetic damage that can trigger cancer. They also found that vanillin influenced 64 genes with a role in cancer, including genes that control how cancer cells grow and die.

Sickle cell anemia. This inherited and incurable disease warps the round, flexible shape of oxygen-carrying red blood cells into rigid, sticky "sickles"—curved slices of cells, like crescent moons. The misshapen cells snag and stall in the bloodstream, choking the flow of blood and oxygen and producing the disease's main symptoms: intense pain and fatigue.

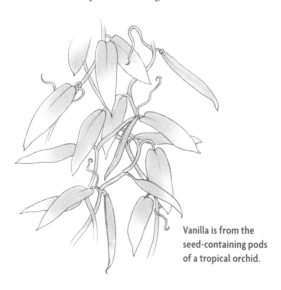

Vanilla is from the seed-containing pods of a tropical orchid.

Researchers at the Children's Hospital of Philadelphia tested a vanillin-derived drug on mice bred to develop sickle cells, and found the compound "significantly reduced" the percentage of sickled cells. The compound, they concluded in the *British Journal of Haematology*, could be a "new and safe anti-sickling agent for patients with sickle cell anemia."

Getting to Know Vanilla

The name *vanilla* is derived from the Spanish *vainilla*, or "little pod," a reference to the thin, seed-containing pods of the tropical orchid, or what we now call the "vanilla bean." Once grown only in Mexico (because the flower is naturally pollinated by a local species of bee), the world-wide crop of vanilla is now hand pollinated, a painstaking process that accounts in part for the spice's expense (second only to saffron).

Vanilla was first used as a culinary spice in confections by Europeans in the 17th century. Today, it's ubiquitous as a flavoring in pie fillings, ice cream (50 percent of the vanilla imported into the US is used to make ice cream), cakes, cookies, mousses, soufflés, rice desserts, and alcoholic drinks.

How to Buy Vanilla

Vanilla has a pervading, sweet fragrance that varies depending on where it's grown. It's sold in two forms: as a dried whole bean and as an extract. Both are available in most supermarkets. For the best taste, favor the bean. They come in several varieties:

French vanilla, also called *bourbon vanilla*, is arguably the best bean, containing the strongest aroma and the most vanillin. French beans are grown in Madagascar, Réunion Island, and the Comoro Islands, in the Indian Ocean. The majority of vanilla beans imported to the US are French beans; they're the bean you'll find in most markets.

Mexican vanilla lacks the depth of flavor found in French vanilla, say connoisseurs, though some vanilla mavens prefer it.

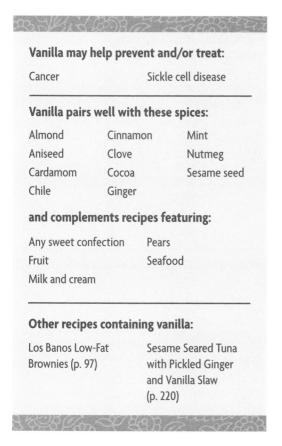

Vanilla may help prevent and/or treat:

Cancer   Sickle cell disease

Vanilla pairs well with these spices:

Almond	Cinnamon	Mint
Aniseed	Clove	Nutmeg
Cardamom	Cocoa	Sesame seed
Chile	Ginger	

and complements recipes featuring:

Any sweet confection	Pears
Fruit	Seafood
Milk and cream	

Other recipes containing vanilla:

Los Banos Low-Fat Brownies (p. 97)	Sesame Seared Tuna with Pickled Ginger and Vanilla Slaw (p. 220)

Indonesian vanilla, also known as *New Guinea vanilla*, is full-bodied, but has a spotty reputation when it comes to quality.

Tahitian vanilla is produced (not surprisingly) in Tahiti, but it's also produced in Hawaii and other Pacific islands. It contains less vanillin and therefore less of the classic vanilla flavor than either French or Mexican beans. However, demand for the Tahitian bean is rising, as its unique flavor has made it popular among chefs.

West Indian vanilla is grown on the French Caribbean island of Guadeloupe. Because of its low vanillin content it's not considered suitable as a spice, and is sold mainly to the cosmetics industry.

Vanilla beans are typically sold in cylindrical tubes, usually in quantities of three. Look for beans that are dark brown (almost black), moist

to the touch, and pliable, like a piece of licorice. You may spot a dusting of sugar powder, called *givre*, on the surface of some beans. It's a sign of a top-quality bean.

If you don't buy the bean, buy pure (or natural) vanilla extract. To create extract, beans are chopped, soaked in alcohol, aged, and strained. The alcohol content is important to the quality: the higher the alcohol, the stronger the flavor. (By federal law, the alcohol minimum is 35 percent.)

Store vanilla beans or extract in an airtight container in a cool, dark place. Both keep for up to 18 months.

What about imitation vanilla extract, which contains no vanillin? This synthetic product mimics but doesn't perfectly duplicate the flavor of true vanilla, and is considered a second-rate addition to the kitchen by vanilla connoisseurs. Be that as it may, there's plenty of imitation vanilla extract out there: the demand for natural vanilla outstrips its availability.

Vanilla is also sold as a paste, which is used mainly in making ice cream and in restaurants.

Vanilla seeds, removed from the bean, are the most expensive form of vanilla. They have the deepest and strongest aroma.

Both paste and seeds can be purchased from specialty vanilla retailers, which you can find online. See the "Buyer's Guide" on page 309 for a list of top-quality online spice retailers.

In the Kitchen with Vanilla

Vanilla is usually found in sweet treats, though vanilla itself isn't very sweet. (It's the sugar in the confections that supplies the sweetness.) In fact, in Africa and other tropical nations, vanilla is used more frequently in savory stews than in sweet dishes. Western chefs have discovered this tasty use of the spice, and you'll now spot vanilla sauces on entrée menus, mostly accompanying fish. Consider experimenting with vanilla in savory dishes in your kitchen.

When using fresh beans, slit along the middle and scrape out the seeds. Both the seeds and the pods are used in cooking.

Spicy Vanilla Rice Pudding

If served cold, this will keep in the refrigerator for two days.

1 cup basmati rice
2 cups water
1 three-inch cinnamon stick
1 teaspoon salt
3 cups whole milk
1½ cup half and half
⅔ cup sugar
¼ teaspoon ground clove
1 teaspoon ground cardamom
1 vanilla bean, split lengthwise
Freshly grated nutmeg

1. Rinse the basmati rice with cold water until water runs clear. (Put the rice in a bowl, cover with water, and run it through a mesh strainer three times.) Put the water, rice, cinnamon stick, and salt in a heavy saucepan over medium-high heat and bring to a simmer. Reduce the heat to low and cover. Simmer until the water is absorbed, about 10 minutes.

2. Add the milk, half and half, sugar, cloves, and cardamom. Scrape in the seeds from the vanilla bean, then add the bean. Increase the heat to medium and cook, uncovered, stirring occasionally until the mixture thickens and becomes creamy, about 40 minutes.

3. Remove the pudding from the heat, remove the cinnamon stick and the bean, and discard. Divide among four dessert bowls and grate fresh nutmeg over the top.

Makes 4 servings.

There is no need to discard the pod after using it. Let it dry out and bury it in a canister of sugar. You can reuse it several times before it completely gives up its flavor, putting it back in the sugar each time. (You can use the vanilla-scented sugar, too.)

Here are some sweet and savory ways to get more vanilla in your diet:

- Vanilla is exceptional with lobster, shrimp, or scallops. Make a cream sauce and spike it with vanilla beans.
- Vanilla marries well with butter. Sweeten butter sauces for savory dishes featuring fish or chicken with a little vanilla.
- Use vanilla to round out stronger flavors in salsas, chutney, and curries.
- Steep a split vanilla bean in coffee, cover, and chill. Serve with whipped cream and nutmeg.
- Add vanilla to fruit compotes featuring apples, gooseberries, and rhubarb.
- Add a drop or two of vanilla extract to holiday eggnog, or when you are whipping fresh cream.

WASABI *Hot Ally against Cancer*

Wasabi is a Japanese condiment best known for gracing a picture-perfect plate of sushi—and for being hot. *Real* hot. Just a dab on the edge of a chopstick is all that is needed to deliver its one-of-a-kind pungent flavor, which tastes somewhat like Chinese hot mustard. That fiery flavor is a sign of a healing spice at work.

Wasabi is also called Japanese horseradish, and it's in the same botanical family as horseradish: the *brassica*, which includes cruciferous vegetables such as cabbage, broccoli, brussels sprouts, and kale. Crucifers are loaded with compounds called *isothiocyanates* (ITCs), which research shows are anti-cancer. The ITCs uniquely found in wasabi are responsible for its sinus-clearing heat—and may have the power to protect you against cancer.

Making It Too Hot for Cancer

Animal and test tube studies show that wasabi might be as tough on cancer as other notable cancer-fighters in the cruciferous family, such as broccoli.

Breast cancer. Japanese researchers found that an ITC in wasabi could stop the growth of breast cancer cells in a test tube, and also kill the cells. The wasabi ITC, the researchers concluded, "is a new possible candidate for controlling cancer cells." The results were in *Cancer Detection and Prevention*.

Stopping metastasis. Metastasis is the spread of cancer from its original site to other sites in the body. When Japanese researchers injected the lungs of experimental animals with skin cancer cells, they found that pretreating with an ITC from wasabi stopped the growth of those cells by 82 percent. "Wasabi appears to not only inhibit tumor cell growth, but also tumor metastasis," wrote the researchers in the journal *Cancer Detection and Prevention*. "Wasabi is apparently a useful dietary candidate for controlling tumor progression," they concluded.

Stomach cancer. In another Japanese study, researchers induced stomach cancer in experimental animals and divided them into two groups, giving one group wasabi. The non-wasabi animals developed four times as many tumors. Stomach cancer "was suppressed by the administration of wasabi," wrote the researchers in the journal *Nutrition and Cancer*.

Colon cancer. In test tube research, scientists from Michigan State University found that compounds in wasabi inhibited the growth of colon cancer cells by up to 68 percent, lung cancer cells by up to 71 percent, and stomach cancer cells by up to 44 percent.

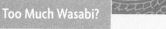
Too Much Wasabi?

Biting into a really hot chile can be tongue-torching experience, but that's nothing compared to an encounter with too much wasabi.

There have been a few reports of serious reactions in people who have naively consumed wasabi as if it were a vegetable rather than a condiment. Though it reportedly can cause pallor, profuse sweating, choking-like cough, and sometimes confusion and even collapse, there is no reported death by wasabi (even though there *is* a movie by that name). An overdose of wasabi, however, is a risk to people with weakened blood vessels, such as those who have had a heart attack or stroke, and people with type 2 diabetes.

If you've literally bitten off more than you can chew, try to stay calm, and begin breathing through the mouth to avoid drawing the irritants into the lungs. The heat dissipates rather quickly and doesn't linger as it does with chile. Nor does it "reheat" if you try to wash it away with water or beer.

Leukemia. Japanese researchers found wasabi could stop the growth of leukemia cells, and concluded the spice was "potentially useful as a natural anti-cancer agent."

Say Sayonara to Disease

There are many other ways that this Japanese spice can protect your health.

Food poisoning. Studies show that wasabi is a natural defender against *E. coli* and *Staphylococcus aureus*, bacteria that cause food poisoning. (Wasabi was first introduced into Japanese cuisine to cut down on the risk of food poisoning from raw fish.)

Ulcers. The bacteria *Helicobacter pylori* are the cause of most stomach ulcers, and a persistent *H. pylori* infection increases the risk of stomach cancer. Several studies show that ITC and other compounds in wasabi kill these bacteria.

High cholesterol. In an animal experiment, Australian researchers found that wasabi could decrease "bad" LDL cholesterol and increase "good" HDL cholesterol.

Tooth decay. Japanese researchers found that the ITCs in wasabi inhibit the growth of the bacteria that cause cavities.

Blood clots. Researchers isolated an ITC in wasabi that is 10 times more powerful than aspirin in preventing blood clots, an artery-plugging cause of heart attack and stroke.

> TO MAKE WASABI PASTE, JAPANESE CHEFS GRIND THE PEELED ROOT ON A SHARKSKIN GRATER CALLED AN OROSHI, THEN SQUEEZE THE GRATINGS INTO A PASTE.

Osteoporosis. In animal research, scientists found that wasabi contains compounds that can increase bone density.

Eczema (atopic dermatitis). An extract of wasabi reduced scratching behavior in animals bred to have an eczema-like condition. The wasabi also cut down on the immune components that produce itching and inflammation. The results were in the *Journal of Nutritional Science and Vitaminology*.

Getting to Know Wasabi

Americans familiar with wasabi know it as a condiment that goes with raw fish served as sushi (with rice) or sashimi (without rice), but in Japan it's used as commonly as ketchup is in the United States.

In Japan, it is used as a condiment on teriyaki dishes and noodles, and it is often added to dips, sauces, dressings, and marinades. A popular pickle called *wasabi zuke* is made by taking all parts of the wasabi plant—leaves, flowers, leafstalks, and the ground roots—and combining them with salt water and sake. You can even find wasabi wine (though it's mostly sold as a novelty), and wasabi liqueur, known for its high alcohol content.

The Japanese prize wasabi for its taste, but also for its aesthetic value. Food presentation is a big part of the Japanese dining experience, and the brilliantly bright green paste is often used to accent the ornamentally sculpted vegetables that adorn a Japanese dinner plate or buffet.

In Japan, making wasabi paste is an art. Chefs peel the root, then finely grate it on a shark-skin grater called an *oroshi*. The root is kept at a 90-degree angle to the grater in order to minimize the release of volatile oils and to produce the best flavor and texture. The gratings are then squeezed to form a paste.

Fresh wasabi is a rare taste treat you'll only find in Japan or fine restaurants in the West. It has a sweet and milder flavor than the paste, and is grated on a variety of dishes just like fresh cheese is grated on pasta in Italian restaurants.

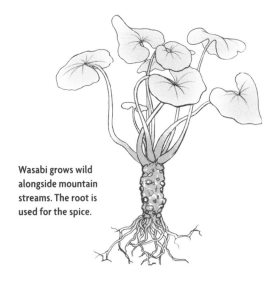

Wasabi grows wild alongside mountain streams. The root is used for the spice.

Wasabi may help prevent and/or treat:

Asthma	cholesterol)
Blood clots	Eczema
Cancer	Food poisoning
Cholesterol problems	Osteoporosis
(high "bad" LDL choles-	Tooth decay
terol, low "good" HDL	Ulcer

Wasabi pairs well with these spices:

Almond	Garlic	Parsley
Bay leaf	Mustard seed	Sesame seed
Coriander	Onion	Sun-dried tomato

and complements recipes featuring:

Meats	Rice
Noodles	Seafood
Raw or cooked fish	

Other recipes containing wasabi:

Sesame Seared Tuna with Pickled Ginger and Vanilla Slaw (p. 220)

The wasabi plant (once referred to as wild ginger) is somewhat rare, growing wild alongside cool mountain streams in parts of Japan where temperatures typically hover in the mid-50s. The popularity of Japanese cuisine during the last 20 years has sparked the interest in cultivating the plant, and wasabi is now grown in Korea, New Zealand, Taiwan, China, and Oregon. New Zealand is developing an excellent reputation for top-notch cultivation of the plant, which is even exported to Japan. A study conducted in New Zealand found the ITC content of New Zealand wasabi was greater than Japanese wasabi.

Because the spice is difficult to cultivate, and because of the time involved in growing a plant to maturity, wasabi is expensive compared to its more common cousin, American horseradish. And (prepare to be disillusioned) because of high cost and high demand, the wasabi served in the typical sushi bar in towns and malls across America is *not* true wasabi. Rather, it is powdered American horseradish, colored with spinach or spirulina, and reconstituted with water. Unless you've been to Japan and eaten in a high-end Japanese restaurant, odds are that you've never tasted true wasabi. It takes an experienced palate—and at least one experience with true wasabi—to recognize the difference between the real thing and the wasabi you get in the typical sushi bar. They both share the same pungency, but that's where the similarity ends.

How to Buy True Wasabi

The "wasabi" sold in the United States comes as a paste in a small tube or powdered in a small tin. The wasabi sold in tubes is American or European horseradish, so your search for true wasabi should be limited to wasabi powder.

The only way you'll be able to tell what you are buying is by checking the label. Wasabi powder made in Japan can be found in Asian markets and in the Oriental section of many major supermarkets. Just because wasabi comes under a Japanese label, however, doesn't mean it is true wasabi. Genuine wasabi products contain *only* wasabi and will not have mustard, horseradish, or dyes listed in the ingredients.

True wasabi can be purchased online. You will find sources for true wasabi in the "Buyer's Guide" on page 309.

In the Kitchen with Wasabi

Wasabi couldn't be simpler to make. Just take a teaspoon of the powder and mix it with a teaspoon or so of water until it is the consistency of paste. Let it sit for at least 10 minutes for the flavor to develop. Keep it covered to retain the flavor. Wasabi is highly perishable, so make only as much as you are planning to use.

There are many ways to enjoy wasabi other

Wasabi Orange Chicken with Toasted Almonds

The amount of wasabi in this recipe sounds like a lot, but the sting dissipates when it is mixed with all the other ingredients. In fact, if you love wasabi and hot food, you might want to add even more, since the amount used here offers only a slight tang. You can serve this over mixed greens garnished with cilantro springs or as a sandwich on a baguette. If the international section of your local market does not have black vinegar, you can find it at an Asian market or substitute balsamic vinegar.

2 cups diced cooked chicken breast
1 eleven-ounce can mandarin oranges,
    drained and diced
4 scallions, green and white parts, thinly sliced
¼ cup chopped cilantro
1 teaspoon canola oil
3 tablespoons sliced almonds
1 teaspoon sesame seeds, preferably black
½ cup low-fat mayonnaise
1½ tablespoons wasabi paste
1 teaspoon black vinegar or balsamic vinegar
½ teaspoon sesame oil

1. Combine the diced chicken, mandarin oranges, scallions, and cilantro in a medium bowl. Heat a small, dry heavy skillet over medium-high heat and lightly coat with ½ teaspoon of the canola oil. Add the almond slices and lightly toast, stirring with a wooden spoon, for one to two minutes. Remove to a plate to cool. Add the sesame seeds to the same skillet and dry roast, shaking the pan back and forth so the seeds do not burn. Remove to a plate to cool. Add to the chicken mixture and stir.

2. In a separate bowl, combine the mayonnaise, wasabi, black vinegar, and sesame oil. Blend into the chicken mixture. Refrigerator at least two hours to let flavors meld before serving.

Makes 4 servings.

than as a condiment for sushi. Here are some suggestions:

- Use it as you would mustard, as a condiment for cooked and cured meats such as ham, pot roast, and corned beef.
- Use it as you would cocktail sauce for raw clams and oysters or for shrimp cocktail. (Just remember to only use a little bit.)
- Spice up the taste of cocktail sauce even more by adding a pinch of wasabi powder.
- Make wasabi mashed potatoes by added wasabi powder to your traditional recipe. Figure about 1 tablespoon wasabi powder per 3 pounds of potatoes.
- Make a wasabi mayonnaise by adding 1 teaspoon of powdered wasabi and a squirt of lemon juice to ½ cup of regular mayonnaise and use it on sandwiches. It is particularly tasty on ham sandwiches.

- Make a wasabi vinaigrette by combining 1 tablespoon wasabi paste with 1 tablespoon each of mayonnaise, mirin, and rice vinegar.
- Substitute wasabi paste for some of the mustard in deviled eggs.
- Make a piquant compound butter by combining ¼ cup each of wasabi powder and dried chives with ½ cup of softened butter. Form into the shape of a cylinder and chill. Slice off butter-pat-sized pieces and melt over grilled tuna or salmon. Or rub into a whole chicken before roasting.
- Try wasabi paste in place of horseradish or Tabasco in a Bloody Mary.
- Snack on wasabi peas. The peas are fried or roasted, then covered with a combination of wasabi and other seasonings and baked until the shell is stiff. Here you know you're getting true wasabi.

PART THREE
Special Spice Combos

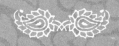

Spice Mixes and Rubs from Around the World:

Easy Combos to Create Delicious Healing Dishes

Spice *mixes* are the best way to enjoy the healing spices—and get the most out of their health and healing potential. There is no better way to develop diverse flavor, intense aroma, and the perception of freshness than by grinding or roasting a batch of spices expertly balanced to accent the taste of food and satisfy the appetite.

The cuisines of the nations renowned for spicy foods get their outstanding and unique taste characteristics as a result of *combining* complementary spices (usually a minimum of four, but often many more) into a flavor unlike any individual spice or food. The world's most famous spice mixes come from India, Southeast Asia, North Africa, Latin America, and the Caribbean, where they have been savored for thousands of years. Spicing is ubiquitous to those parts of the world, and a mix is commonly found on the table, just as Americans always have salt and pepper shakers at hand.

Spice mixtures can be mild or hot, bland or sharp, dry or mixed with wet ingredients to form a paste. They can consist of ground spices or whole spices. Some are pre-roasted, while others are ground and premixed as a convenience to be at the ready when it's time to cook. They can be used as part of a dish, as a condiment to sprinkle on food, or as a marinade to tenderize meat or poultry. They are used to accent flavor, but more often they are used to develop an intensely unique (and delightful) taste.

Generally speaking, no one spice dominates in a well-made spice blend. Spice mixes are balanced to harmonize flavors. (Those with an acute sense of smell may be able to detect the nuances of individual spices.) Even mixes that turn up the fire with additional chile can deliver that hot sensation without the distinct taste of

chile. Jamaican jerk, for example, doesn't taste like chile—but it's spicy hot!

Spice blends also save preparation time. Aromatic dishes such as those that come from the spice nations often call for spices that require roasting and grinding. This can be an arduous task—but only if you do it each time you cook. That's not necessary! Cooks who know their spices make up batches of different spice mixes that store well for months. Such advance planning can turn a recipe with a laundry list of ingredients into a meal you can make in minutes.

There are hundreds of traditional spice mixes, and they can be found all over the world (even in some regions of the United States). However, aside from a few exceptions, you'd be hard pressed to find the exact same recipe for any of these classics from one cookbook to the next, as every chef tends toward personal innovation. But there are specific spices in each mix that make them classic, and this doesn't change. The spices that complement them, and the amount of spice, can be adjusted to suit individual tastes.

The mixes in this chapter are inspired from my well-worn collection of Indian recipes, and from the recipe collections of my co-author, who is trained in French cuisine. We also used creative license, developing these mixes for simplicity, availability of ingredients, and (most importantly) to maximize the use of *healing* spices. They are also designed to complement a wide range of foods and cooking styles. Feel free to improvise—if there is a spice you don't particularly like, use a substitute. You'll find a table of spice substitutes on page 277. Or refer to the "Great Groupings" chart on page 274. Just as long as you stay true to the essential spices in a mix, you should capture the classic flavor.

A Tip on Toasting and Storing

Spice mixes are a convenience for advance preparation, but don't make a blend that you plan to store for a while before its first use. The different components of a blend can have different limitations in freshness, with some turning stale before others, upsetting the balance of the blend. A spice mix is best used within a month (although most last from three to six months, or longer). If you're experimenting, or know you won't be using the blend too frequently, consider cutting the recipe in half. Store these mixes in small, airtight glass containers, kept in a cool, dark place. Be sure to recap them right after use.

Some of the blends call for using whole spices that must be dry roasted and ground. This is easy to do and each recipe instruction indicates how to do it. But it's best to refer to page 8 for more information on the nuances of roasting, grinding, and storing spices.

Many of these blends are also commercially available. You can find them in Indian or Asian markets and via the Internet. However, commercial blends can contain salt, monosodium glutamate (MSG), or other ingredients not found in the traditional blend. When you make your own, you know exactly what you're getting. And because the blends in this chapter emphasize the healing spices, you're guaranteed to get an extra helping of health with every shake of the canister.

Enjoy—or as they say in India, *Bahut bhokh laggi he!*

Masala: Indian Spice

Masala means *spice mix* in India—and the masala is the essence of Indian cooking, with many types and combinations used in a variety of dishes, and with each region renowned for its own blend.

Indian cooks are famous for improvising, adding their own "secret" spice or spices to a classic masala blend and thereby personalizing their recipe repertoire. The range of possible spice combinations is almost endless. But no matter the combination, virtually all combinations of masala include spices with health and healing benefits.

Garam Masala   Heat: Mild

Also called Moghul garam masala, this blend is India's most popular spice mix. It is used in just about everything, in much the same way as Americans use salt and pepper. It is generally used as a final flavoring toward the end of cooking, or sprinkled on top of cooked food just before serving. It is popular for adding a finishing touch to curries. Because the spices are sweet rather than bitter, the mix does not require cooking to mellow the flavor. It can also be sprinkled in stews and soups just before serving, and over rice and vegetables. The spices responsible for the primary flavors are cumin, coriander, black pepper, and brown cardamom. Garam masala originated in the north, birthplace of Moghul cuisine, the haute cuisine of India. Use it as they do in India—in anything you desire.

> 4 tablespoons coriander seeds
> 2 tablespoons cumin seeds
> 1 tablespoon caraway seeds
> 1 tablespoon black peppercorns
> 2 teaspoons brown cardamom seeds
> 1 three-inch cinnamon stick
> 1 whole nutmeg
> 1 teaspoon whole cloves

1. In a small, dry heavy skillet, over medium heat, separately pan roast the coriander seeds, cumin seeds, caraway seeds, peppercorns, and cardamom until they become lightly browned and slightly fragrant. Turn the seeds frequently as they cook so they don't burn. Set aside on a plate to cool.
2. Break the cinnamon stick into small pieces. Put the cinnamon and nutmeg in a spice grinder or mini food processor and process.

Add the roasted seeds and the cloves and process the mixture to a fine powder. The mix will keep in an airtight glass container for up to six months or longer. *Makes about ½ cup.*

Sambaar Masala   Heat: Hot

This mix, popular in South India, is a contrast from the mild masala indigenous to the north. The distinct taste, however, comes from dried legumes, called dals in India. The masala is primarily used in vegetable and lentil dishes, soups, and curries. This makes a small amount, as only a pinch needs to be used. Adjust the chile to turn the heat up or down.

1 tablespoon coriander seeds
2 teaspoons cumin seeds
1 teaspoon brown mustard seeds
1 teaspoon black peppercorns
½ teaspoon fenugreek seeds
½ cinnamon stick, broken in pieces
1 teaspoon turmeric
½ teaspoon ground asafoetida
6 dried red chiles, stemmed and seeded
1½ tablespoon *urad dal* (split white lentils)
1 tablespoon *chana dal* (split yellow peas)

1. In a small, dry heavy skillet, over medium heat, roast the coriander seeds, cumin seeds, mustard seeds, black peppercorns, and fenugreek seeds, until the seeds darken and become slightly fragrant. Stir frequently so they don't burn.
2. Lower the heat and add the cinnamon, turmeric, and asafoetida and continue to cook, stirring constantly for one minute. Remove to a glass dish and cool.
3. To the same skillet, add the chiles and roast, stirring frequently until brown, about two to three minutes. Remove to a separate plate and cool.
4. Add the split lentils and peas to the skillet and roast, stirring frequently, for three to

four minutes, so they don't burn. Transfer to a plate and let cool.
5. Put all the ingredients in a spice grinder or mini food processor and process until the mixture becomes a fine powder. The mix will keep in an airtight glass container for up to six months or longer. *Makes about ⅓ cup.*

Chaat Masala   Heat: Hot

This mix gets its unique flavor from two exotic spices: amchur, the sharp, lemony seasoning that comes from unripe mangoes; and black salt, a pungent condiment popular in India that gives the blend its saltiness. It is frequently used to flavor Indian snacks (many Indians are enthusiastic snackers) and appetizers called chaats, but can be used in soups, stews, or anything that calls for a sharp, hot, and tart flavor.

2 tablespoons cumin seeds
1 tablespoon black peppercorns
2 teaspoons coriander seeds
1 teaspoon ajowan seeds
1 teaspoon aniseed
½ teaspoon dried mint
2 tablespoons black salt
1 tablespoon amchur
1 teaspoon ground ginger
½ teaspoon cayenne
Pinch asafoetida

1. In a small, dry heavy skillet over medium heat, separately roast the cumin seeds, peppercorns, coriander seeds, ajowan seeds, and aniseed until they become lightly browned and slightly fragrant. Turn the seeds frequently as they cook, so they don't burn.
2. Put the seeds and the mint into a spice grinder or mini food processor and process to a fine powder. Mix the powder with the black salt, amchur, ginger, cayenne, and asafoetida. The mix will keep in an airtight container for two months. *Makes about ½ cup.*

Panch Phoron   Heat: Mild

Panch (meaning five) and *phora* (meaning seeds) is a combination of five different aromatic seeds. The key ingredient is black cumin seeds, called kalonji in India. The blend, which comes from Bengal, is used whole, and added to cooking oil at the start of a dish. It is traditionally used in Indian lentil dishes and to flavor vegetables and potatoes, but it can be used to flavor almost any kind of dish. When using, ready a sauté pan with oil as you would for browning or sautéing vegetables. Add about ¼ teaspoon of the mix to the oil, moving the seeds around until they release their fragrance. Add the other ingredients right away.

2 tablespoons mustard seeds
2 tablespoons cumin seeds
2 tablespoons black cumin seeds
1 tablespoon fenugreek seeds
1 tablespoon fennel seeds

1. Put all the seeds into a glass jar with a tight-fitting lid. Shake well to distribute. The mix will keep in an airtight container for a year. *Makes about ½ cup.*

North Africa: Land of the Exotic

Morocco, Tunisia, Algeria, and Ethiopia are well known for their exotic spice mixes, but Moroccan cuisine is the best known to Western palates, possibly because it is the least spicy among them. Tunisian blends tend to be spicy and hot with chiles. There are many famous North African blends. These are some of the best.

La Kama   Heat: Mild

If you've ever visited the northern coastal town of Tangiers you've likely sampled this mix. It is Morocco's most common seasoning and it is used to flavor soups, stews, and the popular slow-cooked dish known as tagine (named after the clay pot in which it is cooked). It is also used as a rub on poultry and lamb. You can make it using ground spices, but do so in small quantity, as it doesn't have a long shelf life.

1 tablespoon ground ginger
1 tablespoon freshly ground black pepper
2 teaspoons turmeric
1½ teaspoons ground cinnamon
1 teaspoon ground nutmeg

1. Combine all the spices. It will keep stored in an airtight container for about a month. *Makes about ¼ cup.*

Ras-el-hanout   Heat: Mild-to-Medium

This is considered the king of spice blends. Its hallmark is its lengthy list of ingredients—sometimes as many as 30 or more—that merge to form a balanced, full-bodied blend. Ras-el-hanout originated as a spice merchant's personal blend of the finest ingredients, and often includes the truly exotic, such as rose petals. It is considered the epitome of combining a diverse collection of spices to form a singular ingredient that is better than any one of its parts. Even though it is mild, ras-el-hanout is considered a full-bodied blend that can substitute for the spices used in everyday dishes. Use it in stews, and add it to the sauté pan when making fish, chicken, or stir-fries. Sprinkled on chicken, it gives nice color and flavor to a roast. In Morocco, it is a popular blend for lamb dishes and couscous. Use about half as much ras-el-hanout as you would other spices in a dish. Though the ingredients vary greatly, the blend almost always includes cardamom, cinnamon, coriander, cumin, ginger, paprika, and turmeric.

2 tablespoons cumin seeds
1 teaspoon green cardamom seeds
1 teaspoon brown cardamom seeds (optional)
1 teaspoon fennel seeds
1 teaspoon caraway seeds

¼ cup mild Hungarian paprika
2 tablespoons ground ginger
1 tablespoon ground coriander
2 teaspoons ground cinnamon
2 teaspoons turmeric
1 teaspoon ground allspice
1 teaspoon ground nutmeg
1 teaspoon ground galangal (Laos powder)
½ teaspoon ground cloves
½ teaspoon ground red chile

1. In a small, dry heavy skillet over medium heat, roast the cumin seeds, green and brown cardamom seeds, fennel seeds, and caraway seeds, until the seeds darken and become slightly fragrant. Stir frequently so they don't burn. Transfer to a plate to cool.
2. Combine all cooled seeds and the rest of the spices in a small bowl and mix well. The mix will keep in an airtight glass container for four to six months. *Makes about 1 cup.*

Tabil   Heat: Hot

Tabil means *coriander*, which is the principal spice in this popular Tunisian blend. It is commonly used in curry dishes, stews, and in stuffings. Or lightly sprinkle it on meat or poultry before grilling.

½ cup coriander seeds
2 tablespoons caraway seeds
1 tablespoon chili powder
1 teaspoon garlic powder

1. Place the coriander and caraway seeds in a spice grinder and grind until smooth. Blend with the chili powder and garlic powder. The mix will keep in an airtight glass container for about six months. *Makes about ½ cup.*

Berbere   Heat: Hot

This is a complex and wet blend from Ethiopia. As in ras-el-hanout, its ingredients can vary, but they revolve around chiles, cloves, and ginger. This blend is excellent for meat, such as steak, chops, lamb roasts, and pork tenderloin. Mix the rub and smother it on the meat two to eight hours before grilling.

3 tablespoons mild paprika
2 tablespoons hot paprika
1 tablespoon ground coriander
1 tablespoon freshly ground black pepper
1 teaspoon chili powder
½ teaspoon ground cardamom
½ teaspoon ground fenugreek
½ teaspoon ground cinnamon
½ teaspoon ground allspice
½ teaspoon hot pepper flakes
¼ teaspoon ground cloves
1 medium onion, diced
4 cloves garlic, diced
2 tablespoons chopped fresh ginger
2 teaspoons salt
1 teaspoon sugar
¾ cup olive oil
¼ cup fresh lemon juice

1. Combine the first 11 ingredients in a small bowl and set aside. Put the onions, garlic, ginger, salt, and sugar in a food processor or blender, and process. Add half the spice mixture. With the processor running slowly, add the olive oil, alternating with the rest of the spices and the lemon juice, until the blend reaches the consistency of a paste. Refrigerated, it keeps for about one week. *Makes about 1½ cups.*

China: Star Spice Master

The cooks of China and the Southeast Asian nations of Malaysia, Thailand, and Vietnam are considered masters at mixing spices, with an emphasis on designing spicy sauces as seasonings, rather than dry mixes. Hoisin, oyster, plum, and fish sauces are just the beginning of a long roster of enticing sauces that make these cuisines some of the most varied in the world. Though there is a clear distinction in the types of sauces and individual spices that set these cuisines apart, they all depend and make liberal use of China's famed "five-spice powder," starring the exotic spice, star anise.

Chinese Five-Spice Powder — Heat: Mild

If you've tried to make Chinese food at home but have not been able to quite duplicate the taste, it could be due to the absence of Chinese five-spice powder. It is what gives Chinese barbequed ribs, dipping sauces, and other specialties their distinctive taste. Many Asian recipes call for five-spice powder, but it is often hard to find (and there is no adequate substitute for the flavor). Star anise and Szechuan peppercorns can be found in Asian or Indian markets, and are starting to become regulars on the spice shelves in many supermarkets. (Black peppercorns bear no resemblance to Szechuan peppercorns and are not a good substitute in this recipe.) If you can't find Szechuan peppercorns, an adequate substitute is equal parts of aniseed and allspice.

    3 star anise
    2 tablespoons Szechuan peppercorns (or 1 tablespoon
        ground aniseed and 1 tablespoon allspice)
    1 tablespoon fennel seeds
    1 tablespoon whole cloves
    1 three-inch cinnamon stick

1. Place all the ingredients in a spice grinder and process to a fine powder. The mix will keep in an airtight container for up to six months. *Makes about ¼ cup.*

Middle East:
Land of Many Spices

The cuisines of the Middle East have been influenced by Iran, India, and Europe. As a result, spice mixes vary widely within the many nations of the area. Here are two of the most renowned.

Baharat — Heat: Medium

Bahar is Arabic for pepper, the principal ingredient in this popular Middle Eastern spice mix. Also known as *advieh*, this mix is an interesting combination of sweet and hot that produces a mellow fragrance. This mix is used extensively in the Gulf States for spicing barbecue, meat stuffings, rice dishes, soups, and stews. It is also used in marinades. Try it as a rub for lamb chops. It is popular in tomato-based dishes, as it helps cut the acidity.

    1 tablespoon black peppercorns
    1 tablespoon coriander seeds
    1 tablespoon cumin seeds
    1 tablespoon cloves
    1 teaspoon black cumin seeds
    10 cardamom pods, seeded
    1 whole nutmeg
    1 four-inch cinnamon stick, broken into pieces
    ½ tablespoon sweet paprika

1. In a small, dry heavy skillet, over medium heat, roast the peppercorns, coriander seeds, cumin seeds, cloves, black cumin seeds, and cardamom seeds separately, until the seeds darken and become slightly fragrant. Stir frequently so they don't burn. Transfer to a plate to cool.
2. Put the nutmeg and cinnamon in a spice grinder or mini food processor and process until coarse. Add the seeds and grind until finely ground. Add the paprika. The mix will keep in an airtight glass container for about two months. *Makes about ½ cup.*

Dukkah — Heat: Mild

All nuts have healing qualities, which makes this tasty Egyptian spice mix a very healthy condiment. A great way to enjoy it: sprinkle it into olive oil and serve as a dip for bread. Or put the dukkah in a small shallow dish next to the olive oil; first dip the bread in the olive oil and then the dukkah. You can also use dukkah as a coating for baked chicken and fish, the same way you'd use bread crumbs.

3 tablespoons sesame seeds
3 tablespoons coriander seeds
2 tablespoons cumin seeds
1 tablespoon black peppercorns
1 teaspoon fennel seeds
½ cup hazelnuts
1 teaspoon dried mint leaves
½ teaspoon dried thyme

1. In a small, dry heavy skillet, over medium heat, individually roast the sesame seeds, coriander seeds, cumin seeds, black peppercorns, and fennel seeds, until the seeds darken and become slightly fragrant. Stir frequently so they don't burn. Transfer to a plate to cool.
2. Put hazelnuts, seeds, mint and thyme in a spice grinder or mini food processor and process until mixture reaches a coarse texture. Do not over-process or the mix will turn into a paste. This mix keeps in an airtight glass jar for about 3 months. *Makes about 1 cup.*

Latin America and the Caribbean: Where It's Hot, Hot, Hot

Say *chile*—and the countries that probably come to mind are south of the American border. However, not all Latin and Caribbean cuisines are fiery—some are mild, revealing a European influence. But if you like your food hot, you'll like Latin and Caribbean cuisines.

Jamaican Jerk Marinade　　　**Heat: Fire**

In Jamaica, *jerk* is a dish, a cooking style, and a way of life. A jerk marinade is a fiery hot wet rub,

customarily made with Scotch bonnet chiles, one of the hottest chiles on the planet. Allspice is the defining flavor. A true jerk is slow-cooked over a low fire, often an hour or longer, depending on the food. For a jerk with less fire, substitute jalapeño or a milder chile for the Scotch bonnet, and use the smallest amount. Jerk is traditionally made with chicken or pork. This mix doesn't keep, so you'll want to make it one recipe at a time.

4 to 8 Scotch bonnet or jalapeño chiles
5 whole scallions, coarsely chopped
1 small onion, peeled and quartered
1 one-inch piece fresh ginger, peeled
4 cloves garlic, peeled
¼ cup white vinegar
2 tablespoons soy sauce
2 tablespoons canola oil
1 tablespoon dark brown sugar
1 tablespoon ground allspice
2 teaspoons dried thyme
1 teaspoon freshly ground black pepper
½ teaspoon ground cinnamon
½ teaspoon ground nutmeg
½ teaspoon salt

1. Add the chiles, scallions, onion, ginger, and garlic to a food processor and process until smooth. With the motor running, add the vinegar, soy sauce, and canola oil, and process until well combined, about 30 seconds.
2. Put the contents into a small mixing bowl and add the brown sugar, allspice, thyme, black pepper, cinnamon, nutmeg, and salt and stir until well combined.
3. Wash and dry the chicken or pork and place in a plastic bag with a zip-lock seal. Pour the marinade into the bag, seal it as airtight as possible, and roll your hands around the outside to make sure all the pieces are covered. Refrigerate for a minimum of four hours. Remove and grill over low heat, until it reaches desired doneness.

Note: To make jerk truly authentic, you need

to grill it over a fire spiked with pimento wood and leaves. Refer to the "Buyer's Guide" on page 309 to find out where you can purchase them.

Makes enough for two pork tenderloins or one cut up chicken.

Adobo   Heat: Mild

Adobo is a popular all-purpose dry seasoning with a garlicky flavor. It is indispensable in the kitchens of Cuba, the Dominican Republic, and Puerto Rico, where it replaces regular table salt and is used on everything. To make it fiery hot, as they do in Mexico, add an extra tablespoon or two of ground red chile.

2 tablespoons black peppercorns
2 tablespoons cumin seeds
2 tablespoons dried oregano
2 tablespoons salt
2 tablespoons garlic powder
½ teaspoon chili powder

1. In a small, dry heavy skillet over medium heat, roast the peppercorns and cumin seeds separately until the seeds darken and become slightly fragrant. Stir frequently so they don't burn. Transfer to a plate to cool.
2. Put the seeds and oregano in a spice mill and process until it becomes the consistency of a fine powder. Combine with the salt, garlic powder, and chili powder and mix well. The mix will keep in an airtight glass container for six months. *Makes about 1 cup.*

Colombo Powder   Heat: Medium

Named after the capital of Sri Lanka, this seasoning is popular in the islands of Guadeloupe and Martinique. The nutty flavor comes from the addition of rice. It is popular in dishes featuring fish, plantains, and sweet potatoes.

¼ cup white rice
¼ cup cumin seeds

1 tablespoon coriander seeds
1 tablespoon black or brown mustard seeds
1 tablespoon black peppercorns
1 tablespoon fenugreek seeds
1 teaspoon whole cloves
¼ cup turmeric

1. Place the rice in a skillet and dry roast it as you would the spices. Separately dry roast the cumin seeds, coriander seeds, mustard seeds, peppercorns, fenugreek seeds, and cloves, and set aside to cool. When cool, combine the rice and other spices in a spice grinder along with the turmeric and grind to the consistency of a fine powder. The mix will keep in an airtight container for up to six months. *Makes about 1 cup.*

Cocoa Rub   Heat: Medium

Cocoa is popular in Mexico, especially as a spicy beverage and as a spice in savory sauces. Cocoa is bitter in the raw but mellows and melds with other spices when it hits the heat. Rub this into pork or the skin of chicken an hour before grilling or add a tablespoon to bread stuffings.

¼ cup unsweetened cocoa powder
¼ cup ground cumin
2 tablespoons paprika
2 tablespoons ground coriander
2 teaspoons chili powder
2 teaspoons coarsely ground black peppercorns
1 teaspoon sea salt
1 teaspoon ground allspice

1. Combine all the ingredients and keep in an airtight container out of heat and light. *Makes about 1 cup.*

France: A Mellow Fare

The French aren't big on spice mixes, believing instead that the natural flavor of the principal food should stand out in a dish. (This is why you don't find French dishes spicy or hot.) There are a few exceptions, however, using herbs and spices to add mellow flavors. These blends originated in the Mediterranean region of southern France.

Quatre Épices   Heat: Mild

Three of the spices in this mix—peppercorns, cloves, and nutmeg—are a constant, but the fourth can be either cinnamon or ground ginger or a combination of both. The peppercorn varies also—either black or white, or a combination of both. I prefer using black because it contains more healthy oils. Use 1 tablespoon of ground ginger in place of the cinnamon. The French use this mix to flavor pates and terrines. It's also used in stuffings, long-simmering stews, and can be added to a glaze for ham or grilled poultry or pork. It will keep well for up to six months.

⅓ cup black peppercorns
1½ tablespoons whole cloves
1 whole nutmeg
1 one-inch cinnamon stick

1. Place all the ingredients in a spice grinder or mini food processor and blend until the spices are the consistency of a fine power. The mix will keep in an airtight container for about 6 months. *Makes ½ cup.*

Spice de Provence   Heat: Mild

For this mix, we've taken a bit of creative license on the French classic *Herbs de Provence*. The only thing missing is lavender and tarragon. If you'd like to add them, use a teaspoon of each. This blend will taste fresher and is much cheaper than purchasing a commercial blend. Use it as you would garam masala—in anything you desire.

4 tablespoons dried thyme
2 tablespoons dried marjoram
2 tablespoons dried parsley

2 teaspoons celery seeds
3 ground bay leaves
2 teaspoons dried rosemary, crumbled

1. Combine all the ingredients and store in an airtight glass container. The mix will keep in an airtight container for 6 months. *Makes about 1 cup.*

Bouquet Garni   Heat: Mild

The purpose of a *bouquet garni* is to infuse a soup or stew with the mellow aroma of fresh or dried spices. The spices can vary, but there is always one constant: bay leaf, almost always crumbled rather than ground. This is why bouquet garni is customarily tied up in a square of cheesecloth, for easy removal at the end of cooking. Use about a tablespoon of the blend for dishes calling for four servings.

4 large bay leaves, crushed into small pieces
3½ tablespoons dried thyme
2 tablespoons dried marjoram
2 tablespoons dried parsley

1. Combine all the ingredients. The mix will keep in an airtight glass container for about six months. *Makes about ½ cup.*

Other Classic Blends

Spice is synonymous with apple pie, pizza, and barbecue, so we don't want to leave them out.

Apple Pie Spice   Heat: Mild

This sweet mix is called for in all forms of pies and pastries. It is a common commercial blend, but making your own guarantees freshness and is less expensive.

1 cinnamon stick, broken into pieces
1 tablespoon whole cloves

1 tablespoon whole allspice
1 tablespoon coriander seeds
1 tablespoon cardamom seeds
1 whole nutmeg

1. In a small, dry heavy skillet over medium heat, roast the cinnamon stick, cloves, allspice, coriander, and cardamom seeds until the seeds darken and become slightly fragrant. Stir frequently so they don't burn. Transfer to a plate to cool.
2. Put the nutmeg in a spice grinder and break up with a few quick turns. Add the cooled cinnamon and seeds and process to a fine powder. The mix will keep in an airtight container for six months. *Makes about ½ cup.*

Pizza Spice Blend   Heat: Mild
You don't need to stop at pizza when using this blend. Put it in anything Italian—tomato sauces, meatballs, lasagna, or as a flavoring on top of spaghetti. Use it as an all-in-one blend for meatloaf. Use about 1 tablespoon of the mix per pound of meat or quart of sauce.

3 tablespoons dried oregano
2 tablespoons dried thyme
2 tablespoons dried basil
1 tablespoon dried marjoram
2 teaspoons dried rosemary, crushed
1 teaspoon garlic powder
½ teaspoon rubbed sage

1. Combine all the ingredients. The mix will keep in an airtight glass container for up to a year. *Makes about ½ cup.*

Basic Barbecue Rub   Heat: Mild
The sugar and salt in this rub will tenderize any cut of meat. It helps seal in the juices, so grilled food stays moist. The rub should be sprinkled on (not rubbed into) red meat steaks, chops, or poultry about two hours before grilling. If temperature permits—that is, if the day isn't too hot and you have air conditioning—let the food soak in the rub at room temperature. If not, refrigerate, taking it out about a half hour before grilling.

1 cup sugar
½ cup mild Hungarian paprika
¼ cup garlic salt
¼ cup celery salt
¼ cup onion salt
3 tablespoons chili powder
3 tablespoons freshly ground black pepper
1 tablespoon ground white pepper
2 teaspoons ground sage
1 teaspoon ground rosemary
1 teaspoon dry mustard
½ teaspoon ground thyme
1 teaspoon garlic powder

1. Combine all the ingredients in a large glass jar with an airtight lid. The mix will keep for a year. *Makes about 3 cups.*

Rosemary Barbecue Rub   Heat: Mild
Rosemary is a powerful antioxidant—so powerful, it can help stop the formation of carcinogenic substances that build up on meat, poultry, and fish when they are grilled or fired at a temperature higher than 352°F. Sprinkle the rub on the food, about two hours before grilling.

2 tablespoons dried rosemary
2 tablespoons black peppercorns
2 tablespoons sea salt
2 tablespoons sweet paprika

1. Mix all the ingredients together. The mix will keep in an airtight glass jar for about six months. *Makes about ½ cup.*

Pickling Spice   Heat: Medium
Anyone into home canning will find that a homemade spice mix will give pickled vegetables

an added dimension in taste. It is best to use whole spices, as the spices will add flavor without leaving a powdery residue. The spice can be tied in a square of cheesecloth and removed at the end of cooking, though some cooks prefer to let the spice roam freely, as it will continue to infuse flavor in the vegetables once they are canned. Use 1 tablespoon of pickling spice per pound of vegetables.

¼ cup yellow mustard seeds

3 tablespoons whole allspice

2 tablespoons black peppercorns

2 tablespoons fennel seeds

2 teaspoons whole cloves

1 cinnamon stick, coarsely ground

1 teaspoon red pepper flakes

1. Combine all the ingredients and store in an airtight glass container. The mix will keep for four to six months. *Makes about 1 cup.*

Mulling Spice   Heat: Mild

Mulled wine or cider and a seat by the fire—it's a combination that's hard to beat on a cold winter's night.

2 cinnamon sticks, broken into small pieces

6 whole nutmegs, coarsely chopped

⅓ cup dried orange peel

⅓ cup dried lemon peel

¼ cup whole allspice

¼ cup whole cloves

2 tablespoons coarsely chopped crystallized ginger

1. Combine all the ingredients. When making mulled cider or wine, take about 1 tablespoon per person and wrap in a piece of cheesecloth.

Secure the bag tightly. Put in a saucepan with the liquid and bring to a simmer. Let the liquid rest for 10 minutes for the spices. Remove the spice bag and serve. *Makes about 1½ cups.*

Chesapeake Bay
Seafood Seasoning   Heat: Medium

Old Bay is a popular spicy seasoning for crab boil in the Chesapeake Bay area. The recipe, developed by a German immigrant by the name of Gustav Brunn about 50 years ago, is supposed to be a deeply guarded secret. But many people have tried to duplicate it, including me. The secret to using this seasoning in a crab or shrimp boil is to use a lot of it. Put ½ cup or more in a pot of a dozen crabs or a pound of shrimp. Sprinkle the shells generously again when you take them out of the water. It makes for messy eating, but people who've tried it never seem to mind.

¼ cup Hungarian paprika

2 tablespoons celery salt

1 tablespoon ground cardamom

1 tablespoon ground cinnamon

1 tablespoon dry mustard

2 teaspoons ground allspice

1 teaspoon celery seed

1 teaspoon chili powder

1 teaspoon freshly ground black pepper

1 teaspoon ground bay leaf

1 teaspoon ground cloves

1 teaspoon ground ginger

1. Combine all the ingredients. Store in an airtight container away in a dry, dark place. Will keep for a year or more. *Makes about 1 cup.*

Great Groupings: Making Culinary Music

Parsley, sage, rosemary, and thyme. Just like the notes from an old melody, certain spices make beautiful culinary music together. There are some old classics (such as basil and tomato, or cinnamon and nutmeg), and some new hits (such as lemongrass and wasabi, or ginger and saffron). And there are many popular imports (such as black cumin and sesame seed, or ajowan and turmeric).

If you are looking for suitable companions for your favorite spices, let this chart help you. Combinations are endless, so consider this a *starting* point. Experiment with different combinations until you find ones that suit your personal taste—and your favorite foods!

AJOWAN	• Celery seed & ketchup • Garlic, ginger & turmeric • Mint, ginger & pomegranate
ALLSPICE	• Almond & cocoa • Cinnamon & nutmeg • Clove, mustard seed & vinegar • Cumin & mint
ALMOND	• Cinnamon, saffron & raisins • Cinnamon & vanilla • Cocoa & mint
AMCHUR	• Ajowan, mint & pomegranate • Cardamom & kokum • Coriander, onion & fermented fish paste • Ginger & kaffir leaf
ANISEED	• Clove & coriander • Cocoa & coconut • Nutmeg & pomegranate • Star anise & savory
ASAFOETIDA	• Ajowan & turmeric • Black pepper, chili powder & fennel seed
BASIL	• Cumin, oregano & cilantro • Curry leaf, garlic & Asian fish sauce • Garlic, oregano & capers • Oregano, olive oil & pine nuts • Scallions & peanuts
BAY LEAF	• Basil, oregano & tomato • Rosemary, garlic & thyme
BLACK CUMIN SEED	• Cinnamon & fenugreek • Poppy seed & sesame
BLACK PEPPER	• Cardamom & coconut milk • Cinnamon, cloves & star anise

CARAWAY	• Juniper berry & paprika • Nutmeg & marjoram
CARDAMOM	• Amchur & kokum • Cinnamon, clove & cumin • Clove & nutmeg • Coriander & cumin
CELERY SEED	• Ginger & soy sauce • Horseradish & tomato • Sage & turmeric
CHILE	• Cilantro, peppercorns & rum • Garlic & ginger • Garlic, lemongrass & shallots
CINNAMON	• Allspice, clove & nutmeg • Black cumin seed & fenugreek seed • Black pepper & hot mustard • Clove & cardamom • Clove, star anise & rice vinegar
CLOVE	• Cardamom, cumin & cinnamon • Cardamom & nutmeg • Cinnamon, nutmeg & star anise
COCOA	• Allspice & red chile • Almond, mint & vanilla • Amchur, coriander & orange zest
COCONUT	• Asafoetida, cumin & ginger • Cinnamon, cocoa & vanilla • Curry leaf, galangal & lemongrass
CORIANDER	• Cardamon & cumin • Chile, garlic, ginger, lemongrass, galangal & kaffir leaf • Lemongrass, shallots, turmeric & peanuts

CUMIN	• Basil, oregano & cilantro • Cardamom, cinnamon & clove • Cardamom & coriander • Cinnamon & saffron • Garlic & ginger • Ginger, sesame seed & cilantro
CURRY LEAF	• Fenugreek seed & turmeric • Galangal & lemongrass • Ginger, lemongrass & kokum • Mustard seed & buttermilk
FENNEL SEED	• Basil & tomato • Black cumin seed & sun-dried tomato • Cocoa & vanilla • Rosemary & kalamata
FENUGREEK SEED	• Black cumin seed & black mustard seed • Clove & onion • Curry leaf & turmeric • Lemongrass, star anise & wasabi
GALANGAL	• Chile & Asian fish sauce • Chile, garlic, ginger, lemongrass & kaffir leaf • Coconut milk, lemongrass & cilantro
GARLIC	• Basil & oregano • Chile, lemongrass & shallots • Cumin, ginger & tomato paste • Ginger, saffron & yogurt • Red chile, oregano & lemon
GINGER	• Capers, oranges & Worcestershire sauce • Chinese mustard & soy sauce • Garlic, lemongrass & shallots or scallion • Garlic, saffron & yogurt • Saffron & vanilla
HORSERADISH	• Black pepper, ketchup & Worcestershire sauce • Celery seed, lemon & tomato • Garlic, scallions & soy sauce
JUNIPER BERRY	• Caraway & paprika • Onion & oregano • Sage & apple

KOKUM	• Amchur & cardamom • Ginger, lemongrass & curry leaf
LEMONGRASS	• Chile, garlic, ginger, galangal & kaffir leaf • Chile, garlic & shallots • Coriander, turmeric & peanuts • Curry, ginger & kokum • Curry leaf & galangal • Fenugreek seed, star anise & wasabi
MARJORAM	• Basil, oregano & pine nuts • Caraway & nutmeg • Garlic, onion & wine
MINT	• Basil & oregano • Fennel seed & tomato • Garlic, cilantro & Asian chili sauce • Mint, cilantro & chives
MUSTARD SEED	• Black cumin seed, cardamom & tamarind • Caraway, clove & horseradish
NUTMEG	• Allspice & cinnamon • Caraway & marjoram • Cardamom & clove • Garlic, cilantro & orange zest
ONION	• Ajowan & coriander • Basil & tomato • Kokum, ginger & turmeric • Marjoram, oregano, rosemary, parsley & sage
OREGANO	• Basil, cumin & cilantro • Capers & black olives • Garlic, red chile & lemon
PARSLEY	• Capers & lemon zest • Chives & tomato
POMEGRANATE	• Amchur & mustard seed • Black cumin seed & turmeric • Chile, cilantro, garlic & onion • Cocoa & mint
PUMPKIN SEED	• Chile & cocoa • Coriander & cumin • Oregano, mint & sun-dried tomato

ROSEMARY	• Ajowan & turmeric • Black pepper & paprika • Oregano & sun-dried tomato • Parsley, sage & thyme
SAFFRON	• Almond, cinnamon & rosewater • Cinnamon & cumin • Coriander, nutmeg & rosewater • Ginger, garlic & yogurt • Ginger & vanilla
SAGE	• Garlic & onion • Ginger & parsley • Mustard seed & cranberries • Tomato, mint & pine nuts
SESAME SEED	• Black cumin seed & poppy seed • Coriander, Asian chili sauce, white wine & honey • Ginger & vanilla
STAR ANISE	• Black pepper, cinnamon & clove • Cinnamon & orange zest • Onion & soy sauce

TAMARIND	• Black mustard seed & turmeric • Coconut & ginger • Red chile & tomatoes
THYME	• Ginger & saffron • Sage & onion
TOMATO	• Basil, black olives & feta cheese • Basil, chives, corn & grated cheddar cheese • Basil & onion • Basil, oregano & fennel seed • Garlic, red pepper flakes & olive oil
TURMERIC	• Coriander, lemongrass, shallots & peanuts • Curry leaf & fenugreek seed
VANILLA	• Almond, ginger & orange • Aniseed, cinnamon & cocoa • Ginger & saffron • Star anise, ginger & sesame seed
WASABI	• Black mustard seed & Dijon mustard • Lemongrass & star anise

The Spice Exchange: Compatible Substitutes

As you'll realize when you start cooking with the healing spices, combining a variety of different flavors imparts its *own* unique flavor. This makes spice cooking very forgiving. If you don't have on hand one of the spices in a recipe, you can skip it or substitute something else. You may get a different flavor—but it will still taste good!

For many of the healing spices, there are substitutes that will deliver the intended flavor, or at least a close imitation. You'll miss out on the healing qualities of the missing spice, but you'll still benefit from the nutrients in the substitute.

This list includes all the healing spices that have adequate substitutes. If you don't find a spice in the list, it doesn't have a substitute. If you don't have the spice or can't find it, just eliminate it from the recipe.

Use equal parts of the substitute, unless otherwise noted.

OUT OF THIS?	THEN USE THIS
Ajowan	Oregano
Allspice	1 part nutmeg and 2 parts each clove and cinnamon
Amchur	1 tablespoon lime juice for 1 teaspoon amchur
Aniseed	Fennel seed or star anise
Asafoetida	Onion powder or 1 tablespoon diced white onion
Basil	Mint
Bay leaf	3–5 black peppercorns or juniper berries per leaf
Black cumin	Black mustard seeds or cumin seeds
Cardamom	Equal parts ground cinnamon and cloves
Cardamom pods, green	½ teaspoon ground cardamom = 10 pods
Celery seed	⅓ cup diced celery per 1 teaspoon celery seed
Chile	Any chile can fill in for another
Cinnamon	Allspice
Clove	Allspice
Cocoa, unsweetened	1 square dark chocolate for 3–4 tablespoons

OUT OF THIS?	THEN USE THIS
Coconut	Ground almonds
Coconut milk	Almond milk
Coriander seeds	Cumin seeds
Cumin	Caraway, cut by half
Curry leaf, fresh	4 or 5 dried curry leaves, or 1 dried bay leaf
Fennel seed	Aniseed
Galangal, fresh	Half the amount of powdered galangal or 1 tablespoon fresh diced ginger per two-inch piece of galangal
Galangal, dried	Ginger, cut by half
Garlic, fresh	1 teaspoon powder for 2 fresh cloves
Ginger, fresh	Dry ginger, cut by two-thirds
Ginger, powdered	Ginger, crystallized
Horseradish	Wasabi, or true wasabi by half
Juniper berry	1 teaspoon gin for every 2 berries
Kokum	1 teaspoon tamarind paste per rind
Lemongrass, fresh	Lemon zest (one 2" x 2" piece) and a few slices of ginger

OUT OF THIS?	THEN USE THIS
Marjoram	Thyme; basil; or Spice de Provence cut by half
Mint, fresh	Cilantro
Mint, dried	Parsley
Mustard, dry	Wasabi powder, cut by half
Nutmeg	Half the amount of ground allspice or clove
Onion, fresh	1 tablespoon of minced dried onion per ¼ cup of diced fresh onion
Oregano	Marjoram, 50 percent more
Parsley	Mint or celery leaf
Pomegranate molasses	Pomegranate jelly
Pumpkin seeds	Sunflower seeds
Rosemary	Thyme
Sage, fresh	¼ teaspoon dried sage per 4 leaves
Sage, dried	Rosemary or poultry seasoning
Scallion	Shallots
Shallots	Onion

OUT OF THIS?	THEN USE THIS
Sesame seeds	Coarsely ground pumpkin seeds
Star anise	Aniseed
Sun-dried tomato	1½ cups drained canned tomatoes per ½ cup sun-dried
Tamarind paste	Kokum, ground
Tamarind pulp	1 tablespoon of molasses diluted with 3 tablespoons of fresh lime juice to an equal amount of tamarind
Tamarind water	Fresh lemon juice
Thyme	Ajowan; or half marjoram and half parsley
Turmeric	1 teaspoon ground yellow mustard and a pinch of saffron
Vanilla bean	2 teaspoons extract to 1 whole bean
Wasabi	Chinese hot mustard or English hot mustard

Currying Flavor

The Secret to Creating Powders and Pastes

Spices are to a curry cook what a paint pallet is to an artist. In fact, making a curry *is* an art, a creative undertaking limited only by the cook's ability to balance flavors and textures. But don't let that "creativity" scare you away. Once you understand the basics, creating a curry—even one of your own design—is as easy as painting by the numbers.

Contrary to popular belief, curry does not connote a single dish made with a common commercial spice called "curry powder." Curry is actually a cooking *style*, characterized by a balanced blend of spices (curry) roasted and ground into a powder that simmers and develops flavor in a sauce. The flavor, consistency, and even the color can vary, but there are two constants: a curry is always savory, and it is always spiced.

The word *curry* comes from the Indian word *kari*, and curry dishes are synonymous with the cuisine of India, where they originated thousands of years ago. Traditional Indian curry—still prepared daily in just about every kitchen—does not have a fixed set of ingredients. But it is typically created using a mixture of the following healing spices: black pepper, cardamom, cinnamon, curry leaf, coriander, cumin, fenugreek seed, mustard seed, and turmeric.

In the distant past, spice traders remembered—and tried to duplicate—the redolent, full-bodied, mouth-watering flavor of Indian curry as they traveled around the world. As a result, curries became a hallmark of cuisines in many Asian countries, including Malaysia, Thailand, Myanmar (Burma), and Indonesia, and also on some Caribbean islands. Even England, a country known for its bland food, developed a taste for curry as a result of its centuries-long occupation of India—and England now boasts more curry restaurants than any nation except India.

Over the centuries, as various non-Indian nations adopted the custom of creating curry, they also altered the dishes to reflect local culinary customs, spices, and foods. Malaysia, Indonesia, and Thailand are well known for their innovative but very different curries. Malaysia's curries are mellow, often flavored with mint and coconut, while Thai curries are fiery, frequently flavored with lemongrass, galangal, and red chile. Indonesian curries are also hot, with coriander, cumin, and chile. Even in India, the flavor of curry changes as you travel. The Punjabis in the north, for example, eat milder curries, accented with cardamom, aniseed, nuts, raisins, and yogurt, while the Tamils in the south eat very hot curries, with mustard seed, tamarind, curry leaf, and chile.

Curry Basics

Curry dishes are made by simmering meat, poultry, fish, seafood, or vegetables in a spiced liquid, in much the same way as a French cook simmers food in wine and herbs. The process begins by frying a blend of spices in hot oil (in India, cooks often use a clarified-type butter called *ghee*) and adding spices again at strategic times during the cooking process. The spices can be a dry mix, or modified by adding liquid to spice mixture and stirring it into a paste.

There are various ways to make a curry, but these are the general directions:

1. Start by sautéing basic fresh flavorings, such as onions and garlic, in oil or some other fat until they are soft. In Indian dishes, chiles and ginger are often added. Starting flavorings are always fresh and well chopped. They can include:

- Garlic
- Ginger
- Lemongrass

- Mango
- Onion
- Potato
- Shallots
- Tamarind
- Other vegetables

They are typically fried in one of the following fats:

- Vegetable oil
- Sesame oil
- Mustard oil
- Ghee

You can also forego the basic ingredients and start with Step 2, by adding nothing but [curr]y powder to the oil. (This is more common [in M]alaysian and Thai curries, which use curry [paste] rather than a dry mix.)

[A]dd a curry powder (not commercial curry [powde]r!) or paste. At this point in the process, [additio]nal spices of the cook's choosing can be [added] as well. This is usually a combination of [milde]r spices—perhaps curry leaves, fenu[greek se]ed, turmeric, nutmeg, cinnamon, or star [anise] that balance the pungency of the ingre[dients u]sed in the initial frying. Let the spices [cook] until they release their aroma. This can [happen] fairly quickly, so be at the ready to add [the rest] of the ingredients.

[The] process of sautéing the spices is very [importa]nt. It should be done over a low flame, [and the] spice or paste should be stirred con[stantly] to prevent sticking and burning. As [the spic]es cook, they will start to darken and [cook.] As they lose their pungency, the fla[vors of t]he different spices blend so that no one [flavor is] discernible. Stronger spices such as [cumin,] turmeric, and black pepper will take a [little mo]re time for their somewhat acrid attri[butes to] mellow.

[Nex]t, add the main ingredient, with enough [liquid to] cover. Legumes, potatoes, or vegeta[bles, if de]sired, can also be added at this point. If the main ingredient is meat or poultry, you have the option to brown it first, then remove it from the pot or pan before starting Step 1. Bring the liquid to a simmer, cover and cook gently for an hour or two, depending on the type and quality of the main ingredient. A thickener can be added during this time, if desired. For a dry curry, simmer in less liquid and uncover about halfway through cooking, so the liquid evaporates. If the liquid evaporates too soon, add some water, so the ingredients do not burn or dry out.

Common liquids used in curries are:

- Broth
- Crushed tomatoes
- Coconut milk
- Milk
- Strained yogurt

Common thickeners include:

- Almond or other nut butters
- Ground seed pastes from fenugreek, mustard, poppy, or sesame
- Pureed onions
- Ground coconut pulp
- Dried Indian legumes, such as *chana dal* (split yellow peas) or *urad dal* (split white lentils)
- Lime or lemon juice
- Tamarind paste
- Vinegar

4. Finish by adding more aromatic spices. This can be a custom blend of freshly roasted or ground spices, or simply add a tablespoon of *garam masala* (page 264). Season to taste. Let the curry rest, covered, for about a half hour. It can be kept longer in the oven at a warming temperature of 250°F. Sprinkle the dish with fresh leaves, if desired, such as cilantro, curry leaf, or mint before serving.

Enjoy your curry!

Curries keep well in the refrigerator, and curry flavor improves with age. Your curries will benefit from making them a day or two in advance.

A curry meal isn't complete without the addition of rice, pickles, chutneys, relishes, and (as in India) lots of breads, such as *naan* or *chapati*. Curries *are* spicy, even if they are not hot. The other dishes in the meal, particularly the rice, are meant to contrast the spiciness.

The Cast of Curry Flavors

Curry dishes and the spicy components that define their flavor are as varied as the cultures of the people who eat them. If your goal is to reproduce the curry of a memorable ethnic meal or favorite cuisine, keep in mind that spice rules—and because the spices are so cleverly blended, you can't depend on your nose to figure out which ones to use. However, I can offer you plenty of help. Here is a country-by-country guide to the key flavorings that differentiate one ethnic curry from another.

India

India is the world's seventh largest country by size and second by population, so it's no wonder that taste preferences vary from region to region. Spice dictates how that taste is delivered. To begin, you want to have a top-quality basic curry powder that includes:

- Black pepper
- Coriander
- Cumin
- Red chile (optional)
- Turmeric

Defining the flavor comes with the additional spices used in the curry. North Indian curries tend to be mild and creamy, with nutty nuances. This can be achieved by using a combination of any of these spices:

- Almond
- Bay leaf
- Black cumin seed
- Cardamom, green or brown

- Cinnamon
- Clove
- Fennel seed
- Fenugreek seed
- *Garam masala* (p. 264)
- Garlic
- Mint
- Onion
- Saffron
- Turmeric

South Indian curries can range from hot to fiery and have a distinct scent of coconut. This can be achieved by using a combination of any of these spices:

- Black pepper
- Coconut and coconut milk
- Curry leaf
- Fennel seed
- Fenugreek seed
- Ginger
- Mustard seed
- Red chile
- Tamarind
- Tomato
- Turmeric

East Indian curries tend to be tangy. This can be achieved by including a combination of any of these spices:

- Asafoetida
- Black cumin seed
- Cilantro (fresh coriander leaf)
- Fenugreek seed
- Green chile
- Mustard seed
- *Panch phoron* (p. 266)
- Tamarind

The curries in West India tend to be hot and more on the sour side. This can be achieved by including a combination of these spices and flavorings:

- Coriander
- Mint
- Red chile
- Saffron
- Vinegar

Sri Lanka

The curries in Sri Lanka, an island off the southern tip of India, are both fiery and exotic. The spices for meat curries are roasted very dark, giving the dishes a deep, dark color. (In fact, they are often referred to as "black curries.") Sri Lankan curries almost always include clove and cinnamon, two spices that are indigenous to the island (clove and cinnamon from Sri Lanka are considered some of the best in the world). To make a Sri Lankan curry, use any combination of these spices:

- Cardamom
- Cinnamon
- Clove
- Coconut milk
- Coriander
- Cumin
- Curry leaf
- Fennel seed
- Fenugreek seed
- Red chile
- Tamarind

Thailand

Thai curries are famous for their fire. This is best achieved by starting with a paste pounded with chiles. Use any chile that you desire, as heat is a matter of personal taste. For a list of chiles according to heat, refer to page 73. The distinct flavor that defines a Thai curry, however, comes from an interesting array of flavorings. To make a Thai curry, include any combination of these:

- Black pepper
- Cilantro (fresh coriander leaf)
- Clove
- Coconut and coconut milk

- Coriander
- Cumin
- Fish sauce
- Galangal
- Garlic
- Lemon and lime zest
- Lemongrass
- Peanuts
- Red chile
- Shallots
- Shrimp paste
- Thai basil
- Turmeric

Malaysia

Malaysian curries—the most delicate and complex of Southeast Asian—are strongly influenced by India, and contain many of the same spices. A Malaysian curry will include a combination of these flavorings:

- Black peppercorns
- Candlenuts
- Cinnamon
- Coconut and coconut milk
- Coriander
- Cumin seed
- Fennel seed
- Galangal
- Ginger
- Lemongrass
- Lime
- Mint
- Onion
- Shallots
- Shrimp paste
- Star anise

Vietnam

Vietnamese curries are an interesting blend of Chinese, Indian, and French influences. They are milder than Thai and Indian curries, and have a sweet and sour taste. To make a Vietnamese curry, use any combination of these flavorings:

At the start of cooking a dish with curry spices, Indian and Asian cooks routinely fry the blend of spices in oil or another fat—a different way of incorporating spices into a dish than is typically used in the US. This step is important: it releases the spices' fragrances, creating an enchanting aroma, and the aroma lets you know that it's time to add the next ingredient. However, doing this technique correctly can take a little practice—and you may lose a batch or two until you perfect it. Here's how to do it:

First, make sure you have the next batch of ingredients close by and prepared to go in the pan. The spices can release their fragrance quickly, so if you're not at the ready with the next ingredients, the spices can burn.

Second, heat the pan or skillet for a few minutes (depending on the type of metal in the appliance) over medium-high heat. Once the appliance is heated, add the oil. Let the oil get hot, to about 350°F.

Now you're ready to add the curry mix. Pour the mix —dry or wet—into the pan and grab a wooden spoon. With your other hand, use a potholder or kitchen mitt to grab the handle of the pan or skillet. Move the pan around, while continuously stirring the spices. If neces-sary, lift the skillet to prevent the spices from browning. (You may need to turn down the heat.)

The process can take anywhere from 30 seconds to a few minutes. You know the spices are ready and it's time to add the next ingredients when you detect the spicy aroma.

If you are using a combination of whole and ground spices, put the whole spices in the pan first, as they will take longer to fry.

If mustard seeds are called for, put them in the pan first. They need to pop, and they don't do so evenly in the presence of other ingredients. Have a lid handy to cover, in case the mustard seeds start to pop out.

Putting many spices in a single dish adds marvelous texture, aroma, and flavor—a flavor that isn't found in any individual spice, and one that is craved by many people after they eat a meal in an Indian, Asian, or other ethnic restaurant noted for its spicy cuisine.

However, don't worry about the exact combination of spices you use. In cooking with the healing spices, there are no hard-and-fast rules. If a recipe calls for nine spices and you only have six, it's no problem that three are missing. You'll still get a delicious dish, though the taste will be different.

- Coconut and coconut milk
- Cilantro (fresh coriander leaf)
- Fish sauce
- Garlic
- Lemongrass
- Mint
- Red chile
- Sugar
- Turmeric
- Vinegar

Indonesia

Curry is quite popular in Indonesia, a vast island nation that includes the Maluku Islands, dubbed the "spice islands" by Dutch colonizers. Virtually every region has its own specialty. Indonesian curries contain some of the most exotic ingredients, such as manioc (cassava), salam leaf, and *trassi*, a type of dried shrimp paste. They often come topped with crispy fried shallots and hard-boiled eggs. Other common flavorings include:

- Caraway seed
- Coconut milk
- Curry leaf (as a substitute for salam leaf)
- Galangal
- Ginger
- Lime leaf
- Nutmeg
- Poppy seed
- Red chile
- Tamarind
- Turmeric

Caribbean

Every island has its own specialties, which vary according to local culinary customs. But most curries in the Caribbean are slightly sour, fruity, and hot. Common flavorings include:

- Allspice
- Black peppercorns
- Clove
- Colombo powder (p. 270)
- Coriander seed
- Cumin seed
- Fenugreek seed
- Ginger
- Mustard seed
- Poppy seed
- Turmeric

Custom Curry Blends

There are hundreds of established curry blends from dozens of countries, all without a fixed set of ingredients, and varying in taste, texture, and intensity. Here are some of the best-known curry powders and pastes.

Powders: Commercial, No; Custom, Yes

Commercial curry powder is *taboo* in true curry cooking, because it guarantees sameness in taste no matter what type of dish is being made. But a top-quality customized curry powder that includes a well-proportioned balance of fragrant spices and ground seeds is *essential* to curry cuisine, because it is what gives a curry its aromatic deliciousness.

For the sake of saving time, and because only a small amount is needed to flavor a dish, curry cooks will make a variety of curry powders in small quantities, as they keep well. Use about 1 tablespoon of curry powder for each pound of meat, fish, poultry, or vegetables used as the main ingredient, or for every 1 to 1½ cups of liquid. All the powders here will keep well in an airtight glass container for up to six months.

Madras Curry Powder

This basic curry powder is a good substitute for commercial curry powder. Because the spices are pre-roasted, this powder can be stirred right into liquids without being cooked first. You don't need to limit its use to curries, however. Use it in any recipe calling for curry powder, rub it into meat roasts before putting them in the oven, or sprinkle it in butter sauces or salad dressings.

½ cup coriander seeds
¼ cup cumin seeds
2 tablespoons black mustard seeds
2 teaspoons black peppercorns
1 teaspoon ground ginger
1 teaspoon chili powder

1. In a small, dry heavy skillet over medium heat, roast the coriander, cumin, mustard seeds, and black peppercorns until they become lightly browned and slightly fragrant. Turn the seeds frequently as they cook, so they do not burn. Transfer to a dish to cool.
2. Put the seeds in a spice grinder or mini food processor and grind until the consistency of fine powder. Mix in the ginger and the chili powder. *Makes about 1 cup.*

Hot Curry Powder

This powder from South India is hot and pungent and goes well with chicken, fish, lamb, and vegetarian curries.

1 cup coriander seeds
½ cup cumin seeds
¼ cup fennel seeds
¼ cup black mustard seeds
2 teaspoons fenugreek seeds
¼ cup dried chiles
2 tablespoons black peppercorns
20 dried curry leaves
1 tablespoon turmeric

Perfectly Browned Onions and Garlic

The secret to thick golden-red curries and tomato sauces is in the *onions*. Indian chefs call the technique brown frying and it serves a multiple purpose, adding color, flavor, fragrance, and thickness to sauce (or what Indian cuisine refers to as *gravy*).

Brown frying takes about 20 minutes and requires careful attention. Fried properly, the onions transform from pungent to a distinctively sweet flavor, as the heated molecules turn to sugar.

Don't allow the onions to burn: they'll turn bitter instead of sweet, and the spectacular sauce will be lost. If you burn the onions, throw them away, clean the pot, and start over again. You won't have to do that, however, if you follow the instructions below. (For every cup of onions, use two tablespoons of fat—one that is low in saturated fat and high in heart-healthy monounsaturated fats, such as olive oil or canola oil.) Here's what to do:

1. Pour the fat into a heavy-bottomed skillet or Dutch oven (depending on what you are making) over low heat for a minute or two until the fat gets hot. Throw in a few onions to test the temperature before adding the whole batch. If the oil is too hot, the onions will not brown evenly. The oil should be hot but not sizzling.
2. Add either thinly sliced or diced onions and mix to coat them with the fat. Turn the heat to medium-high and fry, turning the onions continually with a wooden spoon, as they gradually lose their moisture and release their volatile oils, about five minutes. The onions should be wilted and lightly golden.
3. Continue to cook, turning continually, for another five minutes. The onions may start to clump together as they start to turn a deeper brown. Adjust the heat, if necessary, so they do not burn. If onions begin to burn, add a tablespoon or two of cold water to cool the temperature. Do not remove from the pot or pan from heat, as you should not interrupt the process.
4. Add your diced garlic (or garlic and ginger, as they do in India) and fry another five minutes. It is important to keep turning, so the mixture does not burn. You should have perfect, evenly brown onions with no signs of scorching.

You can prepare browned onions in advance and keep them in the refrigerator. Just bring them to room temperature before putting them in a pan to continue on with a recipe. For browning ahead, figure ¼ cup of browned onions for every cup of raw onions called for in a recipe.

You can also freeze browned onions and defrost them in the refrigerator before using. Freeze them in the amount you typically use in an individual recipe.

---

1. In a small, dry heavy skillet over medium heat, individually roast the coriander seeds, cumin seeds, fennel seeds, mustard seeds, and fenugreek seeds until they become lightly browned and slightly fragrant. Turn the seeds frequently as they cook so they do not burn.
2. Put the seeds, dried chiles, peppercorns, and curry leaves in a spice mill or mini food processor and process to a fine powder. Blend in the turmeric. *Makes about 1½ cups.*

Pastes: Variety in Flavor and Fire

Wet curries—also known as *pastes*—are spices ground with or added to water, oil, vinegar, or coconut milk. Unless otherwise indicated, these pastes should be cooled, if cooked, stored in an airtight glass container, and refrigerated where they will keep for two weeks to one month. They can also be frozen. If freezing, divide into small amounts so you can defrost as needed. Always defrost in the refrigerator.

Here is a sampling of excellent basic pastes, some which call for traditional roasting of the seeds and some made with spices already ground. When using ground, make sure the powder is fresh. Consider 1 to 2 tablespoons of paste per pound of the food used as the main ingredient.

Madras Curry Paste

This paste is quite versatile. In addition to making curries, you can use it as a have-on-hand replacement in recipes calling for garlic, ginger, and similar savory spices. It is designed to enhance the flavor of beef, poultry, and fish curries.

> ½ cup coriander seeds
> ¼ cup cumin seeds
> 2 teaspoons black mustard seeds
> 2 teaspoons black peppercorns
> 1 tablespoon diced fresh ginger
> 1 tablespoon diced garlic
> 2 teaspoon chili powder
> 1 teaspoon salt
> ⅓ cup distilled white vinegar

1. In a small, dry heavy skillet over medium heat, individually roast the coriander, cumin, and mustard seeds until they become lightly browned and slightly fragrant. Turn the seeds frequently as they cook, so they do not burn. Transfer to a dish to cool.
2. Put the seeds and black peppercorns in a spice grinder or mini food processor and grind until the consistency of fine powder.
3. Combine the spice powder, ginger, garlic, chili powder, and salt in a small bowl. Stir in the vinegar until it becomes a smooth paste. Add more if necessary. *Makes about 1 cup.*

Vindaloo Curry Paste

Vindaloo is a hot and sour curry popular in South India. It is perfect paste for pork and game, as its acidity and astringency balance their richness. Vindaloo paste, and the food it's cooked with, is designed to keep for several months under refrigeration.

> 4 tablespoons ground cumin
> 2 tablespoons freshly ground black pepper
> 2 tablespoons ground coriander
> 2 tablespoons ground ginger
> 2 tablespoons turmeric
> 2 tablespoons chili powder
> 2 tablespoons ground mustard
> 2 tablespoons salt
> ½ cup white vinegar
> ½ cup vegetable oil

1. Place the first eight ingredients in a medium-size mixing bowl and combine. Whisk in the vinegar until the mixture form a paste, somewhat like the texture of peanut butter.
2. Heat the oil in a nonstick saucepan over medium-high heat. Add the paste, reduce the heat to low, and vigorously mix with a wire whisk continuously so the spices do not stick and burn. Do not get too close, as the spices give off pungent vapors that could irritate sensitive eyes. Continue to stir until the spices mellow, about 10 minutes. Set aside to cool.
3. Put the cooled paste in an airtight jar and refrigerate until ready to use. *Makes about 2 cups.*

Thai Red Curry Paste

Red curry is Thailand's most famous curry. You can adjust the heat by increasing or decreasing the amount of chiles. Thai cooks use coriander roots, but since they are hard to find, the leaves are an adequate substitute. Shrimp paste can be found in an Asian market or via the Internet. For a list of suppliers, see the "Buyer's Guide" on page 309. You can also use this paste as a rub under the skin of chicken, or add a tablespoon to your favorite meatball or meatloaf mixtures.

> 5–10 dried red chiles
> 1 tablespoon coriander seeds
> 2 stalks lemongrass, outer sheath removed and sliced

1 two-inch piece galangal, coarsely chopped,
   or 1 tablespoon ground (Laos powder)
4 shallots, diced
5 cloves garlic, chopped
¼ cup chopped Thai basil
⅓ cup chopped cilantro
2 teaspoons shrimp paste (optional)

1. Put all the ingredients in a food processor with a metal blade and process to the consistency of a smooth paste. Stop the processor occasionally to scrape down the sides. *Makes about 1½ cups.*

Malaysian Curry Paste

In Malaysia this curry is made with candlenuts, which are indigenous to the area and difficult to find. Macadamia nuts make a fine substitute, but you can also use dry roasted peanuts. This paste goes well with chicken, fish, or seafood.

2 tablespoons coriander seeds
1 tablespoon fennel seeds
1 one-and-a-half-inch cinnamon stick
2 teaspoons black peppercorns
1 tablespoon minced ginger
¼ cup macadamia nuts
4 cloves garlic
4 large shallots
1 teaspoon turmeric
1 teaspoon ground lemongrass
¼ cup distilled white vinegar
¼ cup water
1 teaspoon lemon juice

1. In a small, dry heavy skillet over medium heat, individually roast the coriander seeds, fennel seeds, cinnamon, and peppercorns until they become lightly browned and slightly fragrant. Turn the seeds frequently as they cook so they do not burn. Transfer to a dish to cool.
2. Put the seeds in a spice grinder and process until smooth.

3. Put the ginger, nuts, garlic, and shallots in a food processor and process for 30 seconds. Add the turmeric, lemongrass, the ground spices, vinegar, water, and lemon juice. Process to a smooth paste. Transfer to an airtight glass container. *Makes about 1 cup.*

Caribbean Curry Paste

This recipe delivers a super hot curry paste, which is the custom in many of the islands. It comes from Trinidad, where the cuisine has an Indian influence. If you want to turn down the heat, use a less incendiary chile, such as a jalapeño.

¼ cup coriander seeds
1 teaspoon black peppercorns
1 teaspoon cumin seeds
1 teaspoon black mustard seeds
1 teaspoon fenugreek seeds
1 tablespoon turmeric
1 teaspoon cloves
4 star anise
1 large onion
3 garlic cloves
1 fresh Habanera chile, cut in half and seeds removed
1 1-inch piece fresh ginger
¼ cup oil

1. In a small, dry heavy skillet over medium heat, individually roast the coriander seeds, peppercorns, cumin seeds, mustard seeds, and fenugreek seeds, until they become lightly browned and slightly fragrant. Turn the seeds frequently as they cook, so they do not burn. Transfer to a dish to cool.
2. Put the roasted spices, turmeric, cloves, star anise, onion, garlic, chili, ginger, , and oil in a food processor and process to the consistency of a smooth paste. *Makes about ¾ cup.*

Hot and Healthy:

Healing Tips from the World's Warm Zones

Indian hospitality is legendary—and that hospitality often revolves around *food*. Traditionally, Indians have a sensually sophisticated approach to eating, and an appreciation of the link between good company, good food, and good health.

That tradition is embodied in *Ayurveda*, the ancient Indian system of natural health and healing. (*Ayur* means life or daily living, and *veda* means knowledge.) Ayurveda sees all of life as a cosmic play of five elements—space (or ether), air, fire, water, and earth. Those basic elements are expressed in the human body-mind as three *doshas*: *vatta* (space and air), *pitta* (fire and water), and *kapha* (water and earth). Each dosha controls a set of physical, mental, and emotional functions. Pitta, for example, controls body heat, intelligence, and anger. Everyone has a natural predominance of one dosha. Ayurveda seeks to keep the three doshas *balanced*, for maximum health and healing.

What does all this have to do with spices? Well, one of the principal ways Ayurveda balances the doshas is through food—including the all-important *taste* of food! To balance the doshas, Ayurveda teaches that every meal include an intelligent combination of all six *rasas*, or tastes: sweet, sour, bitter, pungent (spicy), strong (astringent), and salty.

Traditional Chinese medicine (TCM) has a similar philosophy and practice. TCM sees *chi* as the cosmic energy or life-force that flows through the body-mind. An excess or lack of *chi*—too much or too little *yang*, or heat; too much or too little *yin*, or cold—is the cause of disease. And one way chi is kept balanced is through a balance of five tastes: sweet, sour, bitter, spicy (hot), and salty.

In other words, in the ancient traditions of India and China, the meticulous blending of tastes—and spices—is seen as key to maintaining health and healing disease.

Charting Your Way to Spicing Expertise
Along with India and China, many of the warmer zones of the world are famous for a love of spices and an expertise in combining them. Needless to say, those combinations produce the uniquely delicious foods and meals that Americans have come to love when they visit restaurants that feature Thai or Vietnamese or Indonesian— well, you name *your* favorite flavorful "ethnic" cuisine!

But the fact that the peoples of the warmer zones are experts in spicing food is not really surprising. The plants, bushes, and trees that are the source of most of the world's spices are native to those very countries and regions. In the world's warmer zones, spices were medicine, spices were preservatives, spices were flavorings, spices were even money. The equivalence of spices and health—of spices and *life*—was obvious. And it still is.

That's why when you visit a household in many of the "spice nations" you probably won't see a measuring spoon or cup, but you probably will see a mortar and pestle—and a spice cupboard filled not with labeled bottles but with seeds, pods, and powders in a colorful array. And it's not unlikely that your hosts are masters at combining their stock of spices into remarkable (as in the remark, *Delicious!*) flavors.

But you don't have to come from one of the spice-loving countries around the world to specialize in spicing food. Artfully pairing spices in a recipe *is* a skill—but a skill anyone can acquire. All it takes is practice, patience—and knowing this one secret: creatively combining multiple spices in one scrumptious dish calls for (yes, that watchword of Ayurveda and TCM) *balance.*

Spice blends are called *blends* because they balance flavors in a harmonious unity where no one flavor dominates. To help you blend and balance spices for your recipes, we've provided this table "A Taste for Spices" below.

The table places each of the 50 spices in this book into one of six taste categories: sweet, sour, bitter, strong, pungent, and hot. The placement of a particular spice into a particular category is far from arbitrary (garlic *is* hot; vanilla *is* sweet), but it's also not absolute—an individual spice can bridge several tastes. Cumin, for example, is pungent but has a bitter aftertaste. Amchur is both sweet and sour.

As the chart moves from left to right—from sweet to hot—the flavors get stronger. To achieve balance, your combination of spices should roughly equal the percentages indicated on the table.

And, as you'll see, the percentages of sweet/sour/bitter to strong/pungent/hot spices aren't equal. A pungent spice, for example, will overwhelm a sweet spice if you use them in the same amounts, but using more of a sweet spice (or a

Alamelu's Salt Substitute

This superb salt substitute was designed by Alamelu Vairavan, author of *Healthy South Indian Cooking*. It's amazing how well it mimics the real thing—unlike most commercial salt substitutes, there are no chemicals in the blend and no less-than-pleasing aftertaste. It's also very simple to make: Mix equal parts of ground black pepper and ground cumin seeds. (No pre-roasting is necessary.) After preparation, put it in a salt shaker. Use the same amount of this salt substitute as the salt called for in a recipe.

combination of sweet spices) helps you achieve balance.

Whatever you do, remember this: there are no hard-and-fast rules to combining spices, no right way or wrong way. If you want a blend to taste sour or hot, then emphasize more sour or hot spice combinations in the recipe—and add balance with other tastes.

If you want to achieve balance according to the six tastes of Ayurveda or the five tastes of TCM, you'll need to add some salt. If you're required to

A Taste for Spices					
Sweet **30%**	**Sour** **25%**	**Bitter** **20%**	**Strong** **15%**	**Pungent** **5–7%**	**Hot** **3–5%**
Allspice	Amchur	Ajowan	Basil	Asafoetida	Black pepper
Almond	Chile	Cocoa	Bay leaf	Celery seed	Galangal
Aniseed	Juniper berry	Fenugreek seed	Black cumin seed	Clove	Garlic
Cinnamon	Kokum	Turmeric	Caraway	Cumin	Horseradish
Coconut	Lemongrass		Cardamom	Ginger	Mustard seed
Coriander	Pomegranate		Curry leaf	Marjoram	Onion
Fennel seed	Tamarind		Mint	Oregano	Wasabi
Nutmeg			Parsley	Rosemary	
Pumpkin seed			Saffron	Sage	
Sesame seed				Sun-dried tomato	
Star anise				Thyme	
Vanilla					

restrict your salt intake (because of high blood pressure, for example), the salt substitute featured on page 289 is a wonderful option.

As you cook more with spices, making spice blends and even designing your own blends will become more appealing. And a spice blend of your own creation or one from this book makes a great gift for friends. Use "A Taste for Spices" as your guide—and enjoy your new adventure with the healing spices!

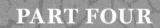

PART FOUR

Spices as
Natural Medicines

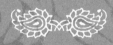

From Arthritis to Ulcers, an A-to-Z Guide to the Therapeutic Potential of the Healing Spices

Perhaps you have heart disease—or a family history of the disease, and you want to prevent it. Or maybe you want to be more proactive in making anti-cancer meals for your family. Or you're trying to find a drug-free way to help relieve arthritis pain. Or you want to balance blood sugar that your doctor says is too high. Whatever your health goal, this at-a-glance chart can help you achieve it—by using more of the healing spices that scientific research shows may help prevent or treat the condition you're concerned about.

However, I need to qualify that statement a bit. This condition-by-condition guide is a list of *ideas*, not of *advice*. The scientific evidence that supports the use of spices to prevent and treat specific health conditions is at many different levels of power and persuasion. Some are test tube studies. Some are on experimental animals. Some were conducted with people, and only some of those were the rigorous "gold-standard" studies that doctors rely on most to judge which treatments really work and which don't. I've included *all* levels of evidence because all of it is promising; but only some of it is proven. The best approach to the healing spices: empha-size those that affect the condition you want to prevent or control, but—as with fruits and vegetables—incorporate as many healing spices as possible into your diet, to employ their full healing power.

Another caveat: never use these spices *instead* of medical care. But do consider them as a possibly powerful adjunct to medical care. And a uniquely effective way to help potentially *prevent* the diseases listed.

That being said, here's the best way to use this guide. Look up the condition you're concerned about in Column 1—and then fill your diet with the spices listed in Column 2! Unlike medicines with their side effects, you can't go wrong adding these culinary spices to your diet.

Column 3 offers specific therapeutic dosages for using spices as *supplements* (such as cinnamon for diabetes) based on one or more studies that have successfully tested the spice at that dosage for that disease. As with all nutritional and herbal supplements, use a spice supplement *only* with the approval and supervision of your medical doctor or another qualified health professional.

Health Condition	Healing Spices	Research-Tested Therapeutic Use
ACNE	Basil Coconut Turmeric	• 500 mg curcumin (turmeric active ingredient), two times a day
AGE SPOTS	Oregano	
AGING	Black cumin seed Garlic Thyme	• For age-related immune decline: Black cumin oil extract (thymoquinone), following the dosage recommendation on the label
ALCOHOL ABUSE	Thyme	
ALLERGIES	Ajowan Black cumin seed Galangal Mint Onion Turmeric	• 40–80 mg of black cumin oil, daily
ALOPECIA AREATA (GENERALIZED HAIR LOSS)	Garlic	
ALZHEIMER'S DISEASE AND NON-ALZHEIMER'S DEMENTIA	Black pepper Cocoa Coconut Curry leaf Fennel seed Marjoram Oregano Pomegranate Saffron Sage Sesame seed Sun-dried tomato Turmeric	• 30 mg saffron, daily • For prevention, drink a cup of cocoa or eat a half ounce of dark chocolate, daily. • For prevention, take aged garlic extract (AGE), following the dosage recommendations on the label.
ANEMIA (IRON DEFICIENCY)	Pumpkin seed	
ANGINA	Pomegranate	• 2 eight-ounce glasses of pomegranate juice, daily
ANXIETY	Lemongrass Mint Nutmeg Rosemary Saffron Sage	• Unsweetened cocoa powder in hot water as a beverage, daily • 300 mg of sage extract, daily • For test anxiety, soak a small piece of cotton with rosemary essential oil, wrap it in a handkerchief, and sniff it before and during test time.
ARTHRITIS, OSTEO-	Bay leaf Celery seed Chile Fennel seed Galangal Ginger	• 1–2 grams of ginger, daily • .025% capsaicin cream (from chile), as directed (Increase to the .075% potency if there is no benefit from the lower dose.)

Health Condition	Healing Spices	Research-Tested Therapeutic Use
(continued) **ARTHRITIS, OSTEO-**	Juniper berry Pomegranate Rosemary Turmeric	
ARTHRITIS, RHEUMATOID	Bay Leaf Black pepper Celery seed Fennel seed Ginger Juniper berry Pomegranate Pumpkin seed Rosemary Turmeric	• 1,200 mg curcumin (turmeric active ingredient), daily
ASTHMA	Ajowan Aniseed Black cumin seed Cardamom Ginger Turmeric Wasabi	• 200 mg cineole oil (active ingredient in cardamom), daily
ATHEROSCLEROSIS	Pomegranate Saffron	• 2 eight-ounce glasses of pomegranate juice, daily
BAD BREATH	Aniseed Cardamom Clove Parsley	
BENIGN PROSTATIC HYPERTROPHY	Amchur Garlic Mustard seed Onion Pumpkin seed	• 160 mg pumpkin seed extract, three times a day, with meals
BLEMISHES	Turmeric	• A traditional Indian remedy for blemishes combines ¼ cup garbanzo (chickpea) flour, with 1 teaspoon turmeric, add 2 drops of vegetable oil, and add water to form a thick paste. Put on blemish and leave until it dries, about 10 minutes. Rinse off. Repeat several times a week until skin is clear.
BLOATING	Coriander	

Health Condition	Healing Spices		Research-Tested Therapeutic Use
BLOOD CLOTS	Cardamom Chile Clove Garlic Marjoram Rosemary Sun-dried tomato Thyme Wasabi		• Garlic oil or aged garlic extract (AGE), daily, according to dosage recommendations on the label. Caution: May interact with blood thinners. Talk to your doctor.
BREASTFEEDING PROBLEMS	Mint		
BRONCHITIS	Horseradish Juniper berry Thyme		• Bronchipret (thyme and ivy formula), following the dosage recommendation on the label
CANCER	Amchur Asafoetida Basil Bay leaf Black cumin seed Black pepper Caraway Chile Cinnamon Clove Coconut Coriander Cumin Fennel seed Fenugreek seed Galangal Garlic Ginger Horseradish Juniper berry	Kokum Lemongrass Marjoram Mint Mustard seed Nutmeg Onion Oregano Parsley Pomegranate Rosemary Saffron Sage Sesame seed Star anise Sun-dried tomato Tamarind Thyme Turmeric Vanilla Wasabi	• These spices may have preventive power, or were proven to have anti-cancer potential in test tube and animal studies. Turmeric (curcumin) is undergoing clinical trials.
CATARACTS	Fenugreek seed Tamarind		
CHOLESTEROL PROBLEMS (HIGH TOTAL CHOLESTEROL, HIGH "BAD" LDL CHOLESTEROL, OR LOW "GOOD" HDL CHOLESTEROL)	Almond Basil Black cumin seed Caraway Celery seed Chile Cinnamon Cocoa Coriander		• A handful of almonds daily, to help prevent and reduce high total cholesterol • 140 mg lemongrass oil (citral), daily • 900 mg standard garlic extract or ½ to 1 clove of garlic, daily

Health Condition	Healing Spices	Research-Tested Therapeutic Use
(continued) **CHOLESTEROL PROBLEMS (HIGH TOTAL CHOLESTEROL, HIGH "BAD" LDL CHOLESTEROL, OR LOW "GOOD" HDL CHOLESTEROL)**	Curry leaf Fenugreek seed Garlic Ginger Horseradish Lemongrass Mustard seed Nutmeg Onion Oregano Pumpkin seed Sesame seed Sun-dried tomato Tamarind Turmeric Wasabi	
CHRONIC OBSTRUCTIVE PULMONARY DISEASE (COPD)	Mint Mustard seed	• To help treat, make a mustard plaster by saturating a poultice (cloth) with mustard seed powder, putting it inside a protective casing, and applying to the chest.
COLD SORES	Clove Juniper berry Sage Star anise Thyme	
COLDS	Garlic Juniper berry Thyme	
COLIC	Aniseed Cardamom Coriander Fennel seed Turmeric	
COLITIS (INFLAMMATORY BOWEL DISEASE)	Black cumin seed Fennel seed Oregano Pomegranate Thyme Turmeric	
COLON CANCER	Cardamom Coriander Curry leaf	
CONJUNCTIVITIS (PINK EYE)	Basil Tamarind	

Health Condition	Healing Spices		Research-Tested Therapeutic Use
CONSTIPATION	Aniseed Black pepper Caraway Cardamom Coriander Parsley Tamarind		• Add a ¼ teaspoon tamarind puree to sweetened cereal in the morning, or about an ounce of tamarind in food throughout the day.
COUGH	Ajowan Mint Thyme		
CROHN'S DISEASE (INFLAMMATORY BOWEL DISEASE)	Coconut		
CYSTIC FIBROSIS	Turmeric		
DEHYDRATION	Aniseed		
DEMENTIA, NON-ALZHEIMER'S	Cocoa Fennel seed Star anise Sun-dried tomato		• For prevention, drink a cup of cocoa or eat a half ounce of dark chocolate, daily. • For prevention, take aged garlic extract (AGE), following the dosage recommendations on the label.
DENTURE PROBLEMS	Clove Pomegranate		
DEPRESSION	Black pepper Nutmeg Rosemary Saffron		• 15 mg saffron, twice a day
DERMATITIS	Black cumin seed Rosemary Sage Turmeric		
DIABETES, TYPE 1	Tamarind		
DIABETES, TYPE 2	Almond Amchur Basil Bay leaf Caraway Chile Cinnamon Cocoa Coriander Cumin Curry leaf	Fenugreek seed Galangal Garlic Juniper berry Lemongrass Mustard seed Onion Parsley Pomegranate Rosemary Sage Turmeric	• ¼ teaspoon of cinnamon (or 1 gram of cinnamon supplement), daily • Bring 1 gram caraway seeds and ½ cup of distilled water to a low boil. Simmer 10 minutes and cool. Drink daily.

Health Condition	Healing Spices	Research-Tested Therapeutic Use
DIABETIC NEUROPATHY	Chile	• Capsaicin (from chile), used topically, as directed by your doctor
DIARRHEA	Ajowan Cardamom Coriander Nutmeg	
DRY EYE SYNDROME	Basil Tamarind	
DYSPHAGIA (DIFFICULTY SWALLOWING)	Black pepper	
EAR INFECTION	Horseradish	
ECZEMA (ATOPIC DERMATITIS)	Black cumin seed Coriander Sage Turmeric Wasabi	
EPILEPSY	Black cumin seed Cumin Lemongrass Nutmeg	
ERECTILE DYSFUNCTION	Pomegranate Saffron	• Dissolve several threads of saffron in warm milk and drink three times a day. • Drink 1 or 2 glasses of pomegranate juice a day.
EYE INFECTION	Basil Tamarind Turmeric	
FALLS	Black pepper	
FATIGUE, MENTAL	Cocoa Mint Saffron Sage	• A cup of cocoa (made with unsweetened cocoa powder) or eating ½ to 1 ounce of dark chocolate • Saffron extract, following the dosage recommendation on the label
FATIGUE, PHYSICAL	Cocoa Pomegranate	
FLATULENCE	Ajowan Aniseed Asafoetida Coriander Turmeric	

Health Condition	Healing Spices	Research-Tested Therapeutic Use
FLU	Asafoetida Garlic Horseradish Juniper berry Pomegranate Star anise Thyme	• For prevention, 1 clove of garlic, daily
FOOD POISONING	Bay leaf Caraway Cinnamon Clove Cumin Horseradish Oregano Wasabi	• These spices have been found to inhibit the bacteria that cause food poisoning, but have not proven to be preventative or curative.
FUNGAL INFECTION	Juniper berry Marjoram	
GALLBLADDER DISEASE	Turmeric	• 20 mg turmeric, daily
GALLSTONES	Fenugreek seed	
GENITAL HERPES	Clove Sage	
GLAUCOMA	Fennel seed	
GOUT	Basil Celery seed Rosemary Turmeric	• Celery seed extract, following the dosage recommendation on the label
GUM DISEASE (GINGIVITIS OR PERIODONTAL DISEASE)	Amchur Clove Mint Pomegranate Turmeric	
HEADACHE, TENSION (SEE ALSO MIGRAINE)	Chile	
HEARING LOSS	Black pepper	
HEART ATTACK	Basil Chile Garlic Ginger Onion Sun-dried tomato Thyme	

Health Condition	Healing Spices		Research-Tested Therapeutic Use
HEART DISEASE	Almond Amchur Black cumin seed Black pepper Cardamom Chile Cinnamon Cocoa Fennel seed Garlic Marjoram	Mustard seed Onion Oregano Parsley Pumpkin seed Rosemary Sage Sesame seed Sun-dried tomato Tamarind Turmeric	• 1 handful of almonds, five times a week • 1 cup of unsweetened cocoa mixed in water, daily • Garlic, liberally added to the diet • 500 mg curcumin, daily • 1 ounce dark chocolate, daily • Tomato and tomato products, daily
HEART FAILURE	Juniper berry		
HEARTBURN (GASTROESOPHAGEAL REFLUX DISEASE, OR GERD)	Caraway Ginger Turmeric		
HEMORRHOIDS	Juniper berry		
HEPATITIS B	Star anise		
HEPATITIS C	Clove		
HIGH BLOOD PRESSURE (HYPERTENSION)	Ajowan Allspice Almond Black cumin seed Black pepper Cardamom Celery seed Cinnamon Cocoa Coriander Fennel seed	Garlic Juniper berry Onion Oregano Pomegranate Saffron Sesame seed Sun-dried tomato Tamarind Turmeric	• 1 gram garlic extract, daily • 1 cup cocoa, with 1 tablespoon unsweetened cocoa powder in water, daily • 200 mg black cumin seed extract, daily
HIRSUTISM (UNWANTED HAIR GROWTH IN WOMEN)	Fennel seed Mint		• 2 cups of spearmint tea a day during and five days following menstrual cycle
HIV/AIDS	Star Anise		
HUNTINGTON'S DISEASE	Sesame seed		
INDIGESTION	Ajowan Aniseed Bay leaf Black pepper Caraway Cardamom	Chile Coriander Ginger Juniper berry Kokum Marjoram Mint	• Enteric-coated peppermint oil, 15 to 30 minutes before meals

Health Condition	Healing Spices		Research-Tested Therapeutic Use
INFECTION, BACTERIAL, FUNGAL OR VIRAL	Ajowan Coconut Fenugreek seed Marjoram Oregano Thyme		
INFECTION, PARASITIC	Oregano		
INFERTILITY, MALE	Pomegranate Saffron Sun-dried tomato		• Dissolve several threads of saffron in warm milk and drink twice a day.
INSOMNIA	Coriander Lemongrass Saffron		
INSULIN RESISTANCE (PREDIABETES)	Almond Cinnamon Cocoa Fenugreek seed Mustard seed Oregano		• 1 gram of fenugreek seed daily, soaked in hot water, to improve insulin sensitivity
IRRITABLE BOWEL SYNDROME	Asafoetida Coriander Mint		• Enteric-coated peppermint oil, three or four times a day
ITCHING	Turmeric		
KIDNEY DISEASE	Juniper berry		
KIDNEY STONES	Fenugreek seed		
	Tamarind		
LEAD POISONING	Coriander		
LIVER DISEASE	Celery seed Coriander Fenugreek seed	Juniper berry Oregano Rosemary Turmeric	
MACULAR DEGENERATION, AGE-RELATED	Saffron Tamarind Turmeric		
MALARIA	Basil		
MEMORY LOSS (AGE-RELATED, MILD COGNITIVE DECLINE)	Black pepper Cocoa Curry leaf Nutmeg Rosemary Saffron Sage		• Saffron extract, following the dosage recommendation on the label

Health Condition	Healing Spices	Research-Tested Therapeutic Use
MENOPAUSE PROBLEMS	Allspice Mint	
MENSTRUAL CRAMPS	Celery seed Fennel seed Juniper berry Mint Saffron	
METABOLIC SYNDROME	Almond Cinnamon Oregano	• 500 mg cinnamon (Cinnulin PF), daily
MIGRAINE	Ginger	• 1 to 2 grams, at first sign of a migraine headache
MONONUCLEOSIS	Star anise	
MORNING SICKNESS	Ginger	• 1 to 2 grams, daily
MOSQUITO BITES	Bay leaf Celery seed Clove	
MOTION SICKNESS	Ginger	• 1 gram of ginger, 30 minutes before travel
MULTIPLE SCLEROSIS	Black cumin seed Saffron	
NASAL CONGESTION	Mint	
NAUSEA	Ginger Mint	• 500 mg to 2 grams ginger, daily
NECK PAIN	Chile	• .025% topical capsaicin cream (from chile), as directed
NERVE PAIN (NEUROPATHY)	Chile	• .025% topical capsaicin cream (from chile), as directed
OSTEOPOROSIS	Cumin Onion Sun-dried tomato Wasabi	
OVERWEIGHT	Almond Black pepper Chile Coconut Fenugreek seed Kokum Oregano Pomegranate Turmeric	• Handful of almonds, five times a week • 350 mg of fenugreek, three times a day, before meals

Health Condition	Healing Spices	Research-Tested Therapeutic Use
PAIN	Ajowan Basil Black cumin seed Coconut Juniper berry Turmeric	• .025% topical capsaicin cream, as directed
PARKINSON'S DISEASE	Saffron Sun-dried tomato Turmeric	
PNEUMONIA, BACTERIAL	Horseradish	
POLLUTION SIDE-EFFECTS	Marjoram Turmeric	• 500 mg curcumin/pepperine, daily
POLYCYSTIC OVARIAN SYNDROME (PCOS)	Cinnamon Mint	• 333 mg cinnamon, three times a day
POSTHERPETIC NEURALGIA	Chili Mint	• .025% capcaisin cream, as directed
PREECLAMPSIA	Cocoa	
PREMENSTRUAL SYNDROME (PMS)	Saffron	
PSORIASIS	Chile Coriander Sage Turmeric	• 0.25% capsaicin cream (from chile), as directed
RASH	Kokum Turmeric	
ROSACEA	Coriander	
SCARS	Onion	
SCLERODERMA	Turmeric	
SEPTIC SHOCK	Star anise	
SEVERE ACUTE RESPIRATORY SYNDROME (SARS)	Bay leaf	
SICKLE CELL DISEASE	Garlic Vanilla	
SINUSITIS	Cardamom Horseradish	• ½ to ¾ drained prepared horseradish in food, such as cocktail sauce, three times a day • 200 mg cineole oil (active ingredient in cardamom), three times a day
SMOKING ADDICTION	Black pepper	
SORE THROAT	Sage	
STAPH INFECTION	Oregano	

Health Condition	Healing Spices		Research-Tested Therapeutic Use
STOMACHACHE	Aniseed Cardamom Coriander		
STREP THROAT	Horseradish		
STRESS	Basil Mint Rosemary		• 1 cup of unsweetened cocoa powder in hot water, daily
STROKE	Almond Celery seed Chile Cinnamon Cocoa Fennel seed	Garlic Ginger Marjoram Rosemary Sage Thyme Turmeric	
THRUSH (ORAL CANDIDA INFECTION)	Garlic Lemongrass Oregano		
THYROID PROBLEMS	Amchur Black pepper		
TOOTH DECAY	Mint Star anise Thyme Wasabi		• CervitecPlus (a tooth varnish containing thymol from thyme and the antiseptic chlorhexidine), used as instructed
TOOTHACHE	Clove		• For pain relief, moisten absorbent gauze with oil of clove and secure it next to the sore tooth.
TRIGLYCERIDES, HIGH	Almond Basil Caraway Cinnamon Curry leaf Fenugreek seed Garlic Ginger Lemongrass Oregano Pumpkin seed Tamarind		• 900 mg standard garlic extract or ½ to 1 clove of garlic daily
TUBERCULOSIS	Caraway Cumin		

Health Condition	Healing Spices		Research-Tested Therapeutic Use
ULCER	Aniseed Basil Bay leaf Black cumin seed Cardamom Celery seed Chile Cinnamon Clove	Coriander Galangal Kokum Marjoram Oregano Parsley Rosemary Sage Thyme Wasabi	
URINARY INCONTINENCE	Pumpkin seed		
URINARY TRACT INFECTION	Horseradish Juniper berry Rosemary		
VAGINAL YEAST INFECTION	Celery seed Cinnamon Coconut Coriander Lemongrass Oregano		
VITILIGO	Black pepper		
WOUNDS	Basil Bay leaf Cinnamon Juniper berry Sesame seed Turmeric		
WRINKLES AND AGING SKIN	Cocoa Garlic Nutmeg Pomegranate Rosemary		

PART FIVE

Resources

A Buyer's Guide to the Healing Spices

You can find most of the spices in this book in the typical supermarket. A few spices that are "exotic" to the American palette, such as kokum, might take a little detective work—but I can help you with that!

You can usually find the spices that aren't yet popular in the US on the shelves of an Asian, Indian, Latin, or Middle Eastern market, depending on the spice's origin, popularity, or use in a culture's cuisine.

If you live in an area with one or more large ethnic populations, you'll probably find such a market nearby. To locate one close to you, check the yellow pages of the phone book, or go online. Many of these markets don't advertise, so there could be one closer than you think. Surveys show that 50 percent of the US population is within driving distance of an ethnic market—often several.

The typical supermarket is limited to generic spices. For example, you can find oregano, but you're not going to find Mexican oregano. Or you'll find pepper, but not necessarily Tellicherry black pepper or white pepper. Or almonds, but not necessarily Majorca almonds. And if you want *genuine* wasabi, you might be hard pressed to find it even in an Asian market!

And that's where this guide comes in handy. The online specialty spice shops featured below—all just a click or a call away—cater to folks who want to go beyond the generic in spices. This guide will help you find even the spices and other ingredients in this book that you may not find in a typical, well-stocked supermarket.

The "Buyer's Guide" is by no means a complete list of every retailer and outlet that carries quality spices or a specific, hard-to-find spice, but it offers more than enough to find what you're looking for.

(Note: The Web sites were current when this book went to press.)

Specialty and Gourmet Spice Retailers

Penn Herb Co.
This Philadelphia retailer and online store carries a full line of traditional spices as well as supplements, essential oils, and natural medicinal remedies.
Web site: www.pennherb.com
Phone: 800-523-9971

Penzys Spices
This family-operated business, headquartered in Duluth, Wisconsin, has more than 40 stores in 24 states. It also has a large online retail business and catalog. Penzys offers approximately 250 varieties of spices, including its own spice mixes. The selection is large, but you may not be able to find some unusual Indian and Asian spices. You can order online or call for a free catalog.
Web site: www.penzeys.com
Phone: 800-741-7787

McCormick & Co.
The world's largest retailer, based in the US, also sells a full range of spices online.
Web site: www.mccormick.com
Phone: 800-632-5847

My Spice Sage
Located in the Bronx, New York, this online-only retailer offers an interesting way to shop: by taste and aroma.
Web site: www.MySpiceSage.com
Phone: 877-890-5244

The Spice House

Founded in Milwaukee, Wisconsin, in 1957 (and now with other retail stores in Evanston, Geneva, and Chicago), this retail business is in its second generation of ownership, and has launched an online business that sells a full line of spices and gadgetry.

Web site: www.TheSpiceHouse.com
Phone: 847-328-3711

The Spicery

This retailer, located in Bath, England, has a large collection of spices, seeds, and spice blends, including the more hard-to-find spices in this book. (You can even buy by the teaspoon!) Shipping is free in the UK, but you'll have to pay for shipping to the US.

Web site: www.thespicery.com
Phone: 01-225-426309

Vanns Spices

This family-owned retailer and wholesaler is headquartered in Baltimore, Maryland, and caters to chefs and cooking enthusiasts. The Web site includes hundreds of spices and spice blends that you can browse by cuisine or style of cooking.

Web site: www.vannsspices.com
Phone: 800-583-1693

Where to Find Hard-to-Find Spices

Ceylon (true) cinnamon

Ceylon Cinnamon Online, based in Sri Lanka, sells true cinnamon from its own groves and caters to everything cinnamon: the spice (whole, quillings, and ground), supplements, oils—even cinnamon toothpicks.

Web site: www.ceylon-cinnamon.com
Phone: 94-777-385793

Chile seeds

The Chile Pepper Institute is a non-profit organization affiliated with New Mexico State University, in Las Cruces, New Mexico, and sells a variety of chile seeds for home gardens.

Web site: www.chilepepperinstitute.org
Phone: 575-646-3028

Cocoa and vanilla

Tharakan and Co. is an Indian-based company specializing in high-grade cocoa and vanilla products.

Web site: www.tharakanandcompany.com

Extra-Virgin coconut oil

Puritan's Pride, a natural supplements and products retailer, carries this item.

Web site: www.puritan.com
Phone: 800-645-1030

Galangal and lemongrass

Based in Issaquah, Washington, this site is a Thai grocery store online that offers a variety of Thai spices, ingredients, cookware, etc.

Web site: www.importfood.com
Phone: 888-618-8424

Indian spices

The Indian Foods Company caters to all Indian cooking needs, offering all the Indian spices, ingredients, and many of the spice blends featured in this book. Free shipping for orders of $75 and over.

Web site: www.indianfoodsco.com
Phone: 866-331-7684

This retailer and wholesaler, distributing out of Wauwatosa, Wisconsin, caters to the "Indian experience," offering groceries, cookware, cookbooks, etc., in addition to a wide range of spices.

Web site: www.iShopIndian.com
Phone: 877-786-8876

Jamaican jerk

A kitchen shop in Minneapolis and an online retailer, Kitchen Window carries a full line of gourmet and hard-to-find items, including Jamaican pimento wood for jerk barbecuing.

Web site: www.kitchenwindow.com

Phone: 888-824-4417

If it's Jamaican and hot, you can find it at this Milwaukee-based online retailer. Items include kitchen, jerk seasonings, and pimento wood chips.

Web site: www.pimentowood.com

Phone: 612-868-JERK

PediaCalm

This natural remedy for colic, featured in the chapter "Fennel Seed," was formulated by pediatrician Sergei Shushunov, MD, a clinical associate professor at the University of Illinois, and director of the Pediatric Intensive Care Unit at Illinois Masonic Medical Center in Chicago. The web site is part of Lev Laboratories, Glencoe, Illinois. Although fennel seed is on the Food and Drug Administration's GRAS (generally regarded as safe) list, for maximum safety, give this product to your baby only with the approval and supervision of your child's pediatrician.

Web site: www.4healthykids.com

Phone: 847-835-5795

Spanish (Majorca) almonds and La Mancha saffron

La Tienda is a family-owned specialty shop in Williamsburg, Virginia, and an online retailer that specializes in everything from Spain—foods, cookware, spices, etc.

Web site: www.tienda.com

Phone: 800-710-4304

Wasabi, pure

Coppersfolly in New Zealand specializes in growing and selling pure wasabi.

Web site: www.coppersfolly.co.nz

Phone: 64-3-325-2166

Index

Note to the reader: You can find references to the use of specific spices for the prevention and treatment of specific diseases in the chart *From Arthritis to Ulcers, an A-to-Z Guide to the Therapeutic Potential of the Healing Spices*, which begins on page 293.

acetylcholine (neurotransmitter)
    in ajowan, and digestive health, 15
    fennel, boosting the activity of, 115
    marjoram, boosting the levels of, 159
    oregano, boosting the activity of, 185
    sage, slowing the loss of, 212
adobos (Latin American spice mixes), 78, 270
advieh (Middle Eastern spice mix), 268
ajowan, 13–18, 274, 277
Ajowan Parathas (Indian bread), 17
Alamelu's Salt Substitute, 289
All-American Chili con Carne, 110
allicin, 127, 176, 180
allspice, 18–21, 274, 277
allyl isothiocyanate (AITC), 141, 142, 167
almond, 21–26, 274, 311
almond butter, 26
almond cocktail snack, 26
alpha-linolenic acid (ALA), 167
Alsatian Pork and Sauerkraut, 148
amchur, 27–30, 274, 277
America, spices in the cuisine of. *See* United States,
   spices in cuisine of
anethole (volatile oil), 4, 30–31, 114, 116, 221
aniseed, 4, 30–33, 274, 277
Anise Kisses recipe, 33
anthocyanins, 176, 191
antioxidants, healing spice sources of
    allspice, 19
    amchur, 27
    black cumin, 47
    chile, 70–71
    curry leaf, 111
    fennel seed, 115
    parsley, 187
    pomegranate, 190–91
    rosemary, 202
    sun-dried tomatoes, 224, 227
    tamarind, 232
    turmeric, 242–43

See also specific antioxidants
antioxidants, vegetable sources of, 159
apigenin, 37, 67, 187–88
Apple Pie Spice, 271–72
Arab nations, spices in cuisine of
    Baharat spice mix, 268
    cardamom, 63, 64
    fennel seed, 117
    See also Middle East, spices in cuisine of
asafoetida, 33–37, 274, 277
A Taste for Spices guide, 289
Ayurvedic medicine, healing spices used in
    almond, 24
    and balancing the doshas, 288–90
    basil, 37, 38
    black pepper, 52
    cinnamon, 83
    coriander, 102
    curry leaf, 111
    fenugreek, 119
    garlic, 127
    kokum, 149–50
    sesame seed, 216
    turmeric, 248
Aztecs, spices used by, 95, 253

Baharat (Middle Eastern spice mix), 268
balancing spices, 288–90
barbecue and rosemary, 201–2
Barbecue Rubs, 272
barbecue sauce, fast and tasty, 231–32
basil, 37–42, 274, 277
Bavarian Apple and Horseradish Sauce, 145
bay leaf, 42–47, 274, 277
Beef Curry, Madras, 106
benni. *See* sesame seed
Berbere (Ethiopian spice blend), 267
beta-carotene, sources of, 27, 47, 111
beverages
    hot chocolate, Mexican, 97